Morality and Health

Morality and Health

◆

Edited by
Allan M. Brandt and Paul Rozin

ROUTLEDGE
New York • London

Published in 1997

Routledge
29 West 35th Street
New York, NY 10001

Published in Great Britain by

Routledge
11 New Fetter Lane
London EC4P 4EE

Library of Congress Cataloging-in-Publication Data

Morality and health : interdisciplinary perspectives / edited by Allan
  M. Brandt and Paul Rozin.
     p.   cm.
  Includes bibliographical references and index.
  ISBN 0–415–91581–3 (hb : alk. paper). — ISBN 0–415–91582–1
(pb : alk. paper)
    1. Health behavior—Moral and ethical aspects. 2. Health
attitudes. I. Brandt, Allan M. II. Rozin, Paul, 1936– .
RA427.25.M67   1997   96-52813
306.4´61—dc21   CIP

Contents

Morality and Behavior in Historical Context

Contemporary Perspectives on Morality and Health

Preface and Acknowledgments

This book emerged from an initiative by the John D. and Catherine T. MacArthur Foundation to investigate the important and complex behavioral, social, and cultural determinants of health and disease. In 1986 the foundation organized an interdisciplinary "network" of behavioral and medical scientists to discuss these problems, and to propose, promote, and support new research initiatives in this area. The MacArthur Network on the Determinants and Consequences of Health Promoting and Health Damaging Behavior was chaired by Judith Rodin. The other members were Nancy Adler, Ralph Horwitz, Solomon Katz, Robert Lawrence, Karen Matthews, Bruce McEwen, Paul Rozin, Eliot Stellar, and G. Terence Wilson, with Grace Castellazzo as coordinator. In the group discussions, the moral concerns of Americans about many illnesses and health-related behaviors frequently emerged. The rapid entry of moral issues into attitudes toward cigarette smoking was particularly notable. This inspired Solomon Katz, one of the members of the group, to examine the emergence and significance of what was widely identified as "secular morality," a morality based on ideas of risk coming out of epidemiology rather than religion. Katz wrote a paper on secular morality that was circulated within the group and focused interest on morality and health. (A revised version of the paper appears as a chapter in this book.) Rozin proposed a book to bring together information and perspectives on this issue from history and other disciplines, and a morality and health initiative was born.

Allan Brandt, Solomon Katz, and Paul Rozin became a committee of three to organize the initiative. Three interdisciplinary MacArthur-sponsored meetings were organized. The third, in Santa Fe, New Mexico, in 1992, was explicitly designed to generate the chapters of this book. Most participants wrote chapters on designated topics, which were distributed before the meeting and discussed at the meeting. The revised and edited chapters constitute this book.

The explorations over the course of the three meetings reinforced and amplified the sense that the interaction between morality and health is both important and pervasive. All cultures seem to have complex and entangling moral and health beliefs. Moral conventions, at different times and places, have a significant influence on the framing of health- and disease-related behaviors. We became more and more aware of the impelling fact that the morality-health link is both very important and little studied. The initial thrust of the meetings was to identify some general principles guiding the manner in which moral-health entanglements occur, and the circumstances under which they grow or disappear. We soon realized that the social processes by which moral explanations for health and disease evolve are, to a substantial degree, culturally and historically specific. Our strategy was to gather information on the nature and origin of moral-health linkages at different times and in different cultures. We hoped, in this way, to situate the problem in its local context and, at the same time, allow important commonalities or principles to emerge from a set of diverse case studies. We recognized, as well, that many scholarly disciplines have valuable perspectives to offer, particularly history, the history of medicine, anthropology, epidemiology, political science, religion, philosophy, psychology, and sociology.

As the book makes clear, no single conceptual disciplinary approach can create a satisfactory account of the complex relations between morality and health. Some authors often point to the historically stigmatizing and alienating aspects of moral judgment; others look to broadly configured moral norms as a critical spur to health promotion and disease prevention. On one thing, however, consensus does emerge: those interested in the problems of health and disease in any culture cannot ignore the power and impact of moral intuitions, reasoning, and judgment. Our hope is that the chapters that follow serve to deepen understanding of the processes by which morals "construct" health; to identify the considerable gaps in our understanding of the relationship of moral discourse and disease; and to identify some general features of human beings and societies that promote or discourage moral-health linkages. The concluding chapter identifies some possible candidates for widely applicable, if not general, principles and relations.

In addition to the authors who contributed chapters to this book, participants in some or all of the three morality and health meetings were Deidre Byrnes, Grace Castellazzo, William Damon, Gordon Defriese, Amitai Etzioni, Claude Fischler, Alan Fiske, Byron Good, Paul Griffiths, Philip Hafner, Jay Katz, Emily Martin, Clark McCauley, Erik Midelfort, Ronald Numbers, Karl Peters, John Pierce, Lee Ross, Thomas Schelling, Barry Schwartz, Martin Seligman, Roxane Silver, George Stone, Paula Treichler, Martha Verbrugge, and Terence Wilson. These individuals have made important contributions to the chapters contained here both as discussants and critics, and we most gratefully acknowledge their counsel.

A number of individuals played a crucial role in the production of this book. Grace Castellazzo has been an exceptional administrator of the MacArthur Network that sponsored this work. She and Deidre Byrnes played a critical role in organizing the conferences. Considerable assistance in the editing and production of the book has also been expertly provided by Deidre Byrnes, Lara Freidenfelds, and Christian Warren. Oona Patrick and Jennifer Chyet did an outstanding job preparing the manuscript for publication. Our editors at Routledge, Philip Rappaport, Ronda Angel and William Germano, have provided both strong "moral" support for the project and excellent editorial advice throughout.

Finally, we thank the MacArthur Foundation for its support of this project from inception through publication. In particular, we thank Laurie Garduque, Idy Gitelson, Denis Prager, and Robert Rose.

Allan M. Brandt   Paul Rozin
Cambridge, Massachusetts Philadelphia, Pennsylvania

Introduction

Allan M. Brandt and Paul Rozin

We live in a time of deep interest in—if not obsession with—the problems of health and disease. In modern Western cultures, a day never passes without announcement of some medical finding, new risks to health, or new treatments for disease. For those who are media vigilant, questions about the consumption of cholesterol (good or bad), alcohol (red wine or white), exercise, diet, and a host of other specified "risk factors" are daily fare. Increasingly, we are told that new knowledge gives us new opportunities to take control of our health. With this new knowledge, however, come new responsibilities and a new set of moral expectations about health and disease. It is this growing recognition of the links between behavior and disease that formed the context for the genesis of the chapters in this book.

Rather than seeing health or disease as random and inevitable, societies have throughout history developed complex and sophisticated explanations for the causes and prevalence of disease. Embedded in these explanatory frames are deeply held, if often unstated, sensibilities about right and wrong, good and bad, responsibility and danger. This book explores—from a wide range of perspectives and disciplines and in diverse contexts—the complex relationship of morality to health.

In this book, morals will be seen operating in many ways and often with considerable ambiguity. Although some authors might celebrate the positive impact that stigmatizing smoking has had on cessation, others recognize the potential for victim-blaming inherent in such strong moral positions emphasizing personal responsibility. It is not unusual for some to argue that medicine and morals should be divorced. Much of the rhetoric of modern medicine advocates the utility of distinguishing fact from value, morals from medicine. Much of modern medicine has reflected the attempt to remove all values from its practice: witness the historical attempts to expunge "bias" from the clinical assessment of new therapies. Medical students are typically taught to be "neutral" and to avoid making value judgments about their patients.

Morals are typically viewed as "warping" or "distorting" medicine, an encroachment on what has become an "objective" domain. The world of medicine is typically configured as the antithesis of the world of morals. Medicine is scientific, objective, and definite—morals are subjective, relative, and indeterminate. Further, moral judgments and their accompanying cultural meanings are often viewed as the source of additional stigma and despair for patients. According to this view, disease should simply be *disease*. We should make no judgments about how it was attained or what illness means. But this view, of course, reflects strong moral assumptions about health and disease as well.

We often see medicine and morals posed as if they were categorically alternative ways of viewing health and disease, the medical versus moral explanatory frameworks. Nonetheless, the essays in this book suggest that medicine and morals are deeply and fundamentally entangled. And, in fact, the view that it would be advantageous to separate them usually reveals a particular moral position. Try though we might to separate medicine from meaning and meaning from values, the history of health and disease reveals their fundamental attachments. Debates about the relationship between moral behaviors and health date to antiquity. They form an important aspect of the Hippocratic corpus, revealing a deeply human need to account for the presence of health and the experience of illness. Morals clearly offered an opportunity to assert a vision of control and practice where the world might otherwise have appeared chaotic.

Even as we have undergone a substantial historical movement in the West, characterized by secularization, morals remain deeply embedded in our considerations of health and disease. And even as powerful medical technologies and institutions have come to play an increasingly dominant role in identifying, defining, and responding to disease, morals continue to be enmeshed in the discourse of science and medicine.

Furthermore, behaviors and dispositions that are associated with health and disease resistance, such as cleanliness, often have moral significance. And the adoption of behaviors or regimes that are presumed to improve health may be easier and more successful if these behaviors and regimes are endowed with moral meaning. Perhaps it is easier to abandon smoking if, in addition to the attendant health risks for the smoker, it is believed to be immoral to smoke.

At the level of society, customary practices and conceptions relating to health—for example, rules about food sharing and food offerings—may bring morality directly into the domain of health. In the United States, there have been many examples of an important linkage between moral positions and health movements. Moral issues may galvanize action, induce commitment, and engage government and institutions. In short, morality may be related to the spread and success of health movements.

The chapters in this book suggest that the processes by which disease becomes a moral issue are, at least in part, determined by historically and culturally specific forces. No doubt, all cultures have developed frameworks for assessing why and how people become ill and suffer. The chapters here suggest, however, that understanding such processes requires careful and specific attention to context. The forces acting on the creation of moral perspectives are highly variable by time and place, by politics and economics, by religion and science. It is clear that there are many frameworks that relate moral and health concerns. But it is also clear that the number of frameworks is limited, and that there are some rather general features that appear in diverse frameworks (health, it seems, is powerfully associated with morality, just as immorality is powerfully associated with illness). Any attempt to learn about ways in which the environment or human nature constrain the formulation of moral-health complexes depends on the explication and understanding of moral-health linkages in their contexts at particular times and places. We hope that the chapters enlighten specific moral-health linkages, as well as suggest our desire to identify more pervasive principles and practices across cultures and historical uses.

One central characteristic of the chapters that follow is that they were written in the shadow of the AIDS epidemic. If there were any questions about the significance of moral perspectives on disease and health, the AIDS epidemic has dispelled them. AIDS has called attention to moral judgments and their impact on disease as few modern diseases could have. The epidemic is a sobering reminder of the important relationship between social and cultural understandings of disease and deeply felt moral ontologies. Explanations of the causes of the epidemic, clinical approaches to those who are sick, and debates about public responses to prevent the spread of the infection have all revealed deep seated—if often unstated—moral assumptions.

Take, for example, the contentious debates about what causes AIDS. Some on the political right have suggested that AIDS is caused by immorality itself. Those who behave morally, according to this reasoning, have nothing to fear in this epidemic. Indeed, by this logic, the epidemic usefully reminds us of moral conventions that are violated only at one's peril.

Alternatively, others have argued that the only acceptable moral position is to view everyone as being at risk of disease. Only by recognizing that we are all vulnerable do we create an environment of compassion and communal caring. Questions about responsibility and risk are at the moral nexus of the debate about the meanings of the epidemic.

There can be little doubt that the social meanings of HIV have been fundamentally dependent on the recognition that those at greatest risk of infection, disease, and death come from socially marginalized and morally stigmatized populations. The close cultural associations of HIV with homosexuality and illicit use of drugs in large measure have determined social responses to the epidemic both in the United States and abroad. AIDS has—since its inception—been a magnet for powerful moral formulations about disease, sexuality, drug use, and responsibility. The epidemic has exposed how powerfully moral notions continue to influence not only what a disease is and what we do about it, but what a disease *means*. According to some constructions of the epidemic, HIV disease *proved* the importance of certain moral norms. In a traditional argument, morality and health were viewed as being synonymous. One need not be concerned about the dangers of disease so long as one maintained a moral life. According to this logic, certain preventive approaches—safer sex techniques, the widespread distribution of condoms, and sterile injection equipment—encourage immoral behaviors. In such arguments, a particular moral calculus becomes apparent: AIDS is a useful tool for demanding moral behavior. Intermediate approaches to preventing infection are *dangerous* because they *promote* immorality. In this framework, moral concerns trump health.

There can be little question now—nearly two decades into the epidemic—that the response to AIDS in the United States and throughout the world has been fundamentally shaped by its particular moral meanings; these impacts range from the personal experiences of illness among individuals to the devastating rates of mortality in particular locales. During its nearly two decades, AIDS has been transformed from a crisis to the routine. In the late 1990s, AIDS has become mundane. The process by which the meanings of AIDS changed so substantially reveals fundamental social perceptions and moral assumptions about the nature of the epidemic. The perception that AIDS has been principally limited to those at highest risk has led to increasing complacency about the epidemic. The calls for isolation and quarantine that characterized the early years of the epidemic diminished as the perception of a "social quarantine" arose. According to this view of the epidemic, the disease was generally confined to the deviant and the criminal—and, in some instances, to their sexual and needle-sharing associates. Attention was typically galvanized by those rare instances in which those perceived to be at high risk spread their infections to those otherwise deemed to be risk free—instances in which the "metaphorical" quarantine was breached. This explains the intense debates about hospital infections—patients and providers now came together in an atmosphere of fear and loathing—bringing new suspicion and bitterness to their encounters. So-called innocent infections laid bare a particular moral approach to the epidemic, invoking guilt, blame, and sympathy, dependent upon one's perceived agency and volition in the communication of the virus.

The very notion of AIDS becoming routine reflects not only a particular set of moral assumptions about the disease in the Western developed world but deeply held values about the nature of disease, poverty, and dependence in the developing world as well, where the epidemic also continues to have devastating effects. Routinization became a vehicle for the healthy and powerful to dissociate themselves from the sick and often impoverished victims of the epidemic.

Our point is that contained in these very "constructions" of AIDS are deeply held moral convictions about the nature of risk and responsibility for disease. And so it has been for other diseases and behaviors at other times. Cultural beliefs and practices about disease are revelatory of a society's most basic moral beliefs and practices. These meanings and moral configurations, in turn, have a dramatic impact on both the care of those who are sick and on broader social and political policies. Indeed, as a number of the chapters suggest, moral beliefs and convention typically have a *material* impact on patterns of disease, clinical care, and the experience of illness.

The chapters are divided into several groupings. The first group offers broad overviews of the dynamic relationship of moral thought to health and disease. These chapters make clear that assumptions about disease causality have traditionally enlisted important moral considerations; nonetheless, they also suggest that seeing such linkages outside particular historical contexts may distort their meanings.

Keith Thomas elucidates the tension between medical systems of belief and religious systems, which are eager to find moral meanings in an individual's "health status." He shows that although "natural" explanations of disease grew in dominance after the seventeenth century, religious and moral explanations of disease persisted or were typically linked to these newly emerging accounts. This critical tension in many respects occurs throughout the essays in this book, albeit in historically or culturally specific examples.

Charles Rosenberg contrasts twentieth-century biomedical reductionism with eighteenth- and nineteenth-century views that integrated mind and body; psychology and physiology; morals and medicine. As he demonstrates, twentieth-century views of disease nonetheless reflected powerful moral views of individual responsibility, especially given the predominance of chronic diseases with clearly identified risk factors. Rosenberg notes the strongly antifatalistic norms and values central in American culture. Accordingly, twentieth-century American science and society has been aggressively committed, he argues, to banishing risk.

Allan Brandt's essay explores related themes by examining notions of risk and responsibility in twentieth-century American culture. Brandt emphasizes that new forms of medical knowledge based on epidemiologic and statistical inference spurred moral assumptions about responsibility for disease based upon individual risks. At times these formulations obscured important social and cultural forces that fostered vulnerability to disease.

David Mechanic pursues related themes from the perspective of medical sociology. Mechanic also notes the increasing emphasis on individual behaviors as they relate to disease. He suggests that there is a growing tendency to view these behaviors outside their broader social and cultural contexts. In Mechanic's view the increasing medicalization of American society has encouraged moral judgments about health and disease.

The second group of chapters demonstrate that analyses of non-Western cultures offer opportunities for appreciating different interpretations of the linkages between morality, behavior, and disease.

Further, they emphasize how such relations are sensitive to local values and beliefs. Such analyses broaden and contextualize our understanding of morality and health. At the same time they suggest an approach to extract widespread or universal features of the way morality and health are related.

Arthur Kleinman and Joan Kleinman expose the moral assumptions underlying the biomedical model of health, with its central focus on the individual. They suggest that alternative explanatory frameworks focusing on sociopolitical models of health also fail to account adequately for the meaning of the illness experience. Using ethnographic data from China on the experiences of neurasthenia, schizophrenia, and possession, the authors argue that the experience of illness can be understood only within a particular web of interpersonal processes; local "moral worlds" are the context in which illness must be understood. They point out that in many areas of the world, high rates of illness are linked to the disruptions of these "worlds."

The chapter by Richard A. Shweder, Nancy C. Much, Monamohan Mahapatra, and Lawrence Park examines both the nature of morality and causal explanations for suffering, across the cultures of the world, with special emphasis on Hindu India. They present an original taxonomy of three moral domains that may encompass all moral systems in the world: autonomy codes, based on rights violations; community codes, based on communal values and hierarchy violations; and divinity codes, based on concepts such as sanctity and purity. The three codes structure the domain of morality as it applies to health and widen the scope of morality-health interactions. The authors summarize prior cross-cultural work on accounts of suffering, supplementing this with their own recent study. This work reveals that the most common explanatory frameworks are interpersonal, moral, and biomedical accounts of suffering. The authors also examine the moral explanations for suffering in an Indian town, where moral imagination emphasizes notions of suffering and responsibility in which individuals know that every act of good or evil that is committed will affect well-being, in contrast with American notions in which illness and suffering may appear random and meaningless.

The next section of the book explores a variety of particular behaviors typically associated with moral views of disease. Warren Belasco and Sidney Mintz evaluate historical and cultural notions of food, consumption, and morality. Mintz demonstrates that abstaining from sugar has historically been connected with large political and social goals; for example, as a means for British citizens to impose economic sanctions against those who kept slaves in the West Indies in the nineteenth century. Forgoing that which is desired became an essential test—not only of will but of moral worth. In the late twentieth century, however, these desires, Mintz suggests, are no longer connected to social objectives and therefore have lost their moral valence.

Belasco follows this theme in his essay on food activists in U.S. history. Tracing debates about adulteration, naturalness, and the alienation of consumers, Belasco argues that in contemporary American culture we no longer see the complex moral and social issues in food choice. The consumer culture, with its emphasis on individual behavior, has unlinked food from critical questions of social responsibility and ecological concern.

In few instances have moral considerations been so persistently invoked as in the case of alcohol consumption. Indeed, the moral fervor that alcohol unleashed in the early twentieth century in the United States led to the dramatic experiment in social engineering of Prohibition. Joseph Gusfield reviews the history of American attempts to control alcohol consumption. Although many have suggested that alcohol use has moved from a moral to a scientific notion of addiction and disease, Gusfield argues that moral norms and values continue to influence the public meanings of drinking significantly. This peculiarly American perspective, he suggests, may be explained by a traditional "temperance sentiment" that emphasizes the continuities between leisure and work, play and control.

Some of the most powerful moral evaluations of behavior in the late twentieth century have focused on the use of illicit drugs. David Courtwright traces the history of the "moralization" of drug use in his essay, demonstrating the effects of socioeconomic status and ethnicity upon the cultural assessment of drug use. Those on the right have typically regarded drug use as a crime, advocating punishment for moral transgression. On the left, drug use is typically constructed as an indicator of deeper social pathologies requiring social interventions. Courtwright argues that drug use is correlated with a low level of religious commitment. He also describes in some detail the different types of Protestantism, and how these differences relate to moral attitudes toward the body. This analysis is relevant to a number of other papers in which the issue of Protestantism arises (for example, the Thomas and Rozin chapters).

Linda Gordon examines the historical evolution of the social meanings of teenage pregnancy and out-of-wedlock births, as well as the reasons for the conflation of these categories in contemporary public debate. Drawing an important distinction between morals and moralism, she demonstrates how parties on both the political right and left have contributed to a harmful moralistic discourse on teenage sexuality. Many currently held perceptions of teen pregnancy and out-of-wedlock birth are based on distorted facts and reveal underlying moral perceptions of race, class, and women's sexuality. She advocates a new moral discussion of teenage sexuality that exposes these historically implicit assumptions.

Moral concerns have not been confined to traditional debates about diet, alcohol and drugs, or sex. In the early twentieth century, even as the new germ theory radically changed assumptions about the environment and susceptibility to disease, important moral considerations about behaviors continued to be articulated. According to Nancy Tomes, the germs of tuberculosis were believed ever-present. Only eternal moral vigilance within the house and community would protect families from this insidious contaminant. Further, she explains how scientific investigation into TB had the effect of furthering moral agendas. Tomes's essay fractures the traditional assumption that scientific and moral paradigms are disconnected. Tuberculosis control demonstrated that science and morality were not dichotomous, but rather were significantly intertwined and difficult, if not impossible, to dissect.

The next section examines a set of contemporary debates about morality and health. Its chapters look particularly at the relative benefits and harms of the moralization of health behaviors and beliefs. The radical transformation of attitudes and practices regarding cigarette smoking offers a crucial case study of the impact of moral arguments relating to disease. Solomon Katz suggests that the history of recent antitobacco campaigns opens an important window on the possibilities for asserting a new "secular morality." This phenomenon—heavily influenced by modern epidemiology and grass-roots advocacy—he believes has great potential for positive social change. Katz demonstrates how morally constituted norms may shape behaviors in the interest of health, and presents a model of the operation of secular morality.

Other authors, however, might caution that the boundaries between a secular morality and secular "moralisms" would be difficult to define in both policy and practice. Lawrence Gostin cautions that the regulation of smoking must be based only on scientifically supported health concerns. Antismoking efforts that overstep either scientific evidence or constitutional protections would, he argues, ultimately delegitimate the movement to control smoking.

Howard Leichter also raises substantial concerns in regard to this new secular morality. Leichter shows how the assertion of a secular morality can lead to an emphasis on "lifestyle" correctness with powerful possibilities for discrimination and stigma. Notions of individual responsibility and control, deeply embedded in American culture and politics, may actually work to augment disparities in health.

In a concluding essay, Paul Rozin identifies the phenomenon of "moralization": the transformation of a morally neutral activity into one with significant moral weight, by individuals or in society. Using the recent moralization of meat eating among some Americans as a principal example, he examines the social and psychological processes by which behaviors come to be "moralized," and discusses the social and personal consequences of "moralization." Drawing evidence from the other chapters he also attempts to extract some causes of moralization that seem to occur frequently, across cultures and times. These include the association of particular behaviors with religious orientations of self-discipline and denial; the effects of the behavior on children; and the association of the behavior with marginalized groups. According to Rozin, these predisposing influences—as well as historically specific political and economic forces—enhance internalization; morally-linked behaviors become more robust, more central to the self, and more consistent with feelings and emotions. This process of moralization is at the heart of this book. Understanding it, no doubt, requires fuller investigation and articulation at both the individual and the group level.

The chapters in this volume are diverse in discipline and in subject matter. All, however, point to the dangers implicit in moral arguments as well as to their potential value. No doubt we need guideposts for thought and action; we rely on cultural values that will shape both our moral discourse and practices. The chapters suggest, above all else, the possibility for understanding in a more sophisticated way the nature of the processes involved in "moralization" and the specific manner in which morals are used in our encounters with health and disease in our everyday lives. The recognition that morality itself differs across cultures and time, that moral-health linkages take many forms, and that morals can invoke stigma, hatred, and the segregation of the sick, as well as compassion, generosity, and care, need not leave us awash in a sea of relativism. Rather, these chapters suggest that the critical illumination of the political, historical, cultural, and psychological forces that create moral categories, thought, and practices offers us an opportunity to shape our world with new ideals and images in the interest of compassion and justice. If and when we do so, perhaps the world will also be a healthier place.

Perspectives on
Morality and Health

Health and Morality
in Early Modern England

Keith Thomas

If thou wilt diligently hearken to the voice of the Lord thy God,
and wilt do that which is right in his sight, and wilt give ear to his
commandments, and keep all his statutes, I will put none of these
diseases upon thee, which I have brought upon the Egyptians: for
I am the Lord that healeth thee. Exodus, 15: 26.

In the United States of the late twentieth century the preoccupation with the preservation of physical health has reached an intensity that may be unique in human history. As Francis Fukuyama has
recently remarked:

In America today, we feel entitled to criticize another person's
smoking habits, but not his or her religious beliefs or moral behavior. For Americans, the health of their bodies—what they eat
and drink, the exercise they get, the shape they are in—has become a far greater obsession than the moral questions that tormented their forebears. (Fukuyama 1992, 306)

This formulation is slightly misleading; it would be a better description of what has happened to say that health itself has been elevated into a major issue of personal morality. To ignore the advice
tendered by doctors and health counsellors is, in the eyes of many,
not just imprudent but morally culpable. John Updike's emblem of
Middle America, Harry "Rabbit" Angstrom, flabby and overweight
after years of junk food and inadequate exercise, suffers his final
and fatal heart attack when engaging in an unaccustomed game of

basketball after eating two dinners on the previous evening. His regimen has been one of guilty defiance. Even his eight-year-old granddaughter reproaches him for buying himself a peanut bar while waiting to meet her at the airport: "Grandpa's been eating candy again, for shame on him." Rabbit knows that people are responsible for their own fates: "Anger is what gives you cancer, he has read somewhere" (Updike 1991, 13, 357, and passim).

The stigma that in modern times attaches to those who indulge themselves at the expense of their health is the latest version of an age-old association between illness and sin. In many simple, so-called primitive societies, illness is merely one of the many forms of misfortune that call for explanation in terms of someone's moral culpability (Currer and Stacey 1986, 57–59). As among the ancient Israelites, the breach of ritual prohibitions is thought likely to be followed by illness or epidemic. The dietary and sanitary rules of Moses or Mahomet had a force that was simultaneously moral, religious, and prudential.

In classical antiquity there developed a body of medical learning that treated illness and disease as purely natural phenomena, capable of explanation in wholly physical terms and of treatment accordingly. The Hippocratic Corpus and the works of Galen were transmitted through the Arabs to medieval Europe and in the age of the Renaissance established themselves as the dominant intellectual tradition within which all medical matters were discussed. According to this tradition the maladies of individuals were caused by humoral imbalance, while large-scale epidemics and endemic diseases were the result of miasma: the defilement of the air caused by stagnant water, human exhalations, putrefying matter, and the malign influence of the stars.

In early modern England, therefore, an intellectual scheme was available that, at least potentially, made it possible to interpret and treat physical illness without any invocation of guilt or personal responsibility. But, side by side with the Galenic tradition, there was the legacy of fifteen hundred years of Christianity. The biblical link between sin and disease and the doctrine that all events on earth were determined by the will of God had shaped the medieval church's teaching on medical matters. Just as saints demonstrated their sanctity by healing miracles, so sinners could expect to be punished by physical illnesses appropriate to their particular form of delinquency. Each of the church's Seven Deadly Sins was conventionally associated in homiletic literature with a pathological condition of the body (Bloomfield 1952, 233, 241–42, 355, 368). Pride, which was a swelling up, was symbolized by tumors and inflammations. Sloth led to dead flesh and palsy. Gluttony meant dropsy and a large belly. Lust produced fluxes and discharges, leprous skin, and, by the sixteenth century, the pox. Avarice was associated with gout or dropsy; envy with jaundice, venom, and fever; wrath with spleen, frenzy, and madness. Of course, these were essentially allegorical or poetic ways of conveying the nature of the sins themselves. But they were also taken literally as indications of the judgments likely to descend upon sinners.

In post-Reformation England the notion that illness was a judgment of God remained ubiquitous. As the Elizabethan Puritan William Perkins observed, "Sicknesse comes ordinarily and usually of sinne" (Perkins 1608–1631, 1:497). When a godly man fell ill, his first instinct was to search himself to determine what it was he had done to bring such an affliction upon himself. Usually, there would be enough on his conscience for it to be easy for him to find an appropriate cause. In this way it was possible for the Presbyterian minister Adam Martindale to decide that the swelling of his sister's face when she died of smallpox was God's way of indicating displeasure at the pride she had taken in her personal appearance (Thomas 1971, 83). Large-scale epidemics were regularly attributed to the prevalent sins of the day such as Sabbath-breaking, covetousness, and playgoing (Mullett 1956, index s.v. 'God's wrath as cause'; Slack 1985, 26).

But, though it was axiomatic that sickness was a symptom of sin, it did not necessarily follow that all illnesses were to be interpreted as divine punishments for misdeeds. It was equally possible that God had sent the affliction as a means of trying an individual's faith. The example of Job, an upright man who suffered an appalling series of afflictions, showed that even the most godly person might be repeatedly tested for no fault of his own. Nor did the divine origin of the disease mean that natural remedies were to be disregarded. On the contrary, it was believed that God usually worked through natural causes and that it was man's duty to employ such natural helps as the divine plan had provided, though without relying upon them exclusively.[1]

What can be seen during the early modern period is a multiple theory of disease causation, with divine providence and Galenic theories being simultaneously invoked. Of course, there were individuals who laid the full burden of explanation upon one or the other, but the most common reaction was to call on both. The epidemics of bubonic plague that struck England in the sixteenth and seventeenth centuries were simultaneously interpreted as punishments for sin *and* as the product of corrupt air and evil humors. Therapy was likewise twofold in character. Pious meditations and calls for repentance did not preclude recourse to physical medicine. "When I had begged God's blessing upon my physic, I took it," recorded a pious seventeenth-century lady (Smith 1901, 314). Prayers and fasts were held at times of danger, but they were also accompanied by an elaborate public health policy involving quarantine regulations and the cleansing of affected areas. The threatened population repented, but they also tried to run away.

Early modern England was thus relatively free from the fatalism that characterized Islamic reactions in the face of epidemic disease. Indeed, the authorities descended firmly upon the occasional zealot who asserted that plague would strike only the reprobate and that no believer would die unless he or she was lacking in faith (Thomas 1971, 87–88; Slack 1985, 49–50, 231–35). Conversely, there was no suggestion that disease would inevitably follow wrongdoing.

Yet, though ministers and public authorities campaigned vigorously against undue readiness to see sickness as evidence of divine judgment and sternly repressed popular tendencies to fatalism, all the evidence suggests that many ordinary people found it difficult to dissociate ill health from moral responsibility. Throughout modern British history, the commonest reaction to severe sickness has been to ask, "What have I done to deserve it?"

Implicit in Protestantism was the doctrine that the human body had been given to man by God and that it was therefore a religious duty to take all reasonable steps to preserve it. In the mid-seventeenth century Thomas Hobbes declared it to be a law of nature that a man was "forbidden to do, that, which is destructive of his life, or taketh away the means of preserving the same; and to omit that, by which he thinketh it may be best preserved." He was merely giving a new formulation to a well-established religious principle (Hobbes 1651/1991, 91). When Protestant divines condemned voluntary suicide as a heinous sin, they did so on the grounds that a person should not do anything to shorten his life when God had given the means to save or prolong it. Those who endangered their health by self-indulgence, overwork, or excessive passion were guilty of indirect self-murder. So were those who failed to seek the best medical advice (Sym 1637, 91–92, 109–11; Cheyne 1725, 3).

Some contemporaries stressed that there were limits to this obligation to do everything possible to protect one's health. As a Jacobean writer remarked, it was no doubt the case that a person would avoid sickness and live longer if he "should be exempt and free from all turmoiling troubles and publique affaires in the Common wealth, livinge onely to himselfe, cherishinge his body and tendringe his health." But, he added, no one could be so "blockish" as to think he was born only for himself and had no obligations to others (Vaughan 1602, sigs. Biij–Biv). Yet, subject to the proviso that life had to be lived in an active and socially responsible way, it was an absolute obligation to do everything reasonably possible to preserve one's health and body.

The religious ban on suicide was not invented by Protestants but was part of traditional Catholic teaching. Medieval Catholicism, however, had also condoned the very different ascetic tradition of utter indifference to the human body, to the extent of regarding extreme acts of bodily neglect as likely evidence of sanctity. Physical illness had been welcomed as a context in which to display spiritual strength. Disease was thought to purify the soul and bring the sufferer closer to God. Holy men were often famous for their personal filthiness and physical decrepitude, while saintly women fasted on such a scale as to have led some modern historians into diagnosing anorexia nervosa (Bell 1985; Bynum 1987, 194–207). The twelfth-century recluse Christina of Markyate, for example, spent four years shut in a tiny cell, sitting on a hard stone; because of her fasting, her bowels dried up and her burning thirst caused little clots of blood to bubble from her nostrils (Talbot 1987, 102). In the Counter-Reformation period Catholics were more cautious about such austerities. As the Jesuit Robert Southwell noted, "I must have care of my health and so temper all my spiritual exercises and bodily afflictions with discretion that I may continue in them still" (Southwell 1973, 40). Protestants sternly emphasized the duty to act as a responsible custodian of one's body; and, in the century after the Reformation, suicide was punished more severely than ever before or afterward (MacDonald & Murphy 1990, 75). Yet even Protestantism was not without its ascetic dimension, and extreme self-denial continued to be practiced by the godly. In 1644 a minister recalled "a religious lady" who "told me of her selfe, that at her first setting out in the way of religion, she had like to have been lost through an illusion, *That no fat person could get to Heaven.* So that she almost had spoiled and wasted her body through too excessive and immoderate fasting" (Torshell 1644, 54).

It was not only ministers of religion who taught that individuals had a moral duty to take good care of their health. The early modern state had an obvious interest in ensuring that the population could supply an efficient fighting force when needed, and local authorities were concerned to reduce the pressure of the indigent and infirm upon the poor rates. Moreover, the Galenic tradition itself carried with it a strong explicit morality of self-care, teaching that it was an obligation to seek a healthy life and that disease was a punishment for neglecting the rules of health (Temkin 1949; 1973, 39–40). During the sixteenth, seventeenth, and eighteenth centuries, there poured from the printing presses a constant stream of medical guidebooks urging the lay public to adopt a regimen that would secure them long life and freedom from serious illness. These works naturally varied somewhat in their detailed prescriptions, but they were decisively shaped by classical teachings. Their overriding theme was that of temperance, and their advice coincided closely with the conventional morality of the day. Indeed, the precepts they offered were as much ethical as medical.

Advice on regimen related to the six so-called nonnaturals, necessary for health, but liable by abuse to become the cause of disease: air, diet, sleep, exercise, evacuation, and the passions of the mind. The regimen to be followed had to be adapted to the physical constitution and circumstances of the person concerned. But the lesson inculcated was invariably one of personal responsibility and moderation. In the words of one early sixteenth-century authority, it was "excesse" in any of the nonnaturals that was "almoste the chefe occasion of all suche diseases as rayne among us nowe a dayes" (Phayer 1546, sig. Miii^v). The doctrine of influential Continental writers on longevity, like Luigi Cornaro (1475–1566), was that human beings were intended by nature to live for a very long time and that it was only their intemperance, particularly in diet, that accounted for the failure of most people to reach their allotted span (Gruman 1961). In many ways this was a secularized version of the old teaching about the Deadly Sins. For what the books on regimen most condemned were gluttony, sloth, lechery, and anger. They did so because these vices were adverse to health, but their readers knew that they were also sinful in themselves.

Gluttony, in particular, was identified as the cause of many diseases. The Elizabethan physician Thomas Cogan declared that the aim of his whole regimen was to discourage "intemperate feeding." Overeating, he asserted, left people "fettered with gowtes, racked with fevers, pierced through with pleurisies, strangled with squinances [quinsy] and finally cruellie put to death oftentimes in youth, or in the flower of their age" (Cogan 1589, 182, 186–87). Other guides urged their readers to avoid "fine junkets and delicious sauces," "voluptuousness and bellychere" (Vaughan 1602, sigs. Biv^v, Fiv).

This doctrine fitted in well with the puritan dislike of self-indulgence and the feeling of those with social consciences that it was wrong for the rich to stuff themselves while the poor were on the brink of starvation. Moderation was also an integral part of the work ethic; hence the resolution by the great judge Sir Matthew Hale, "to be short and sparing at meals, that I may be the fitter for business" (Burnet 1682, 60). His contemporary Slingsby Bethel denounced feasting and hospitality on the grounds that "excess weakens men's bodies, spends vainly their time, dulls their wits, and makes them unfit for action and business" (Bethel 1689, 19). The prohibition of rich food also satisfied nationalistic sensibilities, for it was agreed that English cooking was more "natural" and "wholesome" than the French gastronomy that became fashionable in the later seventeenth century. In the eighteenth century the attack on gluttony was congenial to Tory moralists who wanted to set a limit to consumption by the lower classes, and it echoed the complaints of political writers in the civic humanist tradition that with the growth of material prosperity, the martial valor and patriotic spirit of the English were being undermined by "luxury" and "effeminacy." In his best-selling *Domestic Medicine* (1769), William Buchan remarked that it would be good for mankind "if cookery, as an art, were entirely prohibited" (cited in Rosenberg 1983, 32).

From the later seventeenth century onward, there was increasing stress on the medical advantages of an austere diet based on cold water and vegetables. It was urged that vegetarianism would reduce obesity, keep the blood free from "noxious juices" and conduce to longer life. Though nominally concerned with health and efficiency, this advice had a pronounced ethical dimension. Not for nothing did one of the early vegetarians, Thomas Tryon, urge the foundation of what he called a "Society of Clean and Healthy Livers." Voluntary abstinence from flesh symbolized the triumph of the spirit over the body. The consumption of meat intensified human lusts and introduced undesirable "animal" elements into human nature. It might even be morally wrong to kill fellow creatures to gratify human appetites. These were the arguments that would fuel successive movements for food reform in Britain and North America from the late seventeenth century until the present day (Thomas 1983, 288–300; Smith 1985).

Excessive use of alcohol was also rejected on grounds that were moral as well as medical. Drunkenness, it was thought, rotted the liver, sozzled the brain, killed the memory, and precipitated apoplexy and sudden death. Some authorities rejected wine altogether as "an hurtfull superfluitie" (Bright 1580, 25). But it was very unusual to recommend total abstinence. After all, there was a biblical injunction to "use a little wine for thy stomach's sake" (Tim. 5:23); and many argued on religious grounds that wine was one of God's creations and should therefore be enjoyed (Willet 1631, 205–6; Lord 1630, 47–50). It was also believed that in the English climate it was dangerous to drink cold water (Short 1656, 19–20, 64). The teetotal movement was an invention of the early nineteenth century, not of seventeenth-century Puritanism. When it came, it was driven less by a concern for health than by a moralistic conviction that alcohol was linked to irreligion, poverty, and moral degradation (Harrison 1971, esp. 124; Morris 1976, 137).

The use of tobacco was medically controversial from the start. During the first century after its introduction to Europe, smoking was defended by some as the panacea of all panaceas and attacked by others as physically harmful (Stewart 1967). It was thought to be bad for the teeth and to make the breath smell "worse then the snuffe of a candle" (Aubrey 1980, 1:52; Vaughan 1626, 2:80). More prophetically, the death of the scientist Thomas Harriot in 1621 from cancer of the nose is said to have been linked to his smoking.[2] Once again, there were ethical objections as well as medical ones because smoking was associated with dissolute persons, "guzzling drinkers and company-keeping smokers," as the Quakers called them. Smoking would later become unpopular in evangelical circles (Braithwaite 1919, 509; Kiernan 1991, 104).

It was also thought desirable, both medically and morally, to avoid excessive sexual activity, "specially of them that be students and leane of bodie." Masturbation had long been regarded as "a wol [well] horrible sin:" "these selfe-defilements doe rot and weaken the body, by the curse of God, exceedingly," explained a minister in 1633 (Vaughan 1602, sig. Ui^v; Barnum 1976–, 1(2):58; Capel 1633, 354). Doctors recommended cooling the privates in cold water and drinking water-lily juice, so as to avoid "filthy pollutions" at night. William Vaughan thought sexual intercourse three times a month enough for most people: "Yea, to some, once is to[o] muche" (Vaughan, sig. Uiv^v).

The regimens laid particular stress on the importance for health of regular physical exercise: "strong and vehement walking," for example, until "a man pant and fetche his breath thicke and often with difficultie" (Vaughan 1602, sig. Di). Manual workers who engaged in heavy labor had no need for additional exercise; indeed, they were thought to live longest. But the sedentary classes were advised to take up sports like tennis, despite some doubts as to whether the game was suitable for "grave personages and men much busied with weighty affairs." King Charles II, who enjoyed tennis, once noted that he lost four and a half pounds in weight during a single match (Latham and Matthews 1970–1983, 8:419). Here, too, there was a moral issue. Sloth and inactivity had always been reprehensible. Because it was a duty to keep one's body in working order, preachers taught that recreation was desirable in order to refresh the spirit and renew the zest for labor. John Locke took this principle to an extreme when he argued that the rich, the idle, and all those engaged in sedentary pursuits should safeguard their health by spending three, or preferably six, hours daily in manual labor in "some laborious calling" (Kelly 1991, 2:493–95).[3]

The contrary idea that one might be "worn out" by the stress and wear and tear of a busy life was less evident, perhaps because it conflicted with the Protestant work ethic. Writers in the primitivist tradition attributed greater longevity to simple peoples who supposedly lived carefree and happy lives, and it was accepted that "civilized" society generated many diseases peculiar to it because material luxury weakened the body and competitive emulation put a strain on the mind (Sinclair 1807, 1:15). Yet though people recognized the dangers of overwork, particularly overwork in intrinsically unhealthy occupations, the prevailing view seems to have been that illness was more likely to come from idleness. For this belief, Protestant moralizing about the duty to be active must bear some responsibility.

Finally, all the regimens stressed that it was essential to moderate the passions. Peace of mind was an essential prerequisite for healthy living. "Rabbit" Angstrom's belief that anger gives you cancer echoes centuries of medical warnings about the dangers of excessive joy or indignation. But in modern mythology it is suppressed anger that is dangerous,[4] whereas Christian stoicism discouraged the expression of passion. It also provided a remedy against fearfulness, which, all the commentators agreed, weakened people's resistance at times of epidemic and made them more vulnerable; some were even said to have died of fear alone (see, for example, Kellwaye 1593, 13; Bradwell 1636, 37). Inner cheerfulness and confidence were thus essential psychological attributes. They could be induced by religious faith and a clear conscience. Once again, moral well-being and physical health were closely associated.

There was thus a very close fit between the rules of health set out in the regimens and the rules of everyday morality as expounded by divines. As Sir George Cheyne put it in 1725, "The infinitely wise Author of Nature has so contrived things, that the most remarkable rules of preserving life and health are moral duties commanded to us, so true it is, that godliness has the promises of this life, as well as that to come" (3). The regimen books implied that those who lived in a moderate and temperate way were unlikely to succumb to many of the maladies that afflicted others.

In the early modern period good health was conceived of less as a physical condition, narrowly defined, than as a general state of all-round felicity, of mind and soul as well as body. The very word *health* was used interchangeably to signify both physical wholeness and moral well-being, as in the General Confession in the Book of Common Prayer, where the congregation confesses its misdeeds by saying that "there is no health in us." Conversely, the medical terms for disease had obvious moral overtones. Bad air was *corrupt*, houses were *contaminated*, and epidemics were *pestilent*. The language of the time was certainly capable of distinguishing between physical health and moral purity, but in everyday usage the distinction was frequently blurred. Infection was conceived of as a form of pollution.

Within this framework, some diseases became objects of moral reprobation more readily than others because they were regarded as "unclean," more polluting, more repulsive, more obviously associated with vice. As Susan Sontag has remarked, the most feared diseases are those that transform the body into something alienating (1990, 131). Leprosy, for example, was seen in the Middle Ages as a particularly nauseating instance of physical and moral defilement. Perhaps because of its horrifying symptoms, the disease was wrongly believed to be a venereal infection, contracted in degrading circumstances, for example, by intercourse with a menstruating woman. The leper was stigmatized and separated from society (Brody 1974).

Sufferers from venereal disease were variously regarded according to the observer's point of view. The promiscuous classes tended to refer to "the pox" with a mixture of false jocularity and casual acceptance, though the frequency with which the malady was invoked in casual swearing doubtless reflected an underlying anxiety.[5] To the respectable and the pious, syphilis and gonorrhea were the just judgments of God upon adulterers, fornicators, and prostitutes; if there were no more fornication, the diseases could be eliminated

(Sharrock 1662, 50–51). The words that observers most frequently applied to syphilis were *loathsome* and foul; they carried a sense of physical aversion and moral repugnance (Waugh 1983, 192, 194, 196). The seventeenth-century physician Thomas Sydenham had to begin his essay on venereal disease by rejecting the opinion of those who thought it wrong to teach the cure for a malady brought on by wrongdoing, just as in the twentieth century the discovery of the penicillin cure for gonorrhea was lamented by some as an encouragement to sexual promiscuity (Latham 1848–1850, 2:32–33; Fee 1988). There is some reason to think that in the eighteenth century the attitude toward venereal disease grew more medical and less moral than it had been, but syphilis remained a dreadful family secret until the twentieth century (Quétel 1990, 5). It was because they could conceive of the disease only in terms of illicit female sexuality that British missionaries in Uganda at the end of the nineteenth century failed to appreciate that syphilis was also present in endemic, non-venereally transmitted form. To the missionaries, venereal disease was inextricably linked to sin (Vaughan 1992).

There were other diseases that were commonly attributed to the sufferer's previous way of life. Gout was usually regarded as a predictable reward for over-indulgence in rich food and strong drink, and, therefore, in one eighteenth-century physician's words, "the patient's own fault" (Copeman 1964, 85–86, also 54, 84). Richard Baxter observed that the poor ate simple food and were therefore seldom tormented by it (Powicke 1926, 180). The victims of the sweating sickness that afflicted early Tudor England were thought to be either wealthy idlers or tavern haunters (John Caius, cited in Slack 1979, 271). In the later seventeenth century Thomas Sydenham took the view that chronic diseases were frequently the result of immoderate living (Latham 1848–1850, 2:138).

The hand of God was also perceived in large-scale epidemics. From bubonic plague in the sixteenth century to cholera in the nineteenth, every outbreak was accompanied by a call from religious leaders to repentance. In these cases, however, the sins held responsible were general ones, like selfishness or irreligion, rather than a breach of the rules relating specifically to personal health.

Readiness to impose a moral interpretation upon sickness was greater when the disease was particularly associated with some marginal or deviant sector of society. Syphilis suffered from its origins among the despised indigenous inhabitants of the New World: King James I (1604/1900, 36) called it "a filthy disease, whereunto these barbarous people are . . . very much subiect." Plague was above all a disease of the poor; hence the notion that it could be overcome by purging society of the physical and moral ills associated with poverty: "popular disturbance, drunkenness, filth of all kinds" (Slack 1985, 339). In the nineteenth century the epidemics that afflicted slum dwellers were associated both with their squalid living conditions and with their supposedly immoral character; overcrowding, for example, meant "such negation of all delicacy, such unclean confusion of bodies and bodily functions, such mutual exposure of animal and sexual nakedness, as is rather bestial than human" (John Simon cited in Wohl 1973, 2:613). Leprosy continued to be stigmatized because of Western contempt for the peoples of Africa and Asia among whom it remained prevalent (Gussow and Tracy 1970, 144).

As a final example of the link between health and moral attitudes we may take the complex issue of changing standards of cleanliness.[6] It is well known that the early modern period saw some notable changes in accepted standards of personal hygiene. In the sixteenth and seventeenth centuries it was expected that polite persons would wash their hands and faces regularly but the invisible parts of the body much less often. The normal toilet was a change of clothes and a rubbing down of the body. Only in the late eighteenth century did the upper classes adopt the habit of regular bathing. There were parallel changes in attitudes toward the disposal of waste products of the body. With the introduction of handkerchiefs it ceased to be acceptable to blow one's nose with one's fingers or to wipe it on a sleeve. Water closets made their appearance in the last quarter of the eighteenth century and there was a growing inhibition about urinating in public. Spitting on the floor ceased to be polite; by the nineteenth century even the spittoon was regarded as a barbarism.

Standards of domestic cleanliness also rose. Earth floors covered with rushes gave way to bare boards that could be washed or carpets that could be beaten. Women's clothes became more washable as the material shifted from wool and silk to linen and, in the late eighteenth century, cotton. In the towns improved water supplies made bathing easier, and in the last fifteen years of the eighteenth century the national consumption of soap increased by more than 40 percent (Mitchell and Deane 1962, 265).

Considerations of health played their part in these changes. It was unacceptable to have dead animals, human excrement, and other forms of filth lying around because they were thought to corrupt the air and cause disease. Whenever an epidemic threatened, special efforts would be made to clean up the streets. Dirt was perceived as much through the nose as the eye, and bad odors were regarded as infallible indication of miasma. Florence Nightingale wrote in 1876 that "all foul smell indicates disease" (cited in Rosenberg 1979, 135 n. 30), but long before the Victorian sanitarians, Tudor administrators had struggled to make the streets "clean and sweet" as a preservative against contagion (see Jenner 1991). It was also recognized that "cleanness in houses . . . especially in beds," was "a great preserver of health" (Tryon 1682, 5). Personal cleanliness was also thought of medical importance. As one authority put it in 1588, "The cutting of the heer, and the paring of the nailes, cleane keping of the eares and teethe be not onely thynges comely and honest, but also holsome rules of phisick" (Bulleyn, 1558, fol. xxxiii).

Yet, as this remark reveals, cleanliness was desirable because it was "comely and honest," irrespective of whether it had any medical value. Long ago Norbert Elias (1939) argued that the lengthening chains of social interdependence and the powerful influence of royal courts intensified the pressure on individuals to make their persons agreeable to those with whom they came into close bodily contact. In the conduct books, bodily propriety was commended as a quality that exemplified a noble soul, distinguished the gentleman from his inferiors, and enabled the social aspirant to get on in the world (Bryson 1984, chap. 3; Childs 1984, 201–10).

There was a strong moral element behind the demand for cleanliness; and its associations were middle-class rather than aristocratic. Cleanliness, whether of the person or the household, was a sign of hard work, regularity, and self-discipline. To keep dirt at a distance, particularly the dirt constituted by bodily excreta, was a demonstration of moral purity. Bad smells had an age-old association with hell and the devil.

The first explicit link between cleanliness and godliness is sometimes thought to have been made by John Wesley in a sermon of 1786. In fact, the phrase was proverbial when Wesley quoted it, and the idea had long been implicit in Jewish and Christian teaching (Outler 1986, 249, 392). In Francis Bacon's words, "Cleanness of body was ever deemed to proceed from a due reverence to God, to society, and to ourselves" (Bacon 1857–1859, 3:377). The body was a divine gift and should be kept pure and undefiled. The Elizabethan Catholic Robert Southwell urged that rooms should be kept clean, because "God is delighted in cleanness, both bodily and ghostly, and detesteth sluttishness" (Southwell 1973, 43–44). The

Jacobean Puritan Richard Bernard wrote that "to be cleanly is healthfull to us, delightsome to others, and commendable. God required of his people cleanlinesse" (Bernard, 1628, 255). Protestant controversialists firmly dissociated themselves from such "intolerably ridiculous" medieval notions as the idea that it might be acceptable to God for saintly men to be "nasty and sordid . . . unclean and filthy in their cloathing"; Christianity required purity "not only of soul, but body" (Edwards 1698, 264).

Of course, the new attitudes took time to establish themselves. Protestant Scotland was notorious for its squalor; in England foppish courtiers gave hypercleanliness overtones of triviality and affectation. Richard Bernard deplored the excesses of those who spent "too much time in trimming, washing, and starching" and were too "curiously neate;" and the godly Richard Baxter was brought up to think that "so much washing of stairs and rooms, to keep them as clean as their trenchers and dishes, and so much ado about cleanliness and trifles, was a sinful curiosity, and expense of servants' time, who might that while have been reading some good book" (Bernard 1628, 255; Wilkinson 1928, 137). Among the lower classes cleanliness of the person was regarded with some suspicion as a sign not of industry but of idleness (*Cyvile and Uncyvile Life* 1579, sig. Kl). For working-class men, dirt acquired overtones of macho virility.

Nevertheless, cleanliness had taken on an intensely religious flavor long before Sir Edwin Chadwick set out on his campaign to remove dirt from the cities. It is well known that the Victorian desire to eliminate urban filth stemmed from moral preoccupations that far transcended, and in some ways were even irrelevant to, the immediate requirements of public health. Indeed, the discovery in the later nineteenth century that it was germs, not dirt, that spread disease notoriously caused some initial dismay because it seemed to make illness an accident rather than a consequence of bad behavior. In fact, the germ theory was quickly reconciled with the drive for higher standards of hygiene (cf. Tomes 1990). Cleanliness remained important because of its moral and social implications, not just because it was necessary for health.

Broadly speaking, the tendency between the sixteenth and nineteenth centuries was for impersonal, medical explanations of disease to supersede religious and moralistic ones. Eighteenth-century attitudes toward epidemics, for example, were markedly more secular than Tudor ones. But the trend must not be exaggerated. The

Church of England after 1660 may have had an increasingly naturalistic attitude toward illness, but the Quakers, Methodists, and other Dissenting sects kept alive the tradition of religious healing, and providential explanations of epidemics continued to be urged in Victorian times.

Even when supernatural explanations of illness dwindled, the link between morality and disease was preserved. In a society that set a high value on achievement and active life, illness was bound to be perceived as a form of deviance. It also imposed a burden on others. It is not surprising that the moral obligation to look after one's health is more insisted upon in the twentieth century than ever before. The association between health and "clean living" has been intensified, and though exceptions will be made for diseases seen as the result of heredity or environmental pollution, the likelihood is that when illness strikes, the patients will blame themselves or be blamed by others for not having followed a healthy regimen, perhaps, or for having omitted to consult a doctor sooner, or for having the sort of character that makes them vulnerable to a particular disease (Currer and Stacey 1986, 219, 264, 272, 276; Sontag 1990, 47–48). We have not reached the situation depicted by Samuel Butler in *Erewhon* (1872), where illness is punished as a crime and crime treated as an illness, but his satire has not lost its force.

There has, however, never been a complete coincidence between the dictates of morality and those of health. In the early modern period, the pursuit of moral purity led to rituals of exclusion that had no physical justification, for example, the avoidance of body smells or the separation of menstruating women from certain domestic functions. The preoccupation with conspicuous physical cleanliness was often irrelevant to the needs of health and more concerned with the values of courtesy, civility, and social pretension. The emphasis on the need to participate in the world and to take into acount the interests of others as well as oneself was flatly incompatible with giving absolute priority to personal health. Changing moral standards contributed far less to improvements in health and longevity than did improved nutrition and living conditions or the discovery of new drugs. Nevertheless, illness and moral responsibility were intimately linked throughout the early modern period; and in many areas of life, notably diet and sexuality, the relationship between health and morality was exceedingly close. Perhaps the most enduring codes of morality are those that have an evident biological utility.

Notes

1. John Sym warned that one should "dote not upon, nor trust, or ascribe too much to physicall meanes, but that we carefully looke and pray to God for a blessing by the warrantable use of them" (1637, 14).
2. By John W. Shirley, *Thomas Harriot: A Biography* (1983, 425), though he gives no source for this statement. The link between clay-pipe smoking and cancer of the mouth or nose was known by the 1880s; Kiernan (1991, 219).
3. William Buchan took much the same view (Rosenberg 1983, 26).
4. For a brilliant discussion of this notion, see Susan Sontag (1990).
5. Cf. the (somewhat exaggerated) comments of D. H. Lawrence (1961, 55–57).
6. I have discussed this topic at greater length in my article "Cleanliness and Godliness in Early Modern England" (1994).

References

Aubrey, John. 1980. *Monumenta Britannica*. Edited by Rodney Legg et al. Sherborne, Eng..

Bacon, Francis. 1857–1859. Of the proficiencie and advancement of learning. In *The works of Francis Bacon*, edited by J. Spedding, R. L. Ellis, and D. D. Heath. 7 vols, London: Longmans.

Barnum, Priscilla H., ed. 1976–. *Dives and pauper*. London: Oxford University Press for the Early English Text Society.

Bell, Rudolph M. 1985. *Holy anorexia*. Chicago: University of Chicago Press.

Bernard, Richard. 1628. *Ruths recompence*. London.

Bethel, Slingsby. 1689. *The interest of the princes and states of Europe*. 3d ed. London: Printed for George Graston.

Bloomfield, Morton W. 1952. *The seven deadly sins*. East Lansing: State College Press.

Bradwell, Stephen. 1636. *Physick for the sicknesse, commonly called the plague*. London: Printed for Benjamin Fisher.

Braithwaite, William C. 1919. *The second period of Quakerism*. London: Macmillan.

Bright, Timothy. 1580. *A treatise: wherein is declared the sufficiencie of English medicines, for cure of all diseases, cured with medicine*. London: Printed by Henrie Middleton for Thomas Man.

Brody, Saul N. 1974. *The disease of the soul: Leprosy in medieval litera-ture*. Ithaca: Cornell University Press.

Bryson, Anna Clare. 1984. Concepts of civility in England c. 1560–1685. D. Phil. thesis., Oxford University.

Bulleyn, William. 1558. *A newe booke entituled the governement of healthe*. London.

Burnet, Gilbert. 1682. *The life and death of Sir Matthew Hale*.

Bynum, Caroline. 1987. *Holy feast and holy fast: The religious significance of food to medieval women*. Berkeley: University of California Press.

Capel, Richard. 1633. *Tentations*. London: Printed by T. B. for John Bart-let.

Cheyne, George. 1725. *An essay of health and long life*. 6th ed. Dublin, Ire.: Printed by W. Wilmot for George Ewing.

Childs, Fenela Ann. 1984. Prescriptions for manners in English courtesy lit-erature, 1690–1760, and their social implications. D. Phil. thesis., Oxford University.

Cogan, Thomas. 1589. *The haven of health*. London: Thomas Orwin, for William Norton.

Copeman, W. S. C. 1964. *A short history of the gout and rheumatic dis-eases*. Berkeley: University of California Press.

Currer, Caroline, and Meg Stacey, eds. 1986. *Concepts of health, illness and disease: A comparative perspective*. Leamington Spa, N.Y.: Berg.

Cyvile and uncyvile life. 1579. London.

Edwards, John. 1698. *Sermons on special occasions and subjects*. London: Printed for Jonathan Robinson . . . and John Wyat.

Elias, Norbert. 1939. *Uber den Prozess der Zivilisation*. Basel. Haus zum Falken.

Fee, Elizabeth. 1988. Sin vs. science: Venereal disease in Baltimore in the twentieth century. *Journal of the History of Medicine* 43.

Fukuyama, Francis. 1992. *The end of history and the last man*. New York: Free Press.

Gruman, Gerald J. 1961. The rise and fall of prolongevity hygiene, 1558–1873. *Bulletin of the History of Medicine* 35.

Gussow, Zachary, and George S. Tracy. 1970. Stigma and the leprosy phe-nomenon. *Bulletin of the History of Medicine* 44.

Harrison, Brian. 1971. *Drink and the Victorians*. London: Faber & Faber.

Hobbes, Thomas. 1651/1991. *Leviathan*. Edited by Richard Tuck. New York: Cambridge University Press.

James I. 1604/1900. A counterblaste to tobacco. In *A royal rhetorician*, edited by Robert S. Rait. Westminster: A. Constable.

Jenner, M. S. R. 1991. Early modern English conceptions of "cleanliness" and "dirt" as reflected in the environmental regulation of London, c. 1530–c.1700. D. Phil. thesis., Oxford University.

Kellwaye, Simon. 1593. *A defensative against the plague*. London.

Kelly, Patrick H., ed. 1991. *Locke on Money*. Oxford, Eng.: Clarendon Press.

Kiernan, V. G. 1991. *Tobacco: A history*. London: Hutchinson Radius.

Latham, R., and W. Matthews, eds. 1970–1983. *The diary of Samuel Pepys*. Berkeley: University of California Press.

Latham, R. G., trans. 1848–1850. *The works of Thomas Sydenham*. London: Printed for the Sydenham Society.

Lawrence, D. H. 1961. Puritanism and the arts. In *Selected literary criticism*, edited by Anthony Beal. London: Heinemann.

Lord, Henry. 1630. *A display of two forraigne sects in the East Indies*. London: Imprinted for Francis Constable.

MacDonald, Michael, and Terence R. Murphy. 1990. *Sleepless souls: Suicide in early modern England*. New York: Oxford University Press.

Mitchell, B. R., and Phyllis Deane. 1962. *Abstract of British historical statistics*. Cambridge, Eng.: Cambridge University Press.

Morris, R. J 1976. *Cholera, 1832: The social response to an epidemic*. New York: Holmes & Meier.

Mullett, Charles F. 1956. *The bubonic plague and England*. Lexington: University of Kentucky Press.

Outler, Albert C., ed. 1986. *The works of John Wesley, vol. 3, Sermons 71–114*. Nashville: Abingdon Press.

Perkins, William. 1608–1631. *The workes*. Cambridge, Eng. John Legate.

Phayer, T., trans. 1546. *The Kegiment* [sic] *of life, wherunto is added a treatyse of the pestilence*. London.

Powicke, F. J. 1926. The Reverend Richard Baxter's last treatise. *Bulletin of the John Rylands Library* 10:180.

Quétel, Claude. 1990. *History of syphilis*. Translated by J. Braddock and B. Pike. London: Polity Press in association with Basil Blackwell.

Rosenberg, Charles E. 1979. Florence Nightingale on contagion: The hospital as moral universe. In *Healing and history: Essays for George Rosen*, edited by C. E. Rosenberg. New York: Science History Publications.

———. 1983. Medical text and social context: Explaining William Buchan's *Domestic Medicine. Bulletin of the History of Medicine* 57.

Sharrock, Robert. 1662. *Judicia, (seu Legum Censurae) de Variis Incontinentiae Speciebus*. Oxford, Eng.: H. Hall . . . Thom Robinson.

Shirley, John W. 1983. *Thomas Harriot: A biography*. New York: Oxford University Press.

Short, Richard. 1656. *ΠΕΡΙ ΨΥΧΡΟΠΟΣΙΑΣ Of drinking water*. London: Printed for John Crook.

Sinclair, Sir John. 1807. *The code of health and longevity*. 4 vols. Edinburgh. A. Constable.

Slack, Paul. 1979. Mirrors of health and treasures of poor men: The uses of the vernacular medical literature of Tudor England. In *Health, medicine, and mortality in the sixteenth century*, edited by Charles Webster. New York: Cambridge University Press.

———. 1985. *The impact of plague in Tudor and Stuart England*. Boston: Routledge & Kegan Paul.

Smith, Charlotte Fell. 1901. *Mary Rich, Countess of Warwick (1625–1678): Her family and friends*. New York: Longmans, Green.

Smith, Ginnie. 1985. Prescribing the rules of health: Self-help and advice in the late eighteenth century. In *Patients and practitioners: Lay perceptions of medicine in pre-industrial society*, edited by Roy Porter. New York: Cambridge University Press.

Sontag, Susan. 1990. *Illness as metaphor; AIDS and its metaphors*. New York: Doubleday.

Southwell, Robert. 1973. *Two letters and short rules of a good life*, edited by Nancy P. Brown. Charlottesville: University Press of Virginia.

Stewart, Grace G. 1967. A history of the medicinal use of tobacco, 1492–1860. *Medical History* 11.

Sym, John. 1637. *Lifes preservative against self-killing*. London.

Talbot, C. H., ed. and trans. 1987. *The life of Christina of Markyate*. Oxford, Eng.: Clarendon Press.

Temkin, Owsei. 1949. Medicine and the problem of moral responsibility. *Bulletin of the History of Medicine* 23.

———. 1973. *Galenism: The rise and decline of a medical philosophy*. Ithaca: Cornell University Press.

Thomas, Keith. 1971. *Religion and the decline of magic*. New York: Scribner.

———. 1983. *Man and the natural world: Changing attitudes in England, 1500–1800*. London: Allen Lane.

———. 1994. Cleanliness and godliness in early modern England. In *Religion, culture and society in early modern Britain*, edited by A. J. Fletcher and P. R. Roberts. New York: Cambridge University Press.

Tomes, Nancy. 1990. The private side of public health: Sanitary science, domestic hygiene, and the germ theory, 1870–1900. *Bulletin of the History of Medicine* 64.

Torshell, Samuell. 1644. *The hypocrite discovered and cured*. London: Printed by G. M. for John Bellamy.

Tryon, Thomas. 1682. *A treatise of cleanness in meats and drinks*. London: Printed for the author and sold by L. Curtis.

Updike, John. 1991. *Rabbit at rest*. London: Penguin Books.

Vaughan, Megan. 1992. Syphilis in Colonial East and Central Africa: The social construction of an epidemic. In *Epidemics and ideas: Essays on the historical perception of pestilence*, edited by T. Ranger and P. Slack. New York: Cambridge University Press.

Vaughan, William. 1602. *Naturall and artificial directions for health*. London: R. Bradocke.

———. 1626. *The golden fleece*. London.

Waugh, M. A. 1983. Venereal diseases in sixteenth-century England. *Medical History* 17:192, 194, 196.

Wilkinson, John T., ed. 1928. *Richard Baxter and Margaret Charlton*. London: G. Allen & Unwin.

Willet, Andrew. 1631. *Hexapla in Leviticum*. London: A. Matthews for R. Milbourne.

Wohl, Anthony S. 1973. Unfit for human habitation. In *The Victorian city: Images and realities*, edited by H. J. Dyos and M. Wolff. Boston: Routledge & Kegan Paul.

Banishing Risk

Continuity and Change in the Moral Management of Disease

Charles Rosenberg

We honor randomness in the abstract but seek to manage it in practice, to constrain misfortune in reassuring frameworks of meaning. We want health to make predictive sense, to be based on coherent relationships between behavior and its consequences. Notions about the causation and nature of disease are and have been throughout history inextricably bound up with meaning and identity. Blame, guilt, and anxiety can be harnessed in powerful conjunction—as can the presumed interaction between body and mind. We are what we have done or neglected to do.

These ideas have been articulated countless times and in a variety of forms, from classical antiquity to the present. Throughout the history of Western medical thought, chronic sickness—and predisposition to acute and epidemic ills—was generally understood to be a cumulative product of the longtime interaction between a biologically unique individual and a particular environment. As the body moved through time, it required food and water, sleep and exercise. One was always becoming, thus always at risk. Every circumstance of life and each day-to-day decision was physiologically meaningful. Habits of living once established could lead cumulatively—but with ultimate inexorability—to sickness and death, just as they could, if properly regulated, maintain health well into old age.

It must be recalled that until the mid-nineteenth century the concept of specific disease entities was not understood in the modern sense; a cold could shade into tuberculosis, a bruise into cancer, disorderly eating habits into gout or diabetes. In this sense, a bad habit indulged in over time was—literally—the first stage in a disease process. Lack of disease specificity implied an elusive yet omnipresent nemesis, but one that could be understood, anticipated, and averted. Logically enough, seventeenth- and eighteenth-century guides to health and longevity emphasized the need to control all the aspects of life that a prudent man or woman could control: diet, exercise, sleep, the evacuations, and emotions. In the terminology of the day—and following a tradition that could be traced back to Galen—such factors were termed the "nonnaturals" as opposed to the "naturals," innate factors that might also lead to disease.

> By the term *"non-naturals"* were understood all those things which are *essential to life*, but which *neither enter into the composition of the animal oeconomy, nor form part of the living body*. These comprehend *air, foods and drinks, motion and rest, sleep and wakefulness, secretions, excretions, and retentions, mental emotions, clothing, bathing, &c.* (Pickford 1858)

It is obvious that such concern with day-to-day routine provided an occasion for the enforcing of a society's behavioral norms; there could be no practical distinction between the realms of morality, meaning, and mechanism. The symptoms of moral sickness—sexual promiscuity, gluttony, sloth, uncontrolled emotional excess—inevitably undermined physical health.

Much of this age-old emphasis on regimen will seem enlightened and even prescient to health-conscious late-twentieth-century readers. But too much has intervened between the late eighteenth century and the present; it is no longer possible to share the assumptions of traditional medicine—even if particular elements in that configuration of ideas seem familiar. I would like to emphasize four themes fundamental to this traditional way of understanding health and disease, themes configured so as to constitute a way of thinking about the body antithetical to certain dominant trends in twentieth-century medicine. First, was its aggregate, inclusive, and cumulative quality. In this sense, categorical distinctions between body and mind, physiology and morality were all arbitrary because each was formed and in that process transmuted in the countless ongoing interactions that constituted individuality. Second, was an unquestioned emphasis on idiosyncrasy, not only the individuality of physiological response to drugs and patterning of symptoms in disease but the uniqueness of every man or woman's innate constitution and its particular history since conception.[1] Third, was the physiological centrality of unceasing interactions between body and mind and of the way in which this view of mind incorporated both the treacherous—and potentially pathogenic—passions as well as those "higher" elements involved in decision making. Conscious decisions guided the individual in his or her passage between childhood and death; every aspect of day-to-day life implied choice, and thus volition. Following logically is the fourth element I want to underline, namely, individual responsibility for continued health and—in sickness—the management of recovery, especially in chronic illness. This cluster of ideas can be seen as maintaining a prominent role for volition and responsibility, and thus remaining consistently relevant to the management of randomness.

These linked ideas also constituted a doctrine best suited to the life choices of those who could exercise such choices; contemporaries were well aware of the inequalities in choice mandated by the realities of class and work. A laborer could not easily vary his diet or those of his wife and children; he could not improve his health through regular horseback riding or sea voyages to the Adriatic or West Indies. Nevertheless, then as now, physicians differed, and intellectual positions blurred as contemporaries blamed as well as excused the poor for the sickness that so often followed them through life.

"This Long Disease, My Life"

Emphasis on regimen and lifestyle was somewhat less evident in social constructions of acute and epidemic disease.[2] Chronic illness was a different matter. Each case constituted a unique aggregate of circumstance and responsibility, of morality and imprudence, of countless decisions (and thus behaviors) repeated over time. In chronic ills, not only was one a disease but the disease was oneself. A bout with typhus fever was an episode, for example, not an identity. In flu the patient suffers from but is not flu; one might be attacked by cholera, but if one survived, a man or woman was not defined by cholera in the sense that "dropsy," leprosy, diabetes, or epilepsy become aspects of subsequent identity. (Acute infectious disease could also have long-term consequences, as the examples of polio or smallpox—with its capacity to disfigure and even blind—illustrate in their rather different ways.)

The cure of chronic illness, like its cause, was woven gradually and inextricably into the fabric of life. Recovery or survival was forged over time; one was necessarily more responsible for managing one's own recovery in chronic than in acute ills. "People in acute diseases may sometimes be their own physicians," as the most widely read and reprinted late-eighteenth-century health manual noted, "but in the chronic, the cure must ever depend chiefly upon the patient's own endeavours" (Buchan 1797). Not surprisingly, medical writers of the late-eighteenth and early-nineteenth centuries routinely emphasized a distinction between chronic and acute illness; they were well aware of the very different sort of situation each created for patients, families, and practitioners.

The concept of predisposition that served to explain the selective exactions of acute disease was, as we have suggested, like chronic disease itself, a cumulative aggregate of constitution, circumstance, and regimen. In these instances, too, society articulated a rationalistically framed denial of moral randomness. The glutton, the alcoholic, the anxious and weak of spirit appeared to succumb disproportionately to yellow fever, smallpox, or cholera—as did the malnourished, the dirty, and the economically disadvantaged. In the case of smallpox, of course, nineteenth-century commentators could point to a culpable ignorance in the failure to employ vaccination.

Religious frameworks of meaning coexisted with, supplemented, and interpenetrated such physiological schemes, but by the end of the eighteenth century they could not stand alone. Educated lay people and physicians did tend to believe that culpable errors in behavior—sin—brought temporal punishment, but only through mechanisms built into the human body. Excessive consumption of alcohol caused sickness, not through divine interposition but as an unavoidable consequence of metabolizing an "unnatural" substance. What seems transparently moralistic to a late-twentieth-century sensibility seemed no more than an unmediated reflection of nature's teachings in the late eighteenth century or early nineteenth. The style of these speculative pathologies is, of course, more important than their specific content. They emphasized that mechanisms built into the body guaranteed that only "natural" practices and behaviors would prove consistent with health; not surprisingly, the "natural" overlapped with contemporary notions of the moral. Distilled spirits were unnatural by definition, their consumption necessarily dangerous; monogamy was natural to the species, promiscuity perilous to body as well as soul. Such admonitions—based upon the presumed "design" of living things—were everywhere, in schoolbooks and sermons as well as in medical treatises (Rosenberg 1995).

In the past century and a half, our medical ideas have changed dramatically. We are most comfortable with ills that have a discrete, material, and well-understood basis—a basis demonstrable in the laboratory and at postmortem. Without an understanding of such a mechanism or the presumption that it exists, we are hesitant to grant social recognition to pain and discomfort. Diagnosis can define a social role and often confers social legitimacy; without it, a sufferer may face the malingerer's demeaning and guilt-inducing status. It was inevitable that twentieth-century understandings of pathological mechanism should be made to serve didactic ends paralleling those arguments from design that loomed so prominently in the late-eighteenth and early-nineteenth centuries They are simply too impressive in their explanatory power, integrated too tightly into our way of thinking about the world. They must inevitably bear the burden of meanings that transcend mechanism.

Specificity and Mechanism

The modern view of disease was developed in two stages. The first turned on acceptance of the idea that diseases were specific entities, with characteristic clinical course and underlying pathological basis (physiological, anatomical, or some combination of the two). The second stage in the nineteenth-century history of pathological ideas turned on a revolution in ideas about the causation of infectious disease. I refer, of course, to the germ theory. This new doctrine seemed to underline and confirm the ontological status of those entities (such as typhoid fever, for example) that had already been described by clinicians and clinically oriented pathological anatomists.

There were moral and policy implication as well. Emphasis on the existence of discrete, disease-specific, external causes implied the likelihood that disease might grow out of a chance intersection between individual and etiological agent.[3] Increasingly, it appeared that sickness might become severed from moral agency and thus—as some nineteenth-century commentators feared—from moral order (Stevenson 1955; Rosenberg 1979).

Individual volition and social circumstance threatened to have less and less to do with the explanation of illness. Accepting the necessity of a discrete, particulate cause emphasized the randomness of sickness as well as its mechanism; it was not who but where one was that determined vulnerability. Thus the germ theory undercut the aggregate and cumulative aspect of traditional models of the etiology of disease (in terms, that is, of their emphasis on the prior life course of the sick person both as moral *and* biological individual). The dramatic discoveries of late-nineteenth-century bacteriology thus gradually helped impugn the plausibility of accustomed holistic disease models and endorsed the increasing centrality of a specific, reductionist, and mechanism-oriented understanding of disease. This is a cliche of historical understanding—and like most such truisms reflects a certain measure of truth. But not without modification.

Longtime habits of mind could not be changed overnight. Environmental, constitutional, and occupational factors remained prominent in late-nineteenth-century etiological thinking, especially in explaining the incidence of chronic illness such as tuberculosis. Predispoition and susceptibility still needed to be explained—even if one conceded the necessity of microorganisms to the working out of a particular disease process. The influence of stress, morale, and the passions continued to play a role in medical and lay thinking about health. And likelihoods of intersection with pathogenic organisms could also be seen in social—and thus potentially policy—terms; occupation or origin as distinct from moral status could site an individual in a particular social space and thus explain differential incidences of particular ills. A foundryman or metal polisher, for example, might be particularly susceptible to tuberculosis or other chest ailments—no matter what his personal habits. A poor widow might find it difficult to rent an adequately ventilated apartment, no matter how clean and regular her habits. Predisposition could be social as well as biological.

There was no easy solution to the political and moral dilemma of apportioning social and individual responsibility for the maintenance of health; late-nineteenth-century public health advocates always factored into their thinking the contributory agency of even the most economically and socially disadvantaged victims of disease. One could always find reasons to blame the poverty-stricken and exploited—even in the course of calling for reform in their conditions of life. Workers were routinely accused of alcoholism, poor personal hygiene, and "imprudence," even when it was conceded that they lived in inhumane conditions, worked lengthy hours, and suffered periodic unemployment. The code words *intel-*

ligent and *unintelligent* were often used to explain suceptibility—
and status. The germ theory of infectious disease was to have an
enormous impact, but it could not abolish such deeply felt social
assumptions.

The germ theory had more than intellectual consequences, however. It was soon built into a structure of technical qualification,
laboratory findings, and professional status. This was a world of
credentials and experts increasingly (though by no means consistently) uncongenial to the holistic, individual, and moral understanding of illness that had for millennia helped men and women
deal with its incursions. The germ theory was no mere academic
abstraction; in the last quarter of the nineteenth and first quarter
of the twentieth centuries it would help transform every aspect of
medicine.

One aspect of that transformation lay in the elevation of the
medical profession's social status and in a recasting of the physician's social identity. We have come to expect efficacy and technical
activism as appropriately characterizing the doctor's ministrations
and—as already emphasized—to see medical knowledge in material, mechanism-oriented, and reductionist terms. In the paradoxi-
cally linked yet contradictory elements of art and science that
traditionally constituted medical acumen, the science component
has become increasingly dominant. This style of framing health and
disease also affects how we as patients feel about ourselves, how we
construe our own sickness or continued health.

In terms of our present discussion, however, I want to underline
another and perhaps less familiar aspect of twentieth-century medicine. This is the changed ecology of disease. However we weigh the
relevant variables—however much credit we are willing to allot to
the specific input of scientific medicine and how much to generally
improved standards of living—it is undeniable that the acute infectious diseases have become far less prominent in the course of the
twentieth century.[4]

As we are all aware, men and women have come to live longer
in the Western world and are more likely to live with and ultimately
die from chronic ills that demand social and personal adjustment
and defy one-dimensional etiological explanation. Second, we have
become increasingly wedded to diagnostic categories defined oper-
ationally in terms of laboratory procedures—biochemical and his-
tological, immunological and imaging. Third, we have not only
described a host of new ills but also turned our attention to a variety of proto or incipient ills: the by-products of our effort to moni-

tor and understand the normal and the pathological. I refer to such states as elevated cholesterol level or hypertension. Whatever one thinks about their ultimate prognostic or clinical significance, it is undeniable that once delineated, such states create new emotional agendas. Individuals who harbor in their bodies the immanent menace of an elevated cholesterol or blood pressure reading face years and decades of newly meaningful decisions about every aspect of their day-to-day routine.

Twentieth-century medicine has also created new chronic disease as an unintended by-product of technical change. Therapeutic progress has turned a variety of once rapidly fatal ailments into long-term problems of living. I refer to those individuals who survive as chronic "management" problems—diabetics after the introduction of insulin or sufferers from degenerative kidney disease after dialysis—and whose social and intrapsychic identities have as much as their physiological status to be managed over time. Each such case is clothed with potential moral valence. All of the gradients, choices, and consequent guilts of "lifestyle" management in persons only potentially ill are exacerbated in men and women actually suffering from chronic disease. Are the patients compliant or not? How do they manage themselves? If they suffer from a chronic yet infectious condition such as AIDS or tuberculosis, how responsible are they in seeking available treatment and in avoiding situations in which the ailment might be transmitted?

All of these changes in patterns of morbidity have helped structure a fundamental ambiguity: our general conceptions of disease have become increasingly specific while—as individuals—we have become increasingly likely to suffer from vague, multi-causal and overlapping ailments. As in the twentieth century we have shifted our burden of illness toward the chronic, so have we enlarged our store of specific clinical pictures. And the accepted repertoire of such disease categories constitutes in the social sphere a stock of archetypical narratives—trajectories against which an individual judges his or her prospects for future pain, incapacity, or death. A diagnosis may also place one's past behavior in a very different retrospective light, recasting one's sense of autobiographical self in altered terms. Every clinical entity once articulated and accepted in its several ways in the lay and medical community becomes a factor in doctor-patient relations, in the patient's expectations and self-evaluation, and in intrafamily relationships. A nosology can thus be seen as constituting a culturally available menu of alternative narratives (Rosenberg 1992). How does one arrest or modify the pathological process unfolding in one's body? How does one prevent such illness through an appropriate regimen? It is a contemporary situation subtly different from yet paralleling the general need for physiological prudence and foresight implied by the nonspecific pathologies of traditional medicine. Physicians have always been aware that chronic ills—no matter what their original etiology—implied questions of individual adjustment and social support; time itself and increased lengths of survival imply special problems for society and for the individual patient (e.g., Peitzman 1989; Bates 1992). The omnipresence of chronic disease at the end of the twentieth century (along with what I have called protodisease states such as elevated blood pressure or cholesterol levels) has placed increasing emotional and policy emphasis on lifestyle and individual choice, and thus responsibility. Chronic disease always implies an extended narrative, a "Patient's Progress" of choice and moral self-definition, just as it does a new social role. The metaphors of "narrative" and "social role" express two aspects of—and ways of thinking about—the same lived reality.

It also implies a debate about the locus of responsibility. What is the role of the state in a just—and aging—society? How does one balance individual responsibility against the need for social intervention? How much does the entirely rational attempt to reduce risk through individual suasion serve to blame victims and avoid the necessity of dealing with structural inequities? This drama of contested moral choice and social commitment is one that all twentieth-century societies have acted out in their particular fashion.

Being Sick/Becoming Sick

Recently, the U.S. Department of Health and Human Services published an elaborate position paper, *Healthy People 2000: National Health Promotion and Disease Prevention Objectives*, "a statement of national opportunities." Though calling for an eclectic variety of health-promoting efforts, this document nevertheless highlights the role and responsibility of individuals. As we reach the end of the century, the first page of the introduction notes, "biomedical research has available sophisticated techniques for diagnosing and intervening against disease." Medicine has taught us much about those factors predisposing to sickness and premature death, "and therefore about actions that each of us can take to control our risks for disease or disability. We have learned," the document continues, "that a fuller measure of health, a better quality of life, is within our personal grasp." Cigarette smoking, high-fat foods, alcohol abuse, for example, and sedentary styles of life have all been shown to increase substantially risk of sickness and premature death. Mortality from these causes, the authors contend, "are examples of the impact of personal lifestyle choices on the health destiny of individual Americans and the future of the nation."[5] Three basic elements of a far older view of disease causation are thus linked logically, rhetorically, and emotionally: "personal," "lifestyle," and "choice." Chronic illness becomes in this moral sense an aggregate of cigarettes smoked, seatbelts unfastened, glasses filled and emptied, cheeseburgers devoured.

As in the pre-germ-theory era, habits slide gradually yet finally irreversibly into disease. Our bodies reflect cumulative behaviors and impart worth, with the specter of disease serving as sanction for accepted behavioral norms. The ideal-typical trajectories built into twentieth-century concepts of specific disease imply individual dramas of right and wrong, impulse and denial. Inevitably, such physiologically informed perceptions of self fit easily and consistently into the more general cultural value of control and the achievement of moral stature through the denial of material satisfaction. Eschewing fried foods is resonant with moral as well as biochemical meaning. Exercise brings a sense of worth as well as improved cardiovascular status. And monogamy imparts to believers moral stature as well as risk reduction. Cultural order and thus emotional reassurance remain implicit in a predictable relationship between willed acts and their physiological consequences—as they had in earlier centuries. Self-denial has historically been associated with spiritual stature, and this powerful association correlates nicely with much contemporary understanding of the relationships among diet, exercise, and the etiology of chronic disease.

There are certain other obvious parallels between contemporary and traditional views of chronic disease. One is the omnipresence of what I have already referred to as protodisease states, such conditions as elevated cholesterol or blood pressure levels. Both are artifacts of medicine's reductionist and laboratory-oriented style of practice, yet, ironically, each such problematic physiological status presents a potential site for moral action. Each also represents a diffusion and modification of tightly bounded conceptions of specific disease (and thus harkens back to pre-nineteenth-century conceptions of disease). In hypertension, let us say, the normal melts imperceptibly into the pathological and vice versa; boundaries are not discrete and categorical—unless we choose to create arbitrary, if bureaucratically functional—physiological or biochemical thresholds that legitimate particular diagnoses and trigger associated therapeutic procedures. With our increasing diagnostic capacities, we have provided altered narratives for millions of individuals who might otherwise have lived out their lives in ignorance of a nemesis lurking in their bodies.

We have in the past decades also generated another, psychologically rather than physiologically or biochemically defined, type of protoillness. I refer to such putative entities as the Type A and the addictive personalities. We remain—as our ancestors did—uncomfortable with monolithic etiologies that find no room for psychological and temperamental variables. And these hypothetical "types" are remarkably fluid in their construction; one might well ask whether such personality types constitute sickness, prognostic indicators, self-fulfilling moral judgment, or normal variation. But whatever their role in etiology and diagnosis, such constructs unquestionably do project cultural second thoughts: in the case of Type-A personality, doubts about the unsettling kinds of behavior that so often seem to make the self-made man; in the case of the addictive personality, the fear of loss of control. They also parallel and reaffirm traditional assumptions about the necessary connection between body and mind, health and behavior—as well, of course, as the need to deal with the "passions" if health is to be maintained.

"Psychosomatic medicine" and "holistic medicine" are concepts that have become fashionable in the second half of the twentieth century. Both can be seen as reactions against the categorical claims of the mechanistic reductionist style of medical explanation that dominated the first half of the century. And both are often seen as new and advanced ways of thinking about health and disease. Both, however, would have been seen as orthodox—if not as truisms—by any eighteenth- or early-nineteenth-century physician.

In our universe of accepted disease entities, specificity implies unity of type and predictability of course over time. It implies as well a basis in some particular pathological mechanism. As we have suggested, this cluster of assumptions constituted a fundamental shift away from pre-nineteenth-century ways of thinking about illness. A secure, mechanism-based ontological status implies social legitimacy; the diagnosis of an accepted clinical entity imparts legitimacy to behaviors—and feelings—otherwise ambiguous, conferring the benefits of sick-role status in such contested instances. All ailments are not created morally equal. Despite several generations of criticisms of medicine as excessively reductionist and mechanism-oriented, "functional" ills still bear a burden of moral failure, of psychic weakness or even conscious malingering. As a consequence, men and women often seek the ironic comfort of a diagnosis based on "objective"—in practice often immunological—criteria. Thus the familiar contemporary spectacle of patients demanding a particular diagnosis, asking that physicians see in a cluster of vague, continuing, and troublesome complaints a specific and thus legitimate ailment. Chronic fatigue syndrome and mononucleosis, for example, or hypoglycemia have in the recent past constituted such contested cultural goods. Lyme disease has begun to fill this social role as well. And like many such ailments, it has mobilized lay advocacy groups dedicated to establishing the biological, and thus moral, legitimacy of their ailments. "We are working very hard to alert the public about the seriousness of the disease," the director of the New Jersey Lyme Disease Network contended in the *New York Times*. "We are also trying to convince doctors that patients are victims of Lyme disease, not Lyme hysteria" (Stolow 1992; Aronowitz 1991).

Even if such ills are perceived in often rather different terms by physicians and patients, by the educated and less educated, by women and men, they nevertheless constitute compelling ways of thinking about oneself. We must each still negotiate our own understanding of pain and incapacity. But the physician and the diagnoses he or she is empowered to bestow constitute important elements in that negotiation.

Mechanism and Meanings

We all accept multifactorial models of disease causation; but webs of causation (and especially seamless ones) do not always address our need for meaning—although they make intellectual and even aesthetic sense. Likelihoods and multifactorial complexes of causation do not easily fit into most people's way of thinking about themselves and family members. Nor does it fit nicely into the emotional necessities of the doctor-patient relationship; men and women want to know what is to happen next in their own lives or that of family members, not in that of a statistical aggregate; it is no accident that practicing clinicians have been notoriously slow to think in terms of probability. All patients are individuals; all pain is unique. The very words "risk reduction" and their aura of impersonal distance from the coarse realities of sickness, pain, and premature death reflect precisely a contemporary style of reassuring public discourse—while at the same time fostering guilt and the need for control in its traditional emphasis on lifestyle and regimen.

We have come full circle in this era of concern with chronic disease. A life as lived has once again become a subject of analysis and policy debate; constitution, environment, and volition are once again speculatively configured as we evaluate the etiology and prophylaxis of important ills. Contemporary debates over anorexia, AIDS, and lung cancer, for example, all reflect in their particular ways the persistence of this explanatory style. The movement from propensity to habit to pathological mechanism has once again become a central concern of moralists as well as epidemiologists and clinicians. Body and mind, constitution and lifestyle, choice and responsibility are not easily banished from the world of pathogenesis and public health (Rosenberg 1989). The American Institute for Preventive Medicine issued, for example, the following list of ten New Year's resolutions for 1992. The first was stress management. The others, in order, were practice safe sex; stop smoking; avoid secondhand smoke; develop a social support network; be active; control consumption of cholesterol and saturated fat; limit your intake of red meat, eggs, and cheese; moderate alcohol use; and have a sense of purpose (*Philadelphia Inquirer* 1991).

But this is only one aspect of contemporary strategies for dealing with the prospect—and reality—of sickness, for allaying the specter of randomness. Even if we believe that a culturally homogeneous view of the body in health and sickness still existed in 1800, we can hardly entertain the notion of such a unified vision persisting into the present. Many of us do find an unambiguous, reductionist, nonresonant view of disease compelling: from this perspective, the meaning of disease reduces itself to the mechanism that underlies it. And it is a meaning necessarily discerned and defined by the physician as scientist; emotional security thus grows out of faith in the community of physicians and scientists to whom we have willingly ceded this responsibility. Equally appealing, if to a constituency somewhat different from that content with the seemingly value-free truths of the laboratory and the computer correlation, is the logically contrary emphasis on the etiological and therapeutic power of the individual mind and emotions.

I refer to a group of self-help advocates and believers in willed healing.[6] It is comforting, for some of us at least, to believe that emotional repression can, for example, cause cancer and that mind and emotion can cure it—despite the marginal intellectual status of such beliefs in a medical world dominated by the status and reductionist views of scientific medicine. But this emphasis on the therapeutic efficacy of properly directed emotions brings with it a reciprocal social burden: the guilt of those whose disease is exacerbated by a feeling of individual failure. Critics of this view contend that it is bad enough to fall victim to cancer or other life-threatening illness without feeling that one has somehow crafted one's own suceptibility. "In a turnabout of the age-old agonized question asking why bad things happen only to good people, we are now told that—aha!—bad things happen only to good people (so repressed, you know). Cancer cells are internalized anger gone on a field trip all over our bodies. Give me a break," wrote an impassioned cancer victim rejecting one such view of her ailment's etiology. "I want to face the reality of randomness in life, as well. We humans would rather accept culpability than chaos, but randomness is the law of life." (Sigmund 1989). Despite our growing understanding of the mechanisms that constitute the biological substrate of many diseases, we can hardly lay claim to a parallel understanding of the cultural and emotional phenomena surrounding sickness and death. We will continue to impose meanings, stigmatize victims, use the incursions of disease to sanction—and sometimes to undermine—cultural norms and social policies.

Related to such negotiations is the age-old problem of apportioning responsibility between the individual and society. There is no logical need for policies aimed at the modification of individual behavior to compete for funds with efforts to deal with more general social problems. But schematic logic has little to do with it. In practice that debate continues as we often treat individual and social policies as alternative options in a zero sum game—and as we continue our equally traditional practice of both blaming and exculpating those disproportionately at risk.

There is no simple answer. It is hard for most of us to think about health in other than reductionist terms, yet that way of framing our prospects does not consistently satisfy our needs for meaning and certainty. Even in instances in which we can demonstrate correlations between specific risks—cigarette smoking, a high-fat diet, for example, or sexual promiscuity—objective data are inevitably clothed with subjective resonance. Simple correlations are ordinarily far from simple, so long as they concern matters of emotional import. Behavior, guilt, and responsibility are still powerfully linked. These relationships are ancient and in some ways they have only been recast and exacerbated by the accomplishments of modern medicine. Our expectations of health and long life have increased, and the growing dominance of chronic disease makes those expectations seem often no more than ingenuous. We know too much and not enough.

Notes

I am grateful for the criticism of conference participants and, in addition, to Barbara Bates, Chris Feudtner, Renee Fox, Gerald N. Grob, Steven J. Kunitz, and Irvine Loudon, who were kind enough to read and comment on this paper. A somewhat different version of this paper appeared in 1995 in *Perspectives in Biology and Medicine* 39:28–42, and is printed here with permission of the University of Chicago Press.

1. It should be recalled that *constitution* meant something rather different to physicians and laymen in all centuries before the twentieth and acceptance of a fundamental distinction between hereditary and nonhereditary attributes. In earlier eras, constitution was seen as present at conception—yet necessarily reflecting and incorporating every subsequent interaction with the environment, both in utero and subsequently. Although disease was not regarded as absolutely transmissible from parents to child, tendencies or weaknesses could be thus inherited. And chronic diseases—such as cancer, mental illness, gout, or tuberculosis—were generally regarded as reflecting such constitutional ("diathetical") components in their etiology. For a more detailed discussion, see Rosenberg (1974).

2. The density of social resonance surrounding even acute disease varies according to ailment character. Influenza is brief, ordinarily not life threatening, and recovery is normally complete; not surprisingly, it is comparatively unburdened with an aura of guilt and stigma. Cholera or plague represent very different instances, although neither constituted the same sort of social phenomenon as that of a chronic illness such as epilepsy or diabetes. The phrase "This long disease, my life" is from Alexander Pope's "Epistle to Dr. Arbuthnot" and was used as an apt title in Nicholson and Rousseau (1968).

3. Obviously, there were certain kinds of ailments—most prominently the venereal—in which the newer knowledge of etiology seemed entirely

consistent with the teachings of traditional morality. But then again, no one had ever doubted the contagiosity of such ills, which tended, like smallpox, to be seen as unambiguously contagious by means of a specific reproducible matter.

4. In referring to the weighing of variables, I refer, of course, to the so-called McKeown controversy and to a related and even more elaborate discussion in demographic and development circles of the factors relevant to the "health transition." Thomas McKeown, an English professor of social medicine, focused on the decline of tuberculosis, which was well marked in the second half of the nineteenth century and first quarter of the twentieth, well before effective chemotherapy was available. On McKeown, see, for example, McKeown 1979; Szreter 1988; and Wilson 1990.

5. The document in its entirety underlines the need to contend with social as well as individual "risk factors." But it does reflect the assumption that modifying individual behavior in an era of chronic disease (and accidents) constitutes the most direct and effective tactic for altering patterns of morbidity and mortality.

6. Perhaps most prominent among such advocates are Norman Cousins and Bernie Siegel, the latter of whom has perpetrated the aphorism that there are no incurable diseases, only incurable patients. See Cousins 1979; Siegel 1986.

References

Aronowitz, R. 1991. Lyme disease: The social construction of a new disease and its social consequences. *Milbank Quarterly* 69:79–112.

Bates, B. 1992. *Bargaining for life: A social history of tuberculosis, 1876–1938.* Philadelphia: University of Pennsylvania Press.

Buchan, W. 1797. *Domestic medicine: Or, a treatise on the prevention and cure of diseases by regimen and simple medicines.* Philadelphia: Thomas Dobson.

Cousins, N. 1979. *Anatomy of an illness as perceived by the patient: Reflections on healing and regeneration.* New York: Norton.

McKeown, T. 1979. *The role of medicine: Dream, mirage, or nemesis?* Princeton: Princeton University Press.

McKeown's *The Role of Medicine.* 1977. *Milbank Quarterly* 55:361–428.

Nicholson, M., and G. S. Rousseau. 1968. *"This long disease, my life":*

Alexander Pope and the sciences. Princeton: Princeton University Press.

Peitzman, S. 1989. From dropsy to Bright's disease to end-stage renal disease. *Milbank Memorial Fund Quarterly* 67 (Supp. 1): 16–32.

Philadelphia Inquirer. 1991. December 30, E-1.

Pickford, J. H. 1858. *Hygiene, or, health as depending upon the conditions of the atmosphere, foods and drinks, motion and rest, sleep and wakefulness, secretions, excretions, and retentions, mental emotions, clothing, bathing, &c.* London: John Churchill.

Rosenberg, C. E. 1974. The bitter fruit: Heredity, disease, and social thought in nineteenth-century America. *Perspectives in American History* 7:189–235.

———. 1979. Florence Nightingale on contagion: The hospital as moral universe. In *Healing and history: Essays for George Rosen,* edited by Charles E. Rosenberg. New York: Science History Publications.

———. 1989. Body and mind in nineteenth-century medicine: Some clinical origins of the neurosis construct. *Bulletin of the History of Medicine* 63:185–97.

———. 1992. Framing disease: Illness, society, and history. In *Framing disease: Studies in cultural history,* edited by C. E. Rosenberg and J. Golden. New Brunswick: Rutgers University Press.

———. 1995. Catechisms of health: Textbooks of hygiene in the nineteenth-century classroom. *Bulletin of the History of Medicine* 69:175–97.

Siegel, B. S. 1986. *Love, medicine, and miracles: Lessons learned about self-healing from a surgeon's experience with exceptional patients.* New York: Harper & Row.

Sigmund, B. B. 1989. I didn't give myself cancer. *New York Times,* December 30, op-ed page.

Stevenson, L. G. 1955. Science down the drain: On the hostility of certain sanitarians to animal experimentation, bacteriology, and immunology. *Bulletin of the History of Medicine* 29:1–26.

Stolow, C.1992. Letter to the editor. *New York Times,* June 6.

Szreter, S. 1988. The importance of social intervention in Britain's mortality decline c. 1850–1914: A re-interpretation of the role of public health. *Social History of Medicine* 1:1–37.

Wilson, L. G. 1990. The historical decline of tuberculosis in Europe and America: Its causes and significance. *Journal of the History of Medicine* 45:366–96.

Behavior, Disease, and Health in the Twentieth-Century United States

The Moral Valence of Individual Risk

Allan M. Brandt

Who gets sick? and why? These are among the most profound human questions. Every society has attempted to develop some way to account for the phenomena of disease and death. What are the causes of mortality? and when, in the course of life, does death come? In part, these questions reveal deep moral and philosophical ideals, but they have also engaged other powerful cultural values and beliefs, as well as specific social, medical, and scientific investigation. The nature of morbidity and mortality has historically been subject to dramatic shifts, even over relatively short periods of time.

In the course of the past century, patterns of health and disease in the United States underwent a radical transformation. This change is reflected in major demographic indicators, the nature of the practice of medicine, and cultural norms and values concerning health and disease. Not only do Americans live longer—life expectancy has risen from 47 in 1900 to more than 75 in 1993—they now die from different causes (see Fries 1980; also Helzlsouer and Gordis, 1993). Although these changes have been widely noted and often celebrated, their larger implications for the ways Americans think about health and disease have gone largely uncharted. Nevertheless, as this chapter will suggest, changing perceptions about what *causes* disease—the nature of risk, behavior, and responsibility—reflect powerful moral beliefs. In turn, these beliefs implicitly and explicitly, affect patterns of social behavior and the organization and delivery of health care. This chapter will attempt, in somewhat speculative fashion, to examine the cultural implications and meanings of this "health transition," to explore how theories of disease causality may reflect powerful social and political ideologies concerning risk and responsibility (Douglas and Wildavsky 1982).

At the beginning of the twentieth century, infectious diseases constituted the predominant causes of death. The widespread occurrence of serious epidemics of malaria, smallpox, yellow fever, and cholera throughout the eighteenth and nineteenth centuries had created a shared sense of vulnerability. Epidemics, with their sudden onset and often disastrous impact, created a perception of a world not clearly under human control. Efforts to arrest these contagions through sanitation, quarantine, or medical intervention often failed to have any influence on the course of disease (Ackerknecht 1948; Rosenberg 1962/1987). As late as 1918, an epidemic of Spanish influenza underscored the devastation that disease could wreak in a short time. Worldwide, flu claimed the lives of perhaps as many as twenty million people (550,000 in the United States) (Crosby 1976, 207; also Osborn 1977). If epidemic disease did not result in fatalism, it did at least suggest the limits of human intervention to alter fundamental biological processes. Although explanatory models of disease before the late nineteenth century often centered attention on religious meanings and responses, this reflected in part a deeper recognition of human limits in the face of severe biological constraints.

Epidemics merely represented the fluctuation in more basic patterns of endemic infections. Tuberculosis and pneumonia actually constituted a more serious risk to life than did the intense but time-limited epidemics. Infant mortality (deaths during the first year of life), for example, which remained prevalent into the twentieth century, was typically caused by diarrheal diseases from common enteric infections of newborns. As late as 1900, infant mortality in the United States remained at more than 100 per 1,000 live births. By the mid-1930s, the prevalence of infant mortality had fallen precipitously to approximately 60 per 1,000 (McDermott 1969, 7–28).

Recognizing that diseases were selective in their targets—some suffered and died; others, socially and geographically proximate, were spared—led to medical theories that often emphasized the hereditary quality of susceptibility to particular diseases (Rosenberg 1989). Physicians often stressed the importance of an individual's "constitution" or "diathesis." During most of the nineteenth century, for example, physicians and public health officials emphasized the nature of familial vulnerability to tuberculosis, the most prevalent disease causing death. While physicians and social critics debated the relationship of moral turpitude and disease, the nature of the worthy and the unworthy poor, both epidemic and endemic disease were sorry reminders of the precariousness of life.

By the late nineteenth century, the development of the germ theory of disease had radically altered both medical and social meanings of disease. The preeminent axioms of the germ theory were Robert Koch's "postulates": the rules to live by in modern biological science. Koch, after discovering the tubercle bacillus in 1882, had concluded that a single pathogen was invariably associated with a specific disease; that the organism could be isolated from a lesion and grown in a pure culture, then used to reproduce the disease. The power of these "postulates," and their experimental elegance, transformed the biological sciences. The search for disease-causing microorganisms began in earnest; by 1900 nearly thirty "causal" organisms had been definitively identified under microscopic scrutiny (Dowling 1977; Rosen 1958; also, Winslow 1943/1980).

Soon after the discovery of a number of these organisms, researchers came to understand that it was possible for individuals to be infected but to remain free of disease. This paradox of the "healthy carrier" undermined the conceptual clarity of the germ theory. It soon became clear that the pathogenic agent was a necessary but not a sufficient cause of disease. In fact, this was particularly true with tuberculosis. Researchers found that in many urban areas, a majority of inhabitants were infected yet remained healthy. As René Dubos later pointed out, "Infection is the rule and disease is the exception." Although the notion of specific etiology, the very basis of the "biomedical model," became the focus of medical investigation and treatment, according to Dubos, "few are the cases in which it has provided a complete account of the causation of disease" (Dubos 1959; see also Mishler 1981). Other important anomalies, instances where for one reason or another scientists failed to satisfy the rigor of the postulates in spite of the presence of an organism and its association with a disease, also came to be recognized. With the focus on the organism as the cause of disease, the significance of the social environment was diminished. Other critics suggested that medical science began to focus on the specific aspects of pathogenesis, losing a perspective on the "whole" patient.

Although biomedicine—and the germ theory in particular—led to a far more complete understanding of the causes and nature of many diseases, it did not lead to immediate or effective therapeutic modalities. Nevertheless, infectious diseases did decline, and, in fact, as more demographic data was sifted, it eventually became clear that most important infectious diseases were declining even before the elucidation of the germ theory (McKeown 1979, 1988). The leading causes of death in 1900 were tuberculosis, pneumonia, and diarrhea. In 1990 heart disease, cancer, and stroke constituted the principal causes of death; cancer and heart disease alone now account for almost 60 percent of all deaths (McKeown 1979; also McDermott 1969). To what can this truly revolutionary change in patterns of disease be attributed? Although many associated this epidemiologic and demographic shift with the rise of the germ theory and "scientific" medicine, most data suggest that it was well under way before medicine developed any decisive technologies that would alter basic patterns of disease and death. Changes in the material conditions of life—sanitation, nutrition, and rates of birth—led to important changes in patterns of infection and longevity (see especially McKeown 1979).

For any understanding of the relationship of culture and science, the problem of causation is critically important because it reflects directly on the fundamental moral issue of responsibility for disease. Despite the anomalies implicit in the germ theory and the reductionist qualities of the "biomedical model," the bacteriologic revolution had the effect of "depersonalizing" disease. Under the microscope, diseases could no longer possess the same "moral valence" that they had maintained in the past. In the increasingly secularized and rational world of medicine and science, microorganisms came to be viewed—almost unilaterally—as the cause of disease. This offered the possibility of disconnecting disease from its historical associations with sin, moral turpitude, and idleness.[1] There were, of course, a number of diseases that continued to have powerful moral meanings: mental illness, alcoholism, and the sexually transmitted infections, to name but a few (Brandt 1985/1987; Goffman 1963; Grob 1983; Lender and Martin 1982). By the first decades of the twentieth century, however, many diseases came to be seen as the "random" chain of events that brought together a microorganism, a "vector," and human beings. Disease was no longer seen as *necessarily* reflecting the personal attributes of the sick individual. The biomedical model—in this particular iteration—had the effect of depersonalizing and secularizing disease. In this sense we might call the process the "de-moralization" of disease.

It was in this historically specific context that the attribution of "disease" had the effect of reducing individual responsibility. In this biomedical paradigm, disease became a secular and scientific phenomenon, freed from traditional moral linkages. This accounts for the eagerness with which the founders of Alcoholics Anonymous, for example, seized the notion that alcohol dependence was a *disease* (Robertson 1988; also Mendelson and Mello 1985). It was not so much a desire to "medicalize" the phenomenon of habitual alcohol consumption as it was to free alcohol dependence from its moral stigma, to "re-moralize" the behavior (Fox 1977). A similar phenomenon occurred in the early-twentieth-century movement to transform homosexuality from a crime into a disease, an indication of psychopathology. The implication was that those who suffered from the "disease" should be relieved from the traditional culpability associated with their behaviors (Bayer 1981/1987). Disease implied a lack of volition, or, at least, a failure of individual agency. The concurrent move to expand the nature of the insanity defense during the first decades of the twentieth century is yet another example of this significant trend (Kaufman 1982; Tighe 1983).

In the biomedical model, the occurrence of disease came to be seen largely as the result of discrete phenomena. Susceptibility was defined as a lack of antibodies to a particular organism; resistance could be acquired through natural exposure to the organism or through vaccination to stimulate antibody production (Martin 1994). In keeping with this particular paradigm, biomedicine focused on destroying pathogens or inducing resistance to them. With the introduction of sulfa drugs in the 1930s and antibiotics in the 1940s, the germ theory had spawned effective technologies to combat infection. The promise of Paul Ehrlich's "magic bullets," specific chemotherapies that would root out and destroy "invading organisms," had, at last, been realized. Diseases that a mere decade earlier posed a serious threat to life now could be quickly and definitively treated; antibiotics were routinely saving those previously damned. The "golden age" of American medicine had begun (Burnham 1982).

In spite of its acknowledged theoretical limitations, it is not difficult to recognize the appeal of the biomedical model of disease. If disease was *caused* by a single microorganism, then destroying the organism—either in the environment (through sanitation) or in the body (through therapy)—offered the promise of conquering disease through definitive technologies. The elegance of "magic-bullet" medicine has remained one of the most compelling metaphors in modern medicine (see Brandt 1985/1987; Dixon 1978). The possibility of dramatic cures after centuries of stalemate in the battle against disease inspired a new awe regarding scientific investigation and medical intervention (De Kruif 1926).

The rise in life expectancy, the end of infectious epidemics, and the growth of effective and dramatic medical interventions all led to an era of rising status and authority for the medical profession. Medicine came to be distinguished from biomedicine. Medicine was the undifferentiated past, where doctors could offer patients little beyond support and theory; biomedicine was the result of a "revolution" in bacteriologic and immunologic science. The "miracles" of modern medicine, dispensed in doctors' offices as well as technologically sophisticated hospitals, had brought new respect and acclaim to a profession that only a generation earlier been little more than a competitive trade (Rosenkrantz 1985; Rosenberg 1987). In the nineteenth century, as all forms of regulation had eroded, it had become increasingly difficult to distinguish among a wide variety of medical sects, local healers, quacks, and so-called regular physicians who possessed a specialized education. But by the early twentieth century the profession was able to consolidate its authority and power, in large measure as a result of the rise of the germ theory and the increasingly esoteric, "privileged" knowledge of science (Starr 1982; see also Brandt 1983).

During the course of the twentieth century the epidemiologic shift to the predominance of noncommunicable, chronic diseases exposed the problems inherent in "magic-bullet" medicine. For the persistent problems of cancer, heart disease, and stroke, in which it was impossible to specify a single cause, it proved impossible to specify a single solution. And even in the case of infectious disease, specific therapies proved to have limitations: organisms could become resistant to previously effective chemotherapies. Even when effective treatments were available, they could not always be delivered on a timely basis. Moreover, the notion of specific causality neglected the complex interactions between agent, host, and vector (Berkman and Breslow 1983; Evans 1976; also Susser 1973, Dubos 1959). Clearly, some human beings were more vulnerable than others. As a result of heredity, geography, or environment, some individuals were apparently more susceptible to a number of micro-organisms.

Implicit in this shift from infectious to chronic, systemic disease was a transformation in the meaning of disease and assumptions concerning its causes. In this transformation was embedded a fundamental reconfiguration of moral ideas of disease and its origins. Epidemic infectious disease was typically perceived to be the result of external forces. During the nineteenth century, physicians had debated whether disease resulted from environmental decay—miasmas, poverty, pollution—or from foreigners bringing contagion to new soil. In either case, disease was a "visitation" (see, for example, Pernick 1985); it was episodic and it did not originate or reside in the body. The chronic diseases of the late twentieth century were preeminently diseases of the body. Diseases were no longer caught, they were "acquired" (Crawford 1987, 98). In the postwar era the limits of the germ theory to address systemic chronic disease led to a new recognition of environmental and behavioral forces as determinants of disease.

This change in patterns of disease ultimately challenged the ascendancy of the germ theory. By the 1960s the promise of the biomedical revolution had begun to fade. Despite the firepower of magic bullets, these drugs simply could not target the systemic chronic diseases that now accounted for the preponderance of deaths in the United States and other developed countries. The war on cancer, a national commitment to finding a cure for cancer in the laboratory, had stalled as the promise of any definitive victory dissipated (Patterson 1987). The "technological fix" for the remaining problems of disease proved illusory, despite remarkable technological advances. Cure proved the exception in the battle against the chronic diseases of later life.

New epidemiological studies, recognizing these dramatic changes in patterns of disease, began to reevaluate the basic medical principles of causality. As a result of the changing scientific emphasis in identifying the causal agents of diseases during the late nineteenth century, the discipline of epidemiology had undergone fundamental change. During the early nineteenth century, public health reformers such Edwin Chadwick in Great Britain, Lemuel Shattuck in the United States, and Louis René Villermé in France, had collected voluminous social data from communities in an effort to identify the factors—ranging from housing, work, and pollution, to poverty—that might account for particular patterns of disease prevalence.

After the elucidation of the germ theory, however, the new emphasis in public health came to center on finding and destroying (wherever possible) the noxious microbes (Chadwick 1832/1975; Coleman 1984; Rosen 1958; Rosenkrantz 1972). With the bacteriologic revolution, interest and concern about general social conditions as a cause of disease declined, as epidemiologists turned their attention to laboratory diagnosis (see, for example, Cassedy 1962; also Rosenkrantz 1974). Statistical inference seemed a weak tool in comparison to the sophisticated biochemistry and microscopy of the laboratory.

The significant change in patterns of disease that occurred during the first half of the twentieth century, however, encouraged a "new" epidemiology. From tracking microbes that were uniformly seen as the "cause" of disease, researchers began to identify *risks*: the social, environmental, and behavioral variables that were statistically associated with patterns of chronic disease (Lilienfeld and Lilienfeld 1980). The nature of causal inference in the sciences became a contested domain in the context of this demographic transition. Although some researchers continued to explore theories of specific causes of chronic disease, especially hereditary predispositions, the recognition that many factors were likely to contribute to the development of diseases such as cancer and heart disease led to a revolution in epidemiologic technique. The rise of modern biostatistics and the development of controlled prospective trials offered the opportunity to explore the relationship of a host of environmental and behavioral variables to patterns of health and disease. This new epidemiology offered significant potential for the moral categorization of a wide range of behaviors and social phenomena.

The history of the cigarette provides a prime example of this complex historical process of legitimating new approaches to causal inference and the moralization of health behaviors. The recognition that cigarette smoking causes serious disease and the eventual decline in smoking are characteristic of the postwar shift regarding risk, disease, and behavior. It was no simple task to "prove" that cigarettes *cause* disease. By the end of the Second World War, cigarette smoking had become an enormously popular social behavior in American life, an icon of the consumer culture. An unusual and somewhat stigmatized form of tobacco consumption at the turn of the twentieth century, the cigarette had—through creative marketing and industrial consolidation—become a symbol of affluence, leisure, personal power, and attractiveness. From a behavior of waste and idleness, smoking soon became an icon of sexual attractiveness, seduction, and power. After years of particular social reproach and moral opprobrium for the woman smoker, in the context of the new consumerism, she became a welcomed recruit, instantly doubling the potential market. But despite the categoric success of the cigarette, concerns persisted about its impact on health. Rates of lung cancer, a virtually unknown disease in 1900, had begun to rise alarmingly (see Pearl 1938). By the 1940s, the findings of life insurance actuarial studies spurred major prospective studies of the relationship of cigarettes, lung cancer, and mortality in the United States and Great Britain. These studies concluded that cigarettes constituted an enormous risk to health, not only as a cause of lung disease but also as a contributing factor in heart disease and other cancers (Doll and Hill 1952, 1954, 1956; Hammond and Horn 1958).

The epidemiologic studies of cigarette smoking culminated in the Surgeon General's *Report* of 1964. Written by a group of eminent scientists under the auspices of the Surgeon General, it reviewed the epidemiological evidence indicting cigarettes as a cause of disease and concluded that the studies had, in fact, conclusively demonstrated the risks of smoking. Implicit in this research was an influential critique of the whole notion of specific causality (Surgeon General's Report 1964; also Susser 1973). This type of quantitative epidemiology touched off an important debate within the scientific community about the nature of causality, proof, and risk. At stake were the very epistemological foundations of scientific knowledge. How do we know what we know? What is the reliability of causal inference from statistical data? At the basis of the epidemiological argument was the clear limitation of laboratory experimentation for making determinations about probability and risk. The debate about smoking and health revealed an intraprofessional battle between epidemiology and lab science (the science of the germ theory), and their values, assumptions, and expectations.

Pressured by a growing consumer movement concerned about the dangers of unregulated products, and the voluntary health agencies eager to offer the public an approach to controlling chronic disease, the Surgeon General had finally acceded to studying the problem of the relationship of cigarettes to disease. The report made a fundamental contribution to medical studies of causality. Members of the committee realized the complexity of saying simply that smoking causes cancer. Many individuals could smoke heavily throughout their lives and apparently never suffer adverse consequences: "cause" implied a single process in which A, by necessity, would lead to B. Therefore, the report acknowledged the complexity:

> It should be said at once that no member of this committee used the word "cause" in an absolute sense in the area of this study. Although various disciplines and fields of scientific knowledge were represented among the membership, all members shared a common conception of the multiple etiology of biological processes. No member was so naive as to insist upon the mono-etiology in pathological processes or in vital phenomena.

This statement, a clear criticism of the germ theory's emphasis on specific causality, lent new credibility to the entire field of modern epidemiology. The report underscored the social nature of the process of creating scientific proof. This authoritative study now constituted the "proof" that cigarettes "cause" cancer, signaling the beginning of a major battle between the tobacco industry and public health forces in the United States.

Congress responded to the Surgeon General's report by legislatively mandating that cigarette packs be labeled. The Federal Cigarette Labelling and Advertising Act of 1965 required that all cigarette packages carry the warning "Caution: Cigarette Smoking May be Hazardous to Your Health." Given that the Surgeon General had found that smoking *causes* lung cancer, the warning was remarkably weak, indicating the effectiveness of the tobacco lobby on Capitol Hill. It further reflected the relative lack of experience most legislators had with scientific findings, especially if they were contested. At the hearings concerning this legislation, tobacco spokesmen challenged the findings of the Surgeon General. By treating all perspectives as those of "interested" parties to be brokered in the political process, members of Congress sought compromise. Moreover, powerful economic interests, especially those from tobacco-growing states, acted forcefully to moderate any regulatory initiatives (Fritschler 1969). Nevertheless, as scientific studies collected in subsequent Surgeon General's reports continued to indict the cigarette as a major cause of serious disease, Congress took additional action. In 1971 the label was changed to "Warning: The Surgeon General Has Determined that Cigarette Smoking Is Dangerous to Your Health." And in 1985 Congress mandated four rotating labels. Although originally viewed as an educational and regulatory measure, cigarette labeling served the purpose of shifting responsibility for smoking and its risks from the industry to the individual smoker. The clear warnings printed on every pack had made cigarette smoking the preeminent example of a "voluntary" health risk (Brandt 1990). In this regard, the moral valence of cigarette smoking had been substantially augmented.

Subsequent epidemiological studies would expand the question of risk and behavior far beyond the cigarette. Beginning in the early 1950s researchers in Framingham, Massachusetts began to collect longitudinal data on the relation of a whole host of variables including work, diet, and exercise on heart disease and longevity (Dawber 1980; Kannel 1968). In Alameda County, California, epidemiologists created the Human Population Laboratory to assess the problem of causality of morbidity and mortality within a community, to look at a full range of variables as they contributed to both disease and health. Researchers concluded that three meals a day, breakfast every day, no snacking, plenty of sleep, and moderation in alcohol consumption were the keys to good health and long life (Belloc and Breslow 1972; Berkman and Breslow 1983). But just as the germ theory contained powerful cultural norms regarding the meaning and significance of disease, so too, did the new theories, which emphasized statistically configured "risk factors" (Aronowitz, in press). The health morals of *Poor Richard's Almanac* had come home to roost, now with the growing authority of quantitative epidemiological science. These prescriptions had gained the imprimatur of modern quantitative science.

With this logic and a growing body of supporting data the meaning of disease in American culture underwent a radical shift. By the early 1970s an emerging critique of modern biomedicine and medical technology centered attention on the question of responsibility for disease and its prevention. Few could disagree that disease prevention and health promotion were laudable goals. According to critics such as John Knowles, president of the Rockefeller Foundation, American society had reached the point of diminishing returns from its heavy investment in medical high technology and tertiary care. The failure, asserted Knowles, was in prevention of disease. The goal of health and longevity rested firmly with individuals, who in the past decades had forfeited their health in an "orgy" of greed, avarice, and overeating, the "diseases of affluence." As Knowles concluded, "Most people do not worry about their health until they lose it. Uncertain attempts at healthy living may be thwarted by the temptations of a culture whose economy depends on high production and high consumption." Knowles called for a return to Puritan values of self-discipline and moral restraint. Eager to reduce the "dole" implicit in rising health expenditures, Knowles suggested that "the idea of a 'right' to health should be replaced by the idea of an individual moral obligation to preserve one's own health . . . a public duty if you will" (Knowles 1977). According to this perspective, control of the persistent health problems of the United States—the chronic diseases of middle and later age such as cancer, stroke, and heart disease—depended directly on individual behavior and habits. Individuals could no longer rely on public health interventions, the activities of the medical profession, or the health-care delivery system to solve the problems of disease. Rather, the mantle of responsibility in the quest for health would now be carried on the shoulders of individuals.

The emphasis on individual responsibility for health, as well as the epidemiologic studies that demonstrated the significance of specific behaviors such as cigarette smoking, diet, and exercise offered the possibility of *control* over one's health. No longer would disease be viewed as a random event; it would now be viewed as a failure to take appropriate precautions against publicly specified risks, a failure of individual control, a lack of self-discipline, an intrinsic moral failing. By the late 1970s Knowles's views had entered the political mainstream. In 1978 Secretary of Health and Human Services Joseph Califano, eager to find a way to reduce growing health expenditures, explained:

> We are killing ourselves by our own careless habits. . . . We are a long way from the kind of national commitment to good personal health habits that will be necessary to change drastically the statistics about chronic disease in America. . . . Americans can do more for their own health than any doctors, any machine or hospital, by adopting healthy lifestyles. (U.S. Department of Health and Human Services 1979)

The idea that individuals can and should exercise considerable control over their health, of course, has deep historical roots. Good, clean living formed the basis of religious as well as medical ideals; disease, throughout history, has often been viewed as the physical price of sinfulness. In the nineteenth century, health reformers emphasized the importance of natural laws in determining appropriate behaviors and good health. Health promoters such as Sylvester Graham and James Harvey Kellogg defined a new asceticism, a moral economy of prescribed behaviors that promised prosperity and longevity (Nissenbaum 1980). Although often justified on scientific or medical grounds, the Victorian exercise movement reflected deeper moral and religious sensibilities in an increasingly secular society (Whorton 1982; also Green 1986).

Since the Second World War, but especially since the 1960s, the fitness movement departed from its historical focus on general well-being, taking on the trappings of specific prevention of disease. In particular, clinical and basic research led to concrete conclusions about diet and exercise and their relationship to heart disease, stroke, and cancer (Gillick 1984). Epidemiological findings of major prospective studies were repeatedly cited to justify calls for radical alterations in diet, alcohol consumption, and exercise. Although the fitness revolution preceded many of these data, medical science seized the movement and made it its own. The first major medical studies, for example, on the relationship of exercise to cardiologic function did not appear until the early 1970s, but the medical profession soon acted to legitimate the cultural appeal of vigorous exercise. The boom in physical exercise of the 1970s and 1980s constituted a powerful shift in cultural values as well as actual behaviors. According to most surveys, one-third of all Americans reported engaging in vigorous exercise at least three times a week by the late 1980s; more than three times as many as the early 1960s. As many as fifty million people reportedly jogged regularly, up from twelve million in 1976. Similar data were reported for swimming and aerobic exercise. *Jane Fonda's Workout Book* became one of the best sellers of 1976, with some 1.25 million copies sold; her exercise videos soon became among the most popular commodities in that medium (Barsky 1988; Fonda 1981).

Although some observers suggested that the fitness movement possessed an implicit critique of medical authority and intervention, in practice, organized medicine cooperated vigorously with the crusade for physical fitness. After all, two essential epidemiologic markers of health—blood pressure and cholesterol—remained the province of the profession. The "stress test" combined exercise and the evaluation of cardiologic function in the doctor's office. Those who exercised could measure their progress (or failures) only through these fairly sophisticated medical calibrations. In a new twist on the doctor-patient relationship, the doctor became a health "monitor." Exercise became yet another aspect of the "medicalization" of American culture (Fox 1977; Shorter 1985; Zola 1972).

Now, an individual's moral achievements could be closely monitored and quantified.

Not unlike exercise movements of the past, the modern fitness revolution reflected the desire to assert "control," to reduce the risks of disease or premature death. Exercise promised mastery and self-efficacy. The commitment to exercise promised more than health; it promised personal redemption. The "zen" of running was described by a number of its most vocal advocates, cardiologist George Sheehan among them, as offering "rebirth" and "salvation." According to Sheehan (1979), running promised "self-betterment" and psychological strength. The fitness revolution, notably, did not focus on competitive or team sport; the battle was within the individual. The goal was victory over the uncertainties of the body. Running, aerobic exercise, and modifications of diet all required harsh exertion and self-denial. In this respect, fitness could be viewed as a critique of the consumer culture that had eroded the values of discipline and denial. But the consumer culture rediscovered these values and developed a vast array of commodities of fitness: shoes, machines, and health clubs, among others. The effectiveness with which the consumer culture "captured" the fitness revolution is testament to its contemporary tenacity.

The movement for individual health also had major effects on patterns of food and alcohol consumption. Data collected during the 1980s indicated significant shifts in attitudes and behavior regarding nutrition as more findings appeared specifying the health risks of diets high in cholesterol and fats. A majority of Americans reported attempting to reduce fats in their diets; egg consumption declined; and fish, raw vegetables, and whole grains rose dramatically as staples of consumption. Similar shifts in alcohol consumption also occurred. In 1985, according to the Gallup Poll, 55 percent of those surveyed agreed that "using alcohol for enjoyment is generally a bad thing." Moreover, 38 percent contended that the use of alcohol is morally wrong. The number of adults consuming alcoholic beverages declined from more than 70 percent in the midseventies to 56 percent in 1989 (*Attitudes about Alcohol* 1989; *Physical Fitness* 1984; also Barsky 1988).

It would be easy to view this shift from an ethic of behavior and health that emphasized moral rectitude to one freed from such moralism; good behavior could now be grounded in biomedical rationality. But to view this transformation in attitudes and behaviors in this way would obscure important aspects of the current ideology of health and fitness that reflected deep cultural anxieties not only about health, but bodily appearance as well (see, for example, Brumberg 1988; also Haley 1978). If the fitness "revolution" was driven by scientific findings about risk and behavior, it also took on a powerful moral and prescriptive dimension. In this sense, the fitness crusade of the 1970s and 1980s demonstrates striking continuities with the Victorian campaign of the late nineteenth century.

The intense preoccupation with bodily health, in this respect, is surely not an unprecedented phenomenon. At historical moments of rapid change and social disruption, of apparent unpredictability and widespread perceptions of chaos in social values, the assertion of individual control becomes a paramount social goal. Focusing on the body as the object of that control becomes imperative. Such was the case in the late-Victorian United States; the exigencies of industrialization and urbanization, and the massive changes invoked by the radical transformation of society led individuals to turn inward in a search for order, a search for health.[2] And such has been the case in contemporary American culture since the mid-1960s. A period of domestic and foreign violence and war, and the decline of political legitimacy and professional authority led to a resurgence of demands for individual health. The general failure to define technological solutions to a range of social problems including the depletion of natural energy sources, environmental degradation, and especially chronic disease led to an emphasis on establishing individual control over the vagaries and uncertainties of life, an emphasis on control over the body. The potential for the moralization of this discourse runs deep.

The irony is that the process of pathogenesis is so complex and overdetermined that discussion of "cause" necessarily becomes a socially constructed and often contested domain. The environment, behavior, and the relationship of host and parasite all play significant roles in determining patterns of disease and health, in addition to inborn resistances and vulnerabilities. But at particular historical moments one set of causes may well seem decisively more compelling than another, more susceptible to instrumental human manipulation to control disease. Although science has increasingly specified and differentiated disease etiologies—and in so doing has had some dramatic victories over particular diseases—the explanatory process inevitably goes forward. New diseases are revealed by the nature of biologic and demographic change, by changes in the environment and culture, by changes in science and medicine.

At stake in the process by which health risks come to be elucidated and defined in the United States in the twentieth century is a series of critically important political and moral conflicts. In this respect, cultural norms and values are fundamentally related to a series of political conflicts. Is there a "right" to health care or a "duty" to be healthy? How do we distinguish between assumed risk and imposed risk as they relate to patterns of behavior and disease (Fein 1980)? And indeed, these distinctions probably reflect specific (and changing) historical assumptions about the nature of human behavior more than any empiric reality.

Again, the cigarette provides a telling example of the historical issue. Shall we consider smokers ignorant and stupid for maintaining an "unnecessary" behavior that has been clearly defined as highly dangerous, *or* shall we recognize the power of advertising and cultural conventions, as well as the power of the biological and psychologic qualities of addiction that constrain individual choice? Americans, in this respect, came to reject fatalistic explanatory models of disease and its causes during the course of the twentieth century (Mechanic 1989). Social values have underscored norms that suggest that individuals *can* and *should* exert fundamental control over their health through careful and rational avoidance of risks.

As effective as values of moral responsibility may be in serving to define healthful behaviors, they represent an important political and cultural irony. According to this behavioral ethic, those who continue to take risks must be held accountable for the results. But this emphasis on individual responsibility may deny broader social responsibilities for health and disease. Simply identifying individual behavior as the primary vehicle for risk—even with substantial epidemiologic data—negates the fact that behavior itself is, at times, beyond the scope of individual agency. Behavior is shaped by powerful currents—cultural and psychological, as well as biological processes—not all immediately within the control of the individual. Behaviors such as cigarette smoking are sociocultural phenomena, not merely individual or necessarily rational choices.

The emphasis on personal responsibility for risk taking and disease has come at the very moment when cigarette smoking is increasingly stratified by education, social class, and race. In 1985, 35 percent of African-Americans smoked, compared to 29 percent of whites. For college graduates, the proportion of smokers fell from 28 percent in 1974 to 18 percent in 1985; for those without a college degree, the decrease during the same period was from 36 to 34 percent. Thus, to stress individual accountability is to deny that some groups may be more susceptible to certain behavioral risks, that the behavior itself is *not* simply a matter of choice. Nevertheless, individuals who "take"—note the voluntaristic bias—such risks are considered ignorant, stupid, or self-destructive. Identifying disease as an essentially voluntary process demonstrates the cultural imperative for individual control. If disease can be avoided by carefully following a set of prescriptions regarding personal behavior, then individuals can take control over their bodies and, thereby, their lives. By this logic, the persistent (and now, growing) differentials in the burden of disease between blacks and whites, for example, become but an artifact of the vicissitudes of individual behaviors (see Willis 1989). As the rates of smoking declined to about 25 percent of adult Americans, those who continued to smoke were ascribed ever-greater moral responsibility for their insistence on disregarding the new social norm (*New York Times* 1992).

The very nature of these causal frameworks for understanding disease has been to make complex phenomena seem simple. In this process important cultural values are expressed. Take, for example, the well-known "Just Say No" antidrug campaign of the 1980s. Implicit in this educational campaign, whose legitimate goal was to invigorate individual assertion over peer pressures, was the notion that simple self-denial can solve a complex social problem. The pathology of drug abuse is shifted; rather than the problem reflecting certain external social conditions, it now resides *in* the individual. Drug use becomes preeminently an aspect of individual agency. Just Say No.

To evaluate the power of this set of cultural assumptions one need take but a cursory look at the first decade of the AIDS epidemic. AIDS, of course, crossed some of the most basic assumptions of postwar medicine. The era of infectious epidemics, we had assumed, was over. Ours was a time of chronic diseases that struck late in life, debilitating the growing ranks of the elderly. AIDS strikes the young, it is communicable, and it is caused by a deadly pathogenic organism. But despite these characteristics, AIDS has been placed strongly within the paradigm of responsibility. If one "merely" avoids the risk behaviors associated with transmission of the virus—unprotected sexual intercourse and sharing needles for intravenous drug use—one can avoid AIDS. Therefore, infection is a clear—and usually terminal—marker of individual risk taking, of engaging in behaviors typically held to be deviant or criminal. According to this view, those who are infected are *responsible* for their plight. AIDS is *caused* by a moral failure of the individual (see Brandt 1985/1987; Fee and Fox 1988).

Labeling this perspective "victim blaming" is to miss its full historical implications. Certainly, it does hold victims of disease socially accountable for their illness, disability, and even death. But it also underscores implicit cultural values about the nature of behavior, responsibility for disease, and access to care and services. The triumph of a social ideology of individual control marks a powerful denial of our relative lack of control. Because externally imposed risks appear so difficult—if not impossible—to modify, the tendency in the past two decades has been to focus on the risks over which individuals do have some modicum of control. Implicit is a subtle psychological defense against the reality that human vulnerabilities and, indeed, mortality ultimately may lie beyond these efforts of individual reform. When running enthusiast and author Jim Fixx died of a heart attack while running in 1984, it was but a reminder of an essential irony that fitness provides no guarantees against sudden, premature, unanticipated death.

At particular historical moments social forces have eroded the rigid allocation of responsibility for disease. Just as the Great Depression demonstrated that destitution could be the result of powerful forces beyond the control of the individual, so too did contemporaneous attitudes about disease reflect an ideology of randomness. The fact that the major voluntary health insurers have their origins in the depression reveals a social and economic recognition of shared vulnerabilities to sickness and its costs. When Blue Shield and Blue Cross were organized in the 1930s they were committed to the idea of community rating: anyone could join at the same cost. The essential philosophy behind this premise was that risks should be equitably shared by everyone in the community. In an age of "magic-bullet" treatments and heightened expectations of medicine's ability to cure, political sentiment for the "right" to health care intensified. One result of this political impulse was calls for universal insurance and, eventually, enactment of Medicare and Medicaid in 1965 (Fein 1987; Lubove 1982).

If individuals, however, voluntarily "take" risks, according to this view, they should be held responsible for the injuries or diseases they incur. As more and more risks came to be identified as a result of the "new" epidemiology, so too did a higher level of personal accountability. As the cultural assumptions about disease causation and responsibility for health changed, so did the discourse on insurance and access to care. By the mid-1970s, discussions of the "right" to health care had been transformed to the "duty" to be healthy. In this context, full access to medical care was viewed by some as possibly encouraging unhealthful behaviors. As physician-philosopher Leon Kass noted:

> All the proposals for National Health Insurance embrace, without qualification, the no-fault principle. They therefore choose to ignore, or to treat as irrelevant, the importance of personal responsibility for the state of one's health. As a result, they pass up an opportunity to build both positive and negative inducements into the insurance plan, by measures such as refusing benefits for chronic respiratory disease care to persons who continue to smoke (Kass 1975).

By the 1980s, when new voices supported national health insurance, it was more typically with the goal of limiting rocketing health expenditures which then exceeded 12 percent of the gross national product, than out of egalitarian motives. Equality of access came to be seen as a potential windfall of asserting central control over medical costs.

But the moral implications of risk-taking and disease go beyond any simple economic calculus. In this discourse, one's individual moral failings are clearly perceived as having powerful social implications by placing others at risk. In the case of HIV disease this has been made explicit by the construction of the "innocent victim," an identity with significant historical resonances. There has been a fundamental shift from the traditional libertarian ethic that "it's my body and I'll do as I please" to a wider identification of risks posed to the "moral" by the "immoral." The identification of the risks of side-stream smoke, for example, galvanized the antismoking movement in the 1980s, leading to a remarkable reconfiguration of public space and behavior. Americans became increasingly intolerant of risks imposed by "involuntary" smoking (Brandt 1990). The "discovery" of crack babies and maternal liability in the 1980s marked another extension of this ethos. Historically, infant debility and death had typically been viewed as an extremely sensitive marker of social conditions. Now, individual maternal responsibility was vigorously reasserted, often by district attorneys eager to bring charges against morally delinquent mothers. In this light, "lifestyle" becomes a critical part of the contemporary moral discourse, dramatically enhancing the moral valence of individual risk taking. And it is important to recognize that scientific research and findings are fundamentally tied to the "moralization" of these behaviors. In this respect, science and morality cannot be viewed as dichotomous forces.

This chapter has focused on the cultural implications of fundamental demographic and epidemiological change. The way any society comes to understand patterns of health and disease, and their causes reveals basic cultural norms and expectations. Whether these changes are the result of purposeful human insight and intervention—as they rarely have been—or more basic changes in the material conditions of life, they do have a dramatic impact on assumptions about human behavior and notions of responsibility and morality. In the United States in the twentieth century the "good life" came fundamentally to mean freedom from disease; health became the ultimate goal in a pluralistic, secular culture. And freedom from disease came fundamentally to mean assertion of control over the vagaries of one's body. The ephemeral nature of the effort has yet to discourage this intense capacity for moral reform.

References

Ackerknecht, Erwin H. 1948. Anticontagionism between 1821 and 1867. *Bulletin of the History of Medicine* 22: 562–93.

Aronowitz, Robert. In press.

Attitudes about Alcohol. 1989. *Public Opinion* 12 (May/June): 30–34.

Barsky, Arthur J. 1988. *Worried sick: Our troubled quest for wellness.* Boston: Little, Brown.

Bayer, Ronald. 1981/1987. *Homosexuality and American psychiatry: The politics of diagnosis.* Princeton: Princeton University Press.

Belloc, N. B., and Lester Breslow. 1972. The relation of physical health status and health practices. *Preventive Medicine* 1 (August): 409–21.

Berkman, Lisa, and Lester Breslow. 1983. *Health and ways of living: The Alameda County study.* New York: Oxford University Press.

Brandt, Allan M. 1983. The ways and means of American medicine. *Hastings Center Report* 13 (June): 41–43.

———. 1985/1987. *No magic bullet: A social history of venereal disease in the United States since 1880.* New York: Oxford University Press.

———. 1990. The cigarette, risk, and American culture. *Daedalus* 119(4): 155–76.

Brumberg, Joan Jacobs. 1988. *Fasting girls: The emergence of anorexia nervosa as a modern disease.* Cambridge: Harvard University Press.

Burnham, John C. 1982. American medicine's golden age: What happened to it? *Science* 215 (March 19): 1474–79.

Cassedy, James H. 1962. *Charles V. Chapin and the public health movement.* Cambridge: Harvard University Press.

Chadwick, Edwin. 1832/1975. *The sanitary condition of the labouring populations of Great Britain,* edited by M. W. Flinn. Edinburgh: University of Edinburgh Press.

Coleman, William. 1984. *Death is a social disease.* Madison: University of Wisconsin Press.

Crawford, Robert L. 1987. Cultural influences on prevention and the emergence of a new health consciousness. In *Taking care: Understanding and encouraging self-protective behavior,* edited by N. D. Weinstein. New York: Cambridge University Press.

Crosby, Alfred. 1976. *Epidemic and peace, 1918.* Westport, Conn.: Greenwood Press.

Dawber, Thomas Royle. 1980. *The Framingham study: The epidemiology of atherosclerotic disease.* Cambridge: Harvard University Press.

De Kruif, Paul. 1926. *The microbe hunters.* New York: Harcourt Brace.

Dixon, Bernard. 1978. *Beyond the magic bullet: The real story of medicine.* New York: Harper & Row.

Doll, Richard, and A. Bradford Hill. 1952. A study of the aetiology of carcinoma of the lung. *British Medical Journal* 2 (December 13): 1271–86.

———. 1954. The mortality of doctors in relation to their smoking habits: A preliminary report. *British Medical Journal* 1 (June 26): 1451–55.

———. 1956. Lung cancer and other causes of death in relation to smoking. A second report on the mortality of British doctors. *British Medical Journal* 2 (November 1): 1071–81.

Douglas, Mary, and Aaron Wildavsky. 1982. *Risk and culture.* Berkeley: University of California Press.

Dowling, Harry F. 1977. *Fighting infection: Conquests of the twentieth century.* Cambridge: Harvard University Press.

Dubos, René. 1959. *Mirage of health: Utopias, progress, and biological change.* New York: Harper & Row.

Evans, A. S. 1976. Causation and disease: The Henle-Koch postulates revisited. *Yale Journal of Biology and Medicine* 49: 175–95.

Fee, Elizabeth, and Daniel M. Fox, eds. 1988. *AIDS: The burdens of history.* Berkeley: University of California Press.

Fein, Rashi. 1980. Social and economic attitudes shaping American health policy. *Milbank Quarterly* 58: 349–85.

————. 1987. *Medical care, medical costs: The search for a health insurance policy*. Cambridge: Harvard University Press.

Fonda, Jane. 1981. *Jane Fonda's workout book*. New York: Simon & Schuster.

Fox, Renée C. 1977. The medicalization and demedicalization of American society. *Daedalus* 107 (winter): 9–22.

Fries, J. F. 1980. Aging, natural death, and the compression of morbidity. *New England Journal of Medicine* 303: 130–35.

Fritschler, A. Lee. 1969. *Smoking and politics: Policymaking and the federal bureaucracy*. New York: Appleton-Century-Crofts.

Gillick, Muriel. 1984. Health promotion, jogging, and the pursuit of the moral life. *Journal of Health Politics, Policy, and Law* 9 (fall): 369–88.

Goffman, Erving. 1963. *Stigma: Notes on the management of spoiled identity*. Englewood Cliffs, N.J.: Prentice-Hall.

Green, Harvey. 1986. *Fit for America: Health, fitness, sport and American society*. Baltimore: Johns Hopkins University Press.

Grob, Gerald. 1983. *Mental illness and American society, 1875–1940*. Princeton: Princeton University Press.

Haley, Bruce. 1978. *The healthy body and Victorian culture*. Cambridge: Harvard University Press.

Hammond, E. Cuyler, and Daniel Horn. 1958. Smoking and death rates—report on forty-four months of follow-up on 187,783 men. I. Total mortality. *Journal of the American Medical Association* 166 (March 8): 1159–72.

Hays, Samuel P. 1957. *The response to industrialization*. Chicago: University of Chicago Press.

Helzlsouer, Kathy, and Leon Gordis. 1993. *Risks to health in America*. Unpublished manuscript. In *Risk*, edited by Edward J. Burger. Ann Arbor: University of Michigan Press.

Kannel, William B. 1968. *The Framingham study: An epidemiological investigation of cardiovascular disease*. Washington, D.C.: National Institutes of Health.

Kass, Leon. 1975. Regarding the end of medicine and the pursuit of health. *Public Interest* 40: 11–42.

Kaufman, Irving R. 1982. The insanity plea on trial. *New York Times Magazine*, August 8, 16–20.

Knowles, John H. 1977. The responsibility of the individual. *Daedalus* 106 (winter): 57–80.

Lender, Mark Edward, and James Kirby Martin. 1982. *Drinking in America: A history*. New York: Free Press.

Lilienfeld, Abraham M., and David E. Lilienfeld. 1980. *Foundations of epidemiology*. New York: Oxford University Press.

Lubove, Roy. 1982. The right to health care: Ethical imperatives vs. enforceable claims. In *Compulsory health insurance*, edited by R. L. Numbers. Westport, Conn.: Greenwood Press.

Martin, Emily. 1994. *Flexible bodies: Tracking immunity in American culture from the days of polio to the age of AIDS*. Boston: Beacon Press.

McDermott, Walsh. 1969. Demography, culture, and economics and the evolutionary stages of medicine. In *Human ecology and public health*, edited by E. D. Kilbourne, and W. G. Smillie. New York: Macmillan.

McKeown, Thomas. 1979. *The role of medicine: Dream, mirage, or nemesis?* Princeton: Princeton University Press.

———. 1988. *The origins of human disease*. Oxford: Basil Blackwell.

Mechanic, David. 1989. *Promoting health*. Paper presented at the Rockefeller Conference on the Health Transition, American Academy of Arts and Sciences, June.

Mendelson, Jack H., and Nancy K. Mello. 1985. *Alcohol: Use and abuse in America*. Boston: Little, Brown.

Mishler, E. G. 1981. *Social contexts of health, illness, and patient care*. New York: Cambridge University Press.

New York Times. 1992. May 22.

Nissenbaum, Stephen. 1980. *Sex, diet, and debility in Jacksonian America: Sylvester Graham and health reform*. Chicago: Dorsey Press.

Osborn, June E., ed. 1977. *History, science, and politics: Influenza in America, 1918–1976*. New York: Prodist.

Patterson, James T. 1987. *The dread disease: Cancer and modern American culture*. Cambridge: Harvard University Press.

Pearl, Raymond. 1938. Tobacco smoking and longevity. *Science* 87 (March 4): 216–17.

Pernick, Martin S. 1985. Politics, parties, and pestilence: Epidemic yellow fever and the rise of the first party system. In *Sickness and health in America: Readings in the history of medicine and public health*, edited by J. W. Leavitt and R. L. Numbers. Madison: University of Wisconsin Press.

Physical Fitness. 1984. *Gallup Report* 226 (July): 9–12.

Robertson, Nan. 1988. *Getting better: Inside Alcoholics Anonymous*. New York: Morrow.

Rosen, George. 1958. *A history of public health*. New York: MD Publications.

Rosenberg, Charles E. 1962/1987. *The cholera years: The United States in 1832, 1849, and 1866*. Chicago: University of Chicago Press.

———. 1987. *The care of strangers: The rise of America's hospital system*. New York: Basic Books.

———. 1989. Disease in history: Frames and framers. *Milbank Quarterly* 67: 1–15.

Rosenkrantz, Barbara G. 1972. *Public health and the state: Changing views in Massachusetts, 1842–1936*. Cambridge: Harvard University Press.

———. 1974. Cart before horse: Theory, practice, and professional image in American public health, 1870–1910. *Journal of the History of Medicine and Allied Sciences* 29: 55–73.

———. 1985. The search for professional order in nineteenth century medicine. In *Sickness and health in America: Readings in the history of medicine and public health*, edited by J. W. Leavitt and R. L. Numbers. Madison: University of Wisconsin Press.

Sheehan, George. 1979. *Running and being*. New York: Simon & Schuster.

Shorter, Edward. 1985. *Bedside manners: The troubled history of doctors and patients*. New York: Simon & Schuster.

Sontag, Susan. 1976. *Illness as metaphor*. New York: Viking.

Starr, Paul. 1982. *The social transformation of American medicine: The rise of a sovereign profession and the making of a vast industry*. New York: Basic Books.

Surgeon General's Report. 1964. *Smoking and health report of the Advisory Committee to the Surgeon General of the Public Health Service. U.S. Department of Health, Education, and Welfare, Public Health Service*. PHS Publication No. 1103. Washington, D.C.: U.S. Department of Health, Education, and Welfare, Public Health Service.

Susser, Mervyn. 1973. *Causal thinking in the health sciences: Concepts and strategies in epidemiology*. New York: Oxford University Press.

Tighe, Janet. 1983. A question of responsibility: The development of American forensic psychiatry, 1838–1930. Ph.D. diss., University of Pennsylvania.

U.S. Department of Health and Human Services. 1979. *Healthy people: The Surgeon General's report on health promotion and disease prevention*. Washington, D.C.: Government Printing Office.

Verbrugge, Martha H. 1988. *Able-bodied womanhood: Personal health and social change in nineteenth-century Boston*. New York: Oxford University Press.

Whorton, James C. 1982. *Crusaders for fitness: The history of American health reformers*. Princeton: Princeton University Press.

Wiebe, Robert. 1967. *The search for order*. New York: Hill & Wang.

Willis, David P., ed. 1989. *Health policies and Black Americans*. New Brunswick, N.J.: Transaction.

Winslow, Charles-Edward Amory. 1943/1980. *The conquest of epidemic disease: A chapter in the history of ideas*. Madison: University of Wisconsin Press.

Zola, Irving K. 1972. Medicine as an institution of social control. *Sociological Review* 20: 487–504.

The Social Context of Health and Disease and Choices among Health Interventions

David Mechanic

The notion of disease is typically based on two interconnected judgments. In assessing whether a disease exists, the first rule is to identify evidence of pathology or dysfunction, indications that body processes deviate in some way from how they should perform (Wakefield 1992a, 1992b). In many cases we have objective biological markers, but in others the assessment is made on an experiential basis. Second, an assessment is made as to the consequences of such deviations in terms of a particular set of values. Typically, we concern ourselves with deviations that imply likely future risks of pain, disability, and reduced longevity, and these criteria are for the most part widely agreed upon. Yet individuals have differing perspectives on these consequences and may be willing to trade some increment of life, pain, and risk for other valued goals and priorities. People may put greater priority at various points in their life trajectories on economic advancement, a sense of excitement, prestige, commitment to one's family or group, or even loyalty to nation. In everyday life, judgments of consequences are influenced profoundly by local cultures and prevailing values.

Norms and Morality

The core ambiguity in the notion of disease involves the assumptions we make about how the person should "naturally" perform. From a broader concept the focus on body is, in itself, reductionist, neglecting the degree of harmony or integration between persons and their interpersonal and physical environments. Individuals always live in the context of a group with specific structures, cultures, and patterns of valued activities and associations.

There is a great and growing body of research that links individual pathology to family disintegration, impoverished social networks, loss of meaning, and a sense of alienation, hopelessness, and despair. We have no detailed nomenclature that maps pathology from this perspective, but moral conceptions help define the sources of dysfunction we choose to focus on and those we ignore. Poor health outcomes associated with behavior we deem discreditable, such as substance abuse, receive far more attention than neglect of self and dependents due to community commitment, ambition, or other activities deemed worthy.

One might think that establishing norms objectively would be relatively simple. For a start, statistical patterns of response could be mapped, and those most deviant could be identified. But most reactions vary by group context, time, and place, and the fact that some behaviors are common does not establish they are normative or devoid of dangerous consequences. In American society, large proportions of the population are overweight, and average blood pressure is higher than epidemiological studies suggest would be ideal. Thus, the average is not necessarily an appropriate norm. Similarly, most elderly people have disease and incapacities, and the association is so common that such states are commonly seen as a normal function of aging. But scientific studies demonstrate that pathologies characteristic of the elderly are largely a function of disease and not of age. Studies of successive cohorts show remarkable changes in physical function among the elderly of comparable age.

Norms about health and disease arise through a mix of statistical regularities, public conceptions of desirable outcomes, and societal reactions to behaviors and practices perceived as deviant. Scientific understanding of abnormality is dynamic, and at any time characterized by varying degrees of uncertainty and disagreement. Thus, there is much room for moral ideologies to play a role, often in large part because of the emotional investment and capacity for organization and dissemination that moral movements take on. Morality affects concepts of disease and their precursors in at least two ways. First, moral concepts serve to organize, interpret, and make sense of ambiguous and conflicting information, providing a paradigm that gives special coherence to a confusing environment. Second, moral concepts define the processes and end points that are desirable, a definition that science cannot provide. Norms thus result from the interplay between existing behavior and practices and moral conceptions as embodied in formal and informal societal reactions to ongoing behavior.

A Population View of Health and Disease

The diagnosis of disease is a highly focused activity that abstracts from what Verbrugge and Ascione (1987) have called the iceberg of symptoms, most hidden from the formal medical care system. Epidemiological studies demonstrate, in contrast, that most people have symptoms most of the time but normalize or deny them. Indeed, acute symptoms are so ubiquitous that they are impossible to measure reliably, and thus statistical agencies will usually count such symptoms only if the respondent actually took some action in response, such as self-medication or bed rest (Mechanic and Newton 1965).

Doctors of first contact see many of the same problems commonly occurring in the population, and as Kerr White observed some years ago, almost half of the patients seen at first contact may have such vague and ambiguous presentations that they cannot be given a diagnosis that fits categories covered by the International Classification of Disease (White 1970). A substantial proportion of these patients are also depressed, anxious, and fatigued, although estimates vary wildly contingent on definition and on how such assessments are made. Although there are disagreements on the precise figures, there is no disagreement that most medical problems occur in a social context complicated by issues of class, race, gender, work, and family and community ties.

At any point in time, the practice of medicine is a mixture of theories at varying levels of confirmation and a variety of social judgments and prejudices (Mechanic 1978). Physicians seek to identify patterns of symptoms that imply definable disorder; if they do so successfully and the disease theory is relatively firm, they gain abundant information on likely course and etiology, and guidance for how to proceed in treatment. Physician roles substantially transcend the corpus of medical knowledge, and both patients and the societies of which they are part demand that doctors provide assistance even when knowledge is limited. The process should encourage careful observational and listening skills, but it is not unusual for doctors to apply unconfirmed hypotheses rigidly.

Much disease and its course are influenced by social and environmental factors, but medical practice tends to personalize such influences by focusing on their individual manifestations and consequences typically divorced from broader implications. Why this particular emphasis evolved historically may seem natural to us, but it was neither self-evident nor inevitable, and it is even arguable that the approach is particularly well fitted to much of the morbidity that doctors now treat. As Waitzkin (1991) notes: "That this particular format should have arisen is remarkable partly because its effectiveness in improving medical conditions remains unproven" (33).

Waitzkin in a contextual analysis of a sample of doctor-patient contacts observed the numerous ways in which doctors explicitly or inadvertently exercised social control as they acted on moral ideologies relating to family, work, appropriate behavior, age expectations, and the like.

> [T]hrough messages of ideology and social control, and through the lack of contextual criticism, health professionals subtly direct patients' actions to conform with society's dominant expectations about appropriate behavior. . . . [D]octor-patient encounters become micropolitical situations that reflect and support broader social relations, including social class and political-economic power. The participants in these encounters seldom recognize their micropolitical situation on a conscious level. (Waitzkin 1991, 8–9)

In the primary-medical-care literature much attention is focused on the idea of the patient's hidden agenda: the "real" reason for the consultation that becomes apparent late in the transaction if at all (Balint 1957). An alternative to the traditional approach is to give patients greater latitude to tell their stories and to explain what they expect and hope for from the encounter. Waitzkin (1991) comments,

> Most practitioners would acknowledge that the tendencies to interrupt, cut off, or otherwise redirect the patient's story during the PI [evaluation of present illness] derive at least partly from the drive to make a diagnosis. That is, a doctor wants to hear

those words that are consistent with previously defined diagnostic categories. Parts of patients' stories that do not fit neatly into these categories function as unwanted strangers in medical discourse. (31)

A powerful analogy comes from anthropological work on comparative law. In our legal system courts work with an elaborate body of statutes and legal precedents that guide dispute settlements. In cases before the court, the judge's responsibility is to make decisions through the application of preexisting rules and their elaboration through application to specific cases. The judge's role is to ensure that the presentation of the case follows the rules of evidence and that the issues at stake be resolved on legal principles and not on the underlying motives of the parties to the dispute or the social consequences for the litigants and their kinship group. Yet, we also know that in many instances, medical malpractice and divorce being excellent examples, the issues being litigated are often quite different from the primary dispute that brought the parties into court and not reflective of the actual disagreements between them. The legal battle becomes the turf on which the real underlying dispute is played out, often in a way that further polarizes the parties, making future reconciliation impossible. Judges may be fully aware of this, but searching out the underlying dispute once the issue is before the court is not their business.

Consider, in contrast, the judicial process among the Barotse, a Northern Rhodesian tribe studied by Max Gluckman (1965). The Barotse judge explores in depth the nature of disputes, seeking to resolve basic conflicts and disagreements that might extend well beyond the manifest issue. This requires far-reaching inquiry, allowing each disputant to tell his or her story in full, and encouraging the participation of other interested parties in these deliberations. Gluckman maintained that the aim of the judge, particularly in kinship disputes, was to keep kin together and maintain village integrity. The judge, thus, sees the main role as reconciling the parties and reaching a satisfactory compromise judgment.

As patterns of disease have changed, and as medicine is more concerned with chronic and degenerative diseases, and behavioral patterns associated with morbidity, it is appropriate to reexamine optimal approaches in identifying what the problem really is and alternative management strategies. Such an approach, unlike the dominant medical model, makes values and moral issues more salient. The fact that they are at present implicit in most situations make them no less important. It may well be that an approach to the patient, along the lines of the Barotse judge, may be more helpful in getting to the core of essential issues.

The diagnostic disease model, and particularly its applications in Western countries, encompasses a highly individualized conception of the person, one that puts emphasis on individual responsibility for the problem and its remedy and one that treats the transaction as a private, privileged matter between doctor and patient. Whether intended or not, the application of the model conveys the moral view that patients are solely responsible for their own functioning. In recent years, this framework has come under attack from a variety of perspectives. Increasingly, advocates for the disabled make clear that their disabilities are as much a product of social definitions and restrictions on access and opportunities than intrinsic impairments of persons with disabilities. Families associated with the National Alliance for the Mentally Ill assail psychiatric practices that exclude the family from the treatment planning process and the therapeutic alliance. Thus, while the medical process is still fundamentally governed by a morality organized around individual action, families and health organizations increasingly insist on a somewhat different paradigm and approach—one that recognizes the interconnectedness among individuals, social networks, and societal structures.

Persons and groups with varying problems also have become vocal about the moral implications of causal theorizing about the conditions that affect them. The National Alliance for the Mentally Ill has attacked what it perceives as facile and prejudicial psychodynamic conceptions that it asserts stigmatize and damage the mentally ill, engendering guilt and shame. A major goal of this large national advocacy organization is to educate the public regarding the biological basis of schizophrenia and other major mental illnesses.

In many encounters a negotiation process goes on in which doctor and patient agree to focus on one or another aspect of the problem in a way that may help bring the problem into congruence with an intelligible medical definition. But things are not always easy, and despite concerted efforts to identify a meaningful problem formulation, the doctor may fail to arrive at any hypothesis that fits. Physicians get frustrated with persistent and demanding patients who pose such ambiguities and label them as neurotic, "worried wells," hypochondriacs, or "crocks." The failure to locate a suitable hypothesis may tell us as much about the physician's models and approaches as it does about the illness behavior of the patient, but the failure is usually externalized and in an invidious way. When confirmed medical models don't fit, the patient gets a heavy dose of social judgment often disguised as diagnosis. The characteristic intermixture of clinical observations with judgmental ones makes it almost impossible to separate social from technical clinical norms.

Professional political battles over such areas as homosexuality, neurosis, oppositional defiant disorder, and the like make obvious what is implicit in many diagnostic situations (Bayer and Spitzer 1985; Bayer 1987). Many examples of the tendency to classify behavior as diseases devoid of any reasonable medical basis are found in the Diagnostic and Statistical Manual of Mental Disorders (DSM-III; American Psychiatric Association 1980), in which numerous disorders are simply defined in terms of consequences believed to be undesirable, such as inhibited sexual excitement or inhibited female orgasm, with little reference to any underlying epidemiological or biomedical patterns. The DSM-III tells us, for example, that in the case of disorders of impulse control the defining feature is an act "harmful to the individual or others" (291).

But what about addictions, impulses, and adjustments that elicit rewards and prestige? What makes addiction to work, accumulating wealth, risk taking on the stock market, or involvement in sports fundamentally different from high levels of involvement with alcohol, drugs, and sex? One might reasonably argue that differences lie in the personal and social consequences, but even here the comparison remains ambiguous. Overwork or work in dangerous industries with high risk of injury or exposure to toxic substances may pose risks comparable to substance abuse. Some sports activities are associated with more than usual risks of trauma, brain injury, and even death, as in skydiving, racing, boxing, and motorcycle riding. The inclinations to engage in such activities may be biologically influenced by inborn inclinations toward excitement or activity (a hypothesis with some support) (Kagan 1989). Observing biological concomitants of behavior is by itself trivial in that all behavior has such concomitants. The arbitrary selections of what deviations from statistical or normative standards we focus on reveals a great deal about what is socially and culturally meaningful.

The Role of Uncertainty

A major difficulty with the prevailing diagnostic approach, beyond the fact that many conditions do not fit existing theories, is the relatively limited level of confirmation that characterizes many of those most commonly applied. Kerr White (1988), a distinguished pioneer in the development of health services research, recently observed that "it is still the case that only about 15 percent of all contemporary clinical interventions are supported by scientific evidence that they do more good than harm" (9). Thus, there is a great deal of uncertainty and confusion and great dependence on clinical experience.

Clinical experience, however, is notoriously unreliable. Because doctors see only patients who seek care, they have little basis for assessing how those with comparable symptoms fare with different or no treatment at all. Moreover, patients often seek care during periods of high pain and anxiety whose natural course is often improvement. Thus, clinicians are inclined to overestimate the impact of their interventions. Physicians also have needs to believe they are helping their patients, and patients often respond in positive ways because of placebo effects or a desire to please physicians in appreciation for their efforts.

Uncertainty results in extraordinary variations in practice and high levels of inappropriate interventions, as documented in numerous studies (Variations 1984). The magnitude of variation is highly correlated with the level of uncertainty characteristic of treating particular conditions (Wennberg 1984). It should not be surprising that in endeavors so fraught with uncertainty and variability, there are enormous opportunities for value judgments to be played out under the guise of clinical determinations.

Consider an area as prosaic as benign prostatic hypertrophy (BPH), a condition eventually affecting most men as they age, and one involving high rates of variation in surgical intervention from one geographic area to another. As Wennberg (1990) and his colleagues have found, men vary substantially in their concern about symptoms, and some with even severe symptoms prefer watchful waiting to invasive interventions. As he notes, "[N]o objective data derived from physical examination, clinical history, or careful quantification of symptoms can accurately predict the preferences of individual patients for surgery or watchful waiting" (1202). In fact, Wennberg's research shows that physicians are more interventionist than patients, and that on average patients opt for more conservative and less risky strategies. Here is a case where the values physicians typically have about the implications of symptoms associated with aging and the value of aggressive treatment may be quite discrepant from those of their patients who may have different needs, lifestyles, or willingness to assume certain risks. Such differences also have enormous implications for the costs of medical care.

Alternate Paradigms to the Dominant Medical Model

The dominant concept of disease and the medical process of diagnostic inquiry focused on the individual in contrast to broader systems are not inevitable or necessarily the most efficient or effective way of promoting individual health. Diagnosticians of first contact exist in every culture because people seek a place to bring difficult problems for which they seek relief, hope, and reassurance. But the point of clinical intervention is a peculiar vantage point for viewing the production of health and disease.

At the level of populations, the notion that health is shaped by the material and environmental conditions of life and by the sociocultural structures that people create as much as by their genes and individual health behavior is now commonplace. Many positive or damaging health-relevant behaviors arise from the routine activities and conventional patterns of everyday life, only modestly influenced by health-relevant considerations (Mechanic 1990). Behavior dependent on persistent conscious motivation is likely to be unstable. The flow of health outcomes from routine processes, however, is pervasive and powerful. Changing health-damaging behavior thus depends substantially on the ability of communities to restructure conventional activities in a fashion that offers fewer threats to health, a process inextricably entangled with values and moral judgments. The instruments to achieve this are quite varied, including tax policies and other financial incentives, regulation, skillful use of mass media, and education. Possibilities include social policies regulating environmental and workplace risk exposures; the distribution, labeling, and regulation of food, drugs, and other commodities; controls over smoking, drinking, and other high-risk behaviors; highway construction and road and vehicle safety systems; and inducements for exercise, community participation, and social integration.

Focus on the personal level reflects in part the individualistic bias of Western culture. As concern with promoting health has grown, the emphasis has overwhelmingly been on personal health habits in contrast to other levels of intervention. In considering policy options, there are at least four major possible trade-offs: between macro nonhealth interventions that promote health (education, community empowerment and mobilization, social integration, inducing personal efficacy) and more direct health initiatives; between public health efforts and general medical care; between individual preventive versus curative foci; and between primary care and more specialized types of interventions. Most resource investment in the U.S. system is inversely related to the spheres of action most likely to have the largest impact on population health.

The realities, however, are that we will continue to direct more of our efforts toward inducing personal behavioral change in contrast to interventions at a social level that typically confront opposing powerful interests. Successful behavior change requires engaging the individual at the motivational, cognitive, and behavioral levels, with additional inducers needed to trigger motivation and to reinforce behavioral patterns that require repetition. In some significant sense being "health conscious" is akin to being "modern," a concept of considerable importance in understanding how nations move from underdevelopment to becoming developed industrial economies (Inkeles and Smith 1974). In the process of social development a constellation of beliefs and behaviors is essential among key population groups in sustaining the kind of meaning system that induces a sense of efficacy and empowerment. Such a meaning system, which facilitates an ability to work within organized structures on the one hand and to exercise autonomous judgment on the other, appears to be correlated substantially with what we conceive of as positive health behavior.

Inkeles (1983), who has written extensively on the concept of psychological modernity, has outlined a variety of characteristics that fit neatly into the cognitive-motivational-behavioral conception. At the cognitive level, the modern meaning system is associated with belief in the efficacy of science and medicine and the importance of planning one's affairs. Bridging cognition and motivation is an openness to new experience and innovative practices, and an independence from traditional authority. More central to motivation, persons with such a meaning system have ambition for themselves and their children to achieve educational and occupational goals. And, behaviorally, they accommodate their activities around time and schedules, actively engage issues, keep up with the news, and are active in civic and community affairs. In a sense these dimensions define personal empowerment and share a common domain with such popular concepts as mastery, self-efficacy, internal locus of control, and optimism, all correlated with various types of health outcomes (Peterson and Bossio 1991; Seligman 1991).

Schooling links these various concepts and is a powerful predictor across a broad range of health outcomes. Persons with more schooling seek out information more aggressively, and understand and retain more of it (Feldman 1966). Schooling also is the single most important predictor of "psychological modernity," which Inkeles attributes not only to the content of learning but also to socialization effects such as following a schedule and keeping appointments (Inkeles 1983; Inkeles and Smith 1974). Schooling is a complex proxy variable capturing people's information acquisition and processing styles, as well as self-definitions, coping strategies, and more general orientations to the world (Mechanic 1989). Education may be an enabling variable that affects health primarily when it provides access to efficacious technologies.

The value system underlying many of the concepts referred to above gives primacy to personal autonomy and action, concepts predominant in individualistic market-oriented economies. A growing body of research in the American context attests to the fact that persons who are optimistic, who make attributions of events favorable to themselves, and who have a sense of personal efficacy and a willingness to persevere experience a greater sense of well-being and more favorable health outcomes than individuals who lack these orientations (Seligman 1991). They appear to be activated and confident but not necessarily accurate in their appraisals of reality (Seligman 1991, particularly 298), and, by inference, not particularly open to attributing praise and blame fairly in their social relations. The evidence suggests that individuals often do better by distorting reality, as long as the distortions are within reasonable enough bounds to be sustained and not undermine coping effectiveness (Mechanic 1962).

One current popular psychological theory and related therapy encourages teaching patients positive attributions that avoid seeing oneself as responsible for bad events (Beck 1979). Persons who do so may be less likely to become depressed, although depressed patients often see themselves more accurately than those who are particularly optimistic. Similarly, studies of introspectiveness find that persons who pay more attention to internal feeling states experience more physical and psychological symptoms (Mechanic 1979; Hansell, Mechanic, and Brondolo 1986). But introspectiveness is also associated with knowing oneself better and is seen as a valuable attribute of sensitive human beings, a trait that many thoughtful persons cherish and nurture despite some negative consequences. To the extent that medical intervention seeks to minimize symptoms and distress, it potentially may undermine highly valued characteristics that define what we mean by being an empathic and sensitive human being. This is hardly a new idea. Erich Fromm (1941) argued in *Escape from Freedom* that individuals who adjusted comfortably to unjust and totalitarian regimes were in fundamental ways less "healthy" than those who were tormented by obvious injustices.

The literature on social integration suggests a somewhat different and seemingly contradictory notion of the role of autonomy and individuality. There is substantial evidence that persons well embedded in social networks experience health-protective consequences (House, Landis, and Umberson 1988). Moreover, in many situations individualized responses, however competent, are doomed to failure without supportive group structures dependent on cooperation (Mechanic 1974). This becomes particularly true in a complex organizational society.

References to autonomy as an explanatory variable tend to be vaguely specified, particularly because most relevant research occurs in contexts and with populations where individuality and instrumentality are highly valued. In contexts where autonomy is part of a moral ideology, the exercise of such behavior is publicly supported and even celebrated. The meaning of such behavior in cultures that value group solidarity over individual expressiveness may be quite different. Thus, autonomy could be either a socially expected orientation, encouraged and rewarded, or an extreme form of deviance and disrespect for one's peers and kin. Context, hence, is likely to make a large difference.

It is difficult to make much sense of the aggregate data on maternal education and infant mortality without a richer contextual picture. Is autonomy, for example, a health-promoting force when it clashes with group expectations and increases conflict? High rates of infant and child mortality in Islamic nations may be in part a consequence of the negative orientation toward the education of women and the inhibition of female initiative in family decision making. But it does not follow that education and independence in thinking, which may be one of its products, will function in comparable ways when initiative is supported or contested. Indeed, even in traditional cultures those who get more education may be functioning with family supports that allow continuation of schooling, confounding the two. Educational advances may help break the binds of traditional practices that impede appropriate health action involving contraception, immunization, and appropriate prenatal and child care, but those who pursue such advances may have greater support and encouragement from their immediate intimates.

Some cultural and moral systems, in contrast, are health promoting not only because they constrain practices dangerous to health such as smoking, substance abuse, and promiscuous sexual behavior, but also because they encourage a patterned regularity in daily activities and social routines (Geertsen et al. 1975). This is the case, for example, in the Mormon culture, which teaches the importance of family and parenthood and encourages a strong orientation toward environmental mastery, emphasizing active effort, accomplishment, and the acquisition of skills and education (O'Dea 1957). In such circumstances the collectivity orientation and individual efficacy can act consistently and synergistically.

In the aggregate, such behavioral orientations as self-efficacy and autonomous decision making appear to be health enhancing, but these orientations can also clash with cultural expectations and increase certain types of health risks. Some cultural groups restrict behaviors that pose potential health risks, such as smoking, drinking, and sexual behavior outside marriage. With greater personal autonomy, such behavior is likely to increase, and the emancipation of women, for example, is associated with increased smoking, substance abuse, and other high-risk behaviors. Similarly, in highly restrictive settings, deviance when it occurs is often exaggerated. Most Mormons, for example, don't use alcohol, but when they do, they have been more likely to abuse it than do persons in groups more accepting of alcohol use (Straus and Bacon 1953). But despite this apparent link between increased autonomy and deviant behavior in the aggregate, contemporary research suggests that persons with a greater sense of autonomy are less likely to engage in health-damaging behaviors (Pratt 1976). Smoking prevalence, for example, is inversely related to social status (National Center for Health Statistics 1991, table 5b), and self-efficacy increases with social status. It is apparent that the behavioral patterns under discussion are highly complex, particularly when considered across cultures, and single-factor explanations cannot reconcile seemingly conflicting observations.

The Idea of Health

People's conceptions of their health are substantially formed in relationship to their social environment, their associations with others, and their sense of social and psychological well-being. In one analysis, Richard Tessler and I (Tessler and Mechanic 1978) examined the correlates of self-assessment of physical health in four populations: persons participating in two health care plans, students at a large state university, a middle-aged and elderly population in a southern state, and a sample of men in a state prison. In each case, individual physical health assessments were associated with both the magnitude of acute and chronic symptoms on the one hand and psychological well-being on the other. Patients, unlike physicians, see their health in terms of their capacity to function in social roles and preferred social activities, and one's psychological and social well-being is quite central to these tasks. As the RAND Medical Outcomes Study has demonstrated, depressed mood is one of the most disabling of symptoms seen in general medical contexts (Wells et al. 1989).

We became intrigued with how relatively healthy people, who have few chronic conditions, assess their health and were able to examine the constituents of such health evaluations in a longitudinal sample of 1,193 adolescents (Mechanic and Hansell 1987). We predicted that in the absence of chronic disease or serious morbidity, adolescents would appraise their health on the basis of their general well-being and their demonstrated competence in age-relevant areas. We found that adolescents who reported better school achievement and more participation in sports and other exercise assessed their physical health as better over a one-year period than those reporting lower achievement and less participation, controlling for self-assessed health at the beginning of the year. We also found that adolescents who initially had less depressed mood assessed their health more positively. Health, as people view it, is truly a social concept, reflecting well-being and performance in age-appropriate roles.

These subjective health assessments are more than an academic curiosity, as reflected in their powerful predictive capacity. They are among the best general predictors of mortality, morbidity, and use of medical services (Ware 1986), and are significantly related to objective indicators such as physician assessment and medical record data. Idler (1992) reviewed six follow-up studies based on large probability samples that included baseline health self-assessments and objective health-status measures allowing appropriate statistical analyses. These studies consistently show that self-assessed health has stronger prospective associations with mortality than objective health-status measures. Although much about the predictive power of these self-appraisal measures remains unclear, it is apparent that the well-being dimension is an important aspect of the picture. Social and psychological well-being, of course, is substantially linked to psychosocial stressors, coping responses, the quality of social networks and intimacy, and one's sense of mastery. These are all defined in terms of and influenced by prevailing values and norms. Perceptions of stressful events, the definition of appropriate coping responses, and implications for personal associations and self-esteem are all social constructions highly dependent on local culture.

Morality and Chronic Disease

It might be expected that as science advances, moral conceptions would play a lesser role in the identification, treatment, and amelioration of disease, but the opposite may be the case. With the aging of populations and the growing preponderance of chronic diseases, many of which develop slowly over a lifetime, new opportunities arise to attribute instrumentality and blame to those who do not take protective steps. The epidemiological approach of identifying risk factors, many of which are behavioral and theoretically volitional, offers new opportunities to attribute responsibility and blame. Large new groups who adopt high-risk behaviors expose themselves to moral crusades about personal responsibility, exhortation to change their ways, and new social policies that seek to make them pay for the risks they invite. As the costs of medical care mount, placing new obligations on the public purse, risk-taking populations are seen as doubly burdensome.

Opportunities for moral crusades also multiply as the expectations of medicine and medical care change. The value of medical interventions is no longer simply judged by whether patients' symptoms are alleviated but also by whether the outcomes of care are cost-effective and whether treatment results in improved function, independence, and quality of life. Addressing these outcomes depends on understanding and engaging personal aspirations and peoples' living arrangements, and provides abundant opportunities to intrude on value orientations and personal preferences. Moreover, as rationing of medical care becomes more of a reality and is exercised in the broader context of social adaptation in contrast to disease remission, opportunities for conflict multiply.

The boundaries of medicine have expanded enormously to fill in gaps left by the weakening of the family, neighborhood, and religious institutions. Although some areas, such as homosexuality, have been removed from the medical domain, medicine has become hopelessly intertwined with the functions of welfare and social remediation. It engages whatever issues appear on the public agenda, ranging from violence to self-actualization, bringing its own individually oriented perspective to bear. It reflects and helps perpetuate changing public images of threats to health and pathways to the balanced and healthy life. It follows its own technologic imperative but is tolerant toward almost every competing idea from holistic health to behavioral medicine. In short, medicine is perhaps more than ever a mirror to society with its competing lifestyles and moral proclivities. It can be, at the same time, remarkably tolerant and extraordinarily judgmental, with such large areas of uncertainty that moral entrepreneurs have boundless opportunities to ply their trade.

Conclusions

Within traditional medical sociological formulations, illness is deviant behavior that interferes with the capacity of individuals to perform usual and expected social responsibilities (Mechanic 1978). In the Parsonian formulation (Parsons 1951), the profession of medicine is given the power and legitimacy to excuse failures in role performance and provide support during the period of illness and recuperation, and individuals are expected to cooperate in treatment and seek to get well. At the level of social systems, illness is a source of tension with conflict between a need to sustain and support the ill person on the one hand but to limit the magnitude of disability and dependence on the other, and to ensure that the essential tasks of the community are performed. Such tensions are vividly illustrated in controversies involving our disability system (Osterweis, Kleinman, and Mechanic 1987).

In the practice of medicine, however, business proceeds as if moral judgments lie outside its scope. The physician presumably is to make judgments uninfluenced by the individual's class, race, gender, or moral worth. In fact, practice is influenced by such social judgments, but the ideal norm condemns it and serves as a deterrent. Much more difficult are instances where physicians exercise moral judgments in making medical determinations but with no awareness that they are doing so. Halper (1985), for example, quotes a respected British nephrologist who counseled his colleagues that if one wants to get best results with dialysis, one should choose patients employed in a well-chosen occupation. The logic was that only few were comfortable on charity, and charity patients would not be motivated sufficiently for survival.

As one moves beyond the practice of medicine to consider the patient's perspective, it is apparent that perceptions of health and disease are inextricably linked with the capacity to function in social roles and to participate in desired activities. Symptoms are defined as important not simply in terms of their threat to life or comfort but also in terms of their interference in important ways with preferred function. Thus there is often a discordance between what physicians and patients see as important (Mechanic 1978).

As the boundaries of medicine grow, and medicine takes responsibility for problems that were earlier the province of the family, the church, and the neighborhood, medicine becomes increasingly entangled with moral systems and social values. As René Dubos noted,

> Health and happiness are the expression of the manner in which the individual responds and adapts to the challenges that he meets in everyday life. And these challenges are not only those arising from the external world, physical and social, since the most compelling factors of the environment, those most commonly involved in the causation of disease, are the goals the individual sets for himself, often without regard to biological necessity. (Dubos 1959/1987, 26)

References

American Psychiatric Association. 1980. *Diagnostic and statistical manual of mental disorders*. 3d ed. Washington, D.C.: American Psychiatric Association.

Balint, M. 1957. *The doctor, his patient and the illness*. New York: International Universities Press.

Bayer, R. 1987. *Homosexuality and American psychiatry: The politics of diagnosis.* Princeton: Princeton University Press.

Bayer, R., and R. L. Spitzer. 1985. Neurosis, psychodynamics, and DSM-III: A history of the controversy. *Archives of General Psychiatry* 42:187–96.

Beck, A. T., G. Emery, and J. Rush. 1979. *Cognitive therapy of depression.* New York: Guilford.

Dubos, R. 1959/1987. *Mirage of health: Utopias, progress and biological change.* New Brunswick: Rutgers University Press.

Feldman, J. 1966. *The dissemination of health information.* Chicago: Aldine.

Fromm, E. 1941. *Escape from freedom.* New York: Holt.

Geertsen, R., M. R. Klauber, M. Rindflesh, R. L. Kane, and R. Gray. 1975. A re-examination of Suchman's views on social factors in health care utilization. *Journal of Health and Social Behavior* 16:226–37.

Gluckman, M. 1965. *The ideas in Barotse jurisprudence.* New Haven: Yale University Press.

Halper, T. 1985. Life and death in a welfare state: End stage renal disease in the United Kindgom. *Milbank Quarterly* 63:52–93.

Hansell, S., D. Mechanic, and E. Brondolo. 1986. Introspectiveness and adolescent development. *Journal of Youth and Adolescence* 15:115–32.

House, J. S., K. R. Landis, and D. Umberson. 1988. Social relationships and health. *Science* 241:540–45.

Idler, E. 1992. Self-assessed health and mortality: A review of studies. *International Review of Health Psychology* 1:33–54.

Inkeles, A. 1983. *Exploring individual modernity.* New York: Columbia University Press.

Inkeles, A., and D. H. Smith. 1974. *Becoming modern: Individual change in six developing countries.* Cambridge: Harvard University Press.

Kagan, J. 1989. *Unstable ideas: Temperament, cognition, and self.* Cambridge: Harvard University Press.

Mechanic, D. 1962. *Students under stress: A study in the social psychology of adaptation.* New York: Free Press.

———. 1974. Social structure and personal adaptation: Some neglected dimensions. In *Coping and adaptation,* edited by G. Coelho, D. Hamburg, and J. Adams. New York: Basic Books.

———. 1978. *Medical sociology.* 2d ed. New York: Free Press.

———. 1979. Development of psychological distress among young adults. *Archives of General Psychiatry* 36:1233–39.

————. 1989. Socioeconomic status and health: An examination of underlying processes. In *Pathways to health: The role of social factors*, edited by J. P. Bunker, D. S. Gomby, and B. H. Kehrer. Menlo Park, Calif.: Kaiser Family Foundation.

————. 1990. Promoting health. *Society* 27:16–22.

Mechanic, D., and S. Hansell. 1987. Adolescent competence, psychological well-being, and self-assessed physical health. *Journal of Health and Social Behavior* 28:364–74.

Mechanic, D., and M. Newton. 1965. Some problems in the analysis of morbidity data. *Journal of Chronic Diseases* 18:569–80.

National Center for Health Statistics. 1991. *Health, United States, 1990*. Hyattsville, Md.: Public Health Service.

O'Dea, T. F. 1957. *The Mormons*. Chicago: University of Chicago Press.

Osterweis, M., A. Kleinman, and D. Mechanic. 1987. *Pain and disability: Clinical, behavioral and policy perspectives*. Committee on Pain, Disability, and Chronic Illness Behavior, Institute of Medicine. Washington, D.C.: National Academy Press.

Parsons, T. 1951. *The social system*. New York: Free Press.

Peterson, C., and L. Bossio. 1991. *Health and optimism*. New York: Free Press.

Pratt, L. 1976. *Family structure and effective health behavior: The energized family*. Boston: Houghton Mifflin.

Seligman, M. 1991. *Learned optimism*. New York: Knopf.

Straus, R., and S. D. Bacon. 1953. *Drinking in college*. New Haven: Yale University Press.

Tessler, R. C., and D. Mechanic. 1978. Psychological distress and perceived health status. *Journal of Health and Social Behavior* 19:254–62.

Variations in medical practice. 1984. *Health Affairs* (special issue) 3 (summer).

Verbrugge, L., and F. J. Ascione. 1987. Exploring the iceberg: Common symptoms and how people care for them. *Medical Care* 25:539–69.

Waitzkin, H. 1991. *The politics of medical encounters: How patients and doctors deal with social problems*. New Haven: Yale University Press.

Wakefield, J. 1992a. The concept of mental disorders: On the boundary between biological facts and social values. *American Psychologist* 47:373–88.

————. 1992b. Disorder as harmful dysfunction: A conceptual critique of DSM-IIIR's definition of mental disorder. *Psychological Review* 99:232–47.

Ware, J. E., Jr. 1986. The assessment of health status. In *Applications of social science to clinical medicine and social policy*, edited by L. H. Aiken and D. Mechanic. New Brunswick: Rutgers University Press.

Wells, K. B., A. Stewart, R. D. Hays, A. Burnam, W. Rogers, M. Daniels, S. Berry, S. Greenfield, and J. Ware. 1989. The functioning and well-being of depressed patients: Results from the medical outcomes study. *Journal of the American Medical Association* 262:914–19.

Wennberg, J. 1984. Dealing with medical practice variations. *Health Affairs* 3:6–32.

———. 1990. Outcomes research, cost containment, and the fear of health care rationing. *New England Journal of Medicine* 323:1202–4.

White, K. 1988. Foreword. In *Medicine and culture: Varieties of treatment in the United States, England, West Germany, and France*, edited by L. Payer. New York: Holt.

White, K. 1970. Evaluation of medical education and health care. In *Community medicine: Teaching, research and health care*, edited by W. Lathem and A. Newberry. New York: Appleton-Century-Crofts.

Morality and Culture

Moral Transformations of Health and Suffering in Chinese Society

Arthur Kleinman and Joan Kleinman

The Theory of Local Worlds as Mediators and Transformers of Experience

Two opposing positions dominate studies of health and its social sources and consequences (see Kleinman 1995 for a fuller treatment). The biomedical orientation—and the psychological theories (especially cognitive neuroscience) that are increasingly closely related to it (Kosslyn 1992)—centers its analysis on *the individual*, who is further reduced into the *objective* biological structures that underlie bodily processes. Disease is viewed as a diathesis, an entity, a "natural" form that even if it is evoked by stress unfolds into a "natural" course independent of biography or context. It is held to be a *universal*, whose essential properties are invariant. Disease is admitted to have social consequences, but these are regarded to be preventable by technological interventions. The social origins of disease and the human contexts of illness experiences are largely left out of the biomedical discourse.

Over against this perspective stand the sociopolitical and political economic orientations that hold diseases to result from major social changes and to require similar societal transformations for their prevention. Biological and personal mediators are often overlooked or at least deemphasized; coping with suffering and the quest for treatment are discounted, often with a tinge of moral superiority; they are even regarded as mystification. If the former position is a classical illustration of reductionism, the latter is also reductionism, though to different axes of interpretation. Overgeneralized analytic strategies characterize both.

Although each of these perspectives has its own advantages and limitations, the gross division between the individual and the social seriously distorts the conditions of health. This dichotomy greatly restricts the possibilities for understanding the processes that transform illness (Kleinman and Kleinman 1991; Kleinman 1992; Kleinman 1995). In this chapter, we draw upon the East Asian tradition to present a third perspective, one that privileges the *interpersonal processes* that connect the body-self with collective meanings and social institutions (Ware and Kleinman 1992). This approach seeks to dissolve the distorting polarity between "subjective" and "objective" worlds, and to replace it with emphasis on human interconnections. Interpersonal relations are the appropriate domain for exploring the relationship between morality and health (Csordas and Kleinman 1990).

We begin with a theory of social experience in local worlds. We then turn to review research that we have conducted in China and Taiwan that asks the question, how does the social world mediate and transform the variety of forms of suffering? We expand this framework of analysis to consider the pandemic of behavioral and mental health problems internationally whose sources include the breakdown of local moral orders under the pressure of the current, particularly destructive, phase of worldwide socioeconomic and political transformations (Desjarlais et al. 1995; Kleinman and Kleinman 1995). Along the way, we sketch the implications of this middle-level analysis.

The Ethnography of Local Moral Worlds

We begin with the ethnographer's focus on local worlds. These are villages, market towns, urban neighborhoods, social networks. Here everyday living is transacted. Participants engage in the local politics of interpersonal interactions. In local interactions certain things really matter: power, position, prestige, material resources, ethnic identity, social order, ultimately survival. Because vital interests and values are at stake, everyday social activities are *moral*.

Rather than regard the individual actors or the institutional structure of the local world as a whole as primary, we take the processes of interpersonal agency—communication, engagement, transaction, and negotiation—to be fundamental. These interpersonal processes create the flow of *social experience* (Kleinman and Kleinman 1991). They circulate back and forth through the inner space of the body-self and the social space of lived meanings and institutions. So defined, social experience is the medium through which moral commitments and negotiations join the corporeal with the collective (see Csordas 1990). So joined, the rhythms, routines, and rituals of everyday social life mediate existential human conditions. Life-cycle changes—including aging, loss and bereavement, health and illness, death and dying—all exist in the stream of social experience. This medium of "sociosomatic" processes also can transform human conditions, so that healing and transcendence are realized as well in this middle space between the personal and the social.

Viewed in this way, the local medium is what anthropologists refer to as culture. Culture results from both the patterning of social experience by way of language and other symbol systems *and* the emergence of the patterned moral reality of what matters most in everyday social transactions. Local cultural worlds stand between the force of large-scale social changes—for example, economic and political transformations—and their outcomes in survival, mortality, morbidity, suffering, and coping. In the particular historical setting of social experience, certain categories of persons are relatively protected from specific effects, whereas others are made especially vulnerable (Kleinman and Kleinman 1995). Description of how local worlds protect some while risking others should indicate more precise ways of intervening to improve health and health care.

Phenomenologists along with ethnographers have identified several key themes that characterize local worlds, including their overbearing practical relevance; the existential pressure for coherence; the immediacy of their felt quality; their multiplicity; and resistance to life plans; among others (see Dewey 1922/1957, 269, 1925/1989; Jackson 1989, 1–15; Merleau-Ponty 1962). Of course, ethnographers and social historians have also repeatedly demonstrated that local contexts are particular. These worlds legitimate differing forms of experience. Anthropologists have been especially active in arguing that indigenous categories and practices that are close to lived experience—that is, that relate to how people get on with practical affairs of everyday life—offer a more valid analytic strategy for getting at local worlds (see, for example, Geertz 1987; Hallowell 1955/1967); Rosaldo 1980; Schieffelin 1976; among a large number of ethnographers).

Moral Mediation of Suffering in Chinese Society

Chinese Experience-Near Categories of Interpersonal Transactions

There is a tradition among Chinese social scientists of sinicizing the study of interpersonal experience (Hwang 1987; Yang 1987). Influential Chinese scholars criticize Western analytic categories in the study of human behavior, which they regard as overemphasizing individual psychological states and underemphasizing social context. Thus, mind-body interactions, they hold, need to be reformulated as mind-body-in-context. Chinese scholars argue rather that like the paradigmatic differences between biomedicine and traditional Chinese medicine (see Nakayama 1984; Unschuld 1985), an emphasis on *process* needs to complement an emphasis on *structure*; dialectical models must balance single causal models; and an idea of resonance or rhythm is needed to develop an adequate conception of efficacy. (See, among others, Hwang 1987, King 1991, Yang 1987, and You 1994.)

Most notably, these Chinese psychologists and sociologists draw on traditional Chinese categories that give primacy to social relationships. Thus, their analytic models turn on the centrality of alliances or interpersonal connections (*guanxi*) in local worlds. They focus on the local politics of building, sustaining, and using social networks. These networks of persons and families are further understood as based on a particular type of reciprocity (*bao*) in which *renqing* (favor), *lianzi* ("face," moral position), and *mianzi* ("face" as self-affirming social status) are moral resources. These resources, or moral capital, endow social conditions. Success and failure depend on the deployment of moral capital to mobilize networks and foster their effects. Reciprocity of face and favor make human networks into gift relationships in which the exchange of moral capital is emphasized. The network of connections (the social body) can be described by the same terminology of efficacy (*ling*) and energy (*qi*) that is applied to the anatomical body. Networks, like bodies, can be vitalized or devitalized, demoralized or remoralized. Indeed, bodies are networked, networks embodied. "Giving" and "acquiring" face and favor is the moral order of Chinese society. The moral, the physiological, and the social psychological animate the same processes of everyday living.

Thus, in this model, behavior is located in local worlds whose alliances are both political and moral. Behavioral choices are strategic decisions in different fields of power. Action is always in context. Reading, exchanging, and repaying *renqing* are the moral (and political) core of relationships. Elsewhere we have written that in traditional Chinese thought

> balancing emotion and situation is essential to master social relations with others. Demonstrating strong feelings, including the menaced and aggrieved affects of suffering, is dangerous, because it gives others power over relationships and restricts one's flexibility to respond effectively. Ultimately, uncontrolled emotional displays threaten one's position in a world of power. Balance, blandness, control provide greater access to power and protect one from the feared effects of power: loss of resources or status or life. (Kleinman and Kleinman 1991)

We have also noted that

> emotion (*qing* or *zhih*) is not presented as an independent phenomenon, separable from the rest of experience. The Su Wen section of the *Huangdi neijing* (The Yellow Emperor's classic of internal medicine) sets out an indigenous theory of the emotions as they relate to health and illness. Suicidal grief, immobilizing sadness, manic passion and other extreme emotional states are held by the dominant Chinese medical tradition of systematic correspondences up to the present to be etiological factors that cause organic pathology; they are also signs of social pathology. They are *pathogens*, internal etiologic factors (*nei yin*) that create organic dysfunction. In Traditional Chinese Medicine (TCM) emotion is not a general phenomenological descriptor. Instead, there are seven specifically named entities the *qiqing*, seven kinds of situationally embedded emotional reactions, namely joy (*xi*), anger (*nu*), melancholy (*you*) [also translated as anxiety/depression], worry (*si*), grief (*bei*), fear (*kong*), and fright (*jing*). These, if excessive, may become pathological factors. These include excessive joy, anger, and melancholy, over-worrying or thinking too much, and fear. They are said to influence the normal circulation of *qi* (vital energy) and the blood in the internal organs, thereby caus-

ing morbid conditions. In this view, the human body as well as its pathological changes are in a continuous state of adapting to the variations of the "natural environment." This is the concept of *tian ren xiangying*—nature and man adapt to each other—and here "nature" includes the four seasons, the physical and social environment, and the physical structure and physiological processes of the individual himself. Thus, emotional pathology may become both sign and cause of social pathology, and balancing the emotions means harmonizing social relations and vice versa. (Kleinman and Kleinman 1991)

The perspective does not deny individuality or novelty but views them as the outcome of long-term interactions (cf. Bourdieu 1989; Chartier 1988). Health and healing must be viewed in the same way. We will illustrate the analytical use of such experience-near indigenous categories in working through the ethnographic materials that follow.

The Pain, Exhaustion, and Vertigo of Alienation and Resistance

From the late 1950s to the mid-1970s, China was a place of ferocious political repression that went from vise-like social control to chaos, and then back to a greatly oppressive social order culminating in the whirlwind of the Cultural Revolution, which created a universe of accusation and trauma. By the late 1970s the society was undergoing a delegitimation crisis that profoundly affected its core institutions (Tu 1992).

Beginning in 1978, we initiated a series of long-term studies of the experiences of Chinese who had been traumatized during the Cultural Revolution and its predecessors. Research was conducted primarily in the outpatient clinics of the Hunan Medical College in Changsha, Hunan; we also conducted an ethnography of that work-unit (*danwei*) and interviewed selected families.

From 1978 to 1980, there was a period of national preoccupation with victims' accounts of their trauma—the all-too-brief literary flowering that is called the literature of wounds or scars. But by 1980, China's political leaders had determined that these morbid stories, many of which had a critical edge, had gotten out of hand, so they initiated yet another movement, which successfully cracked down on expressions of criticism through stories of terror and hostility. Thus, in the early 1980s we were impressed by the way that retelling narratives of sickness, especially of neurasthenia (a common syndrome of chronic pain, sleeplessness, fatigue, dizziness, and many other somatic symptoms together with sadness, anxiety, and anger), authorized social memory and thereby enabled oblique criticism of the bitter reality of life during the Cultural Revolution and other political movements, which our informants held to be the origin of their conditions. (See Kleinman 1986 for details of the study.)

Content analysis of the thematic structure of these illness narratives indicated that remembrance of physical complaints (bodily metaphors of individual experience) acted as an embodied memory of the social experience of menace and loss and the associated feelings of demoralization, fear, and hatred (cf. Connerton 1989; Kleinman and Kleinman 1994). Three paradigmatic symptoms—*dizziness* (or vertigo), *exhaustion*, *pain*—created an interpersonal space of suffering in which shared personal complaints indirectly expressed social distress and shared criticism. Dizziness—a common though usually unmarked symptom of neurasthenia and other chronic fatigue syndromes in the West—carries particular salience in Chinese society, where the Chinese medical tradition emphasizes balance and harmony as constitutive and expressive of health. To be dizzy is to be unbalanced, out of rhythm, to experience malaise, to be dis-eased. Dizziness was understood by our informants to be the embodiment of alienation, the felt meaning of delegitimation in their local worlds. It was as close as many could come to expressing political opposition and cultural criticism, at a time when overt expression of hidden transcripts carried dangerous political outcomes (cf. Scott 1990).

Dizziness also expressed the felt experience of falling (or fear of falling) from a higher to lower social position. The topsy-turvy cycles of the Cultural Revolution spread this experience across all social positions. One group ascended by means of struggle, was in turn struggled against, and then was passed by.

Exhaustion from sleeplessness, and the paralyzing fatigability and weakness associated with it, recalled shared traumatic events. Months of working frenetically in political campaigns, often at contradictory purposes, convinced sufferers that they and the nation had reached the end of revolution. Vital resources were exhausted. Personal and collective efficacy had been drained. Fatigue and weakness in traditional Chinese medical theory express loss or blockage in the flow of *qi* (vital energy). Devitalization is understood to affect the body-self and the network, the microcosmic local world and the macrocosmic society.

Pain—headaches, backaches, cramps—also re-created the effects of the Cultural Revolution's turmoil on human lives. This lived metaphor was easily extended from personal anatomy to the social body. Pain and inner resentment, outer suffering and social resentment merged. (The seventeenth-century English meaning of *resent* was to feel pain as the embodiment of a social state [O.E.D.]). Each complaint, elaborated in the context of a story that integrated social and bodily suffering, was a moral commentary, first, about a delegitimated local world, ultimately about the delegitimation of Chinese society.

Our informants lived in worlds of pain in work-units and families, where relationships had become poisoned, aspirations obstructed, and bitter accusations and conflicts interminable. The body, exhausted, painful, vertiginous—the body that had lost its social force and moral face—became the grounds for negotiation over jobs, time, responsibilities, and resources.

The symptoms of Chinese sufferers of neurasthenia take on serious interpretive value as the forms of mediation and transformation through which interpersonal processes create the moral core of local worlds (here work-units and family units). Symptoms of social suffering and the transformations they undergo *are* the cultural forms of lived experience. The origins and consequences of these symbolizing sensibilities of distress and criticism reveal what those local worlds are about; how they change; and what significance they hold for the study of health and moral conditions.

Schizophrenia and Stigma

In another series of studies of family and community responses to members suffering from schizophrenia in Taiwan and China, we have learned that the powerful stigma of mental illness affects the patient's and family's circle of social connections such that the afflicted person and the members of his or her network lose face (*lianzi, mianzi*), vitality (*qi*), and efficacy (*ling*), and thereby express and constitute bad fate (*yunqi buhao*)—an ultimate icon of moral failure, a form of evil. Stigma is made visible in the transformation in habitus (literally a fallen face) and in network (which shrinks, a sort of ruins of connections). Inasmuch as connections are held to be the source of power in social life because of the moral favor (*ren-qing*) they bestow and the practical benefits they yield, the "unfavorable" networks of the mentally ill are seen as unavailing: devitalized and devitalizing. Their members drop out, and others hesitate to fill their place, wishing not to be contaminated by bad fate or to have their moral position and social influence questioned. If no longer able to disguise the problem or in other ways to control the damage done by discrediting labels, family members may ultimately seek to permanently institutionalize or abandon a schizophrenic member (see Xiong et al. 1994; Phillips 1993).

The *form* itself of the illness experience (that is, the syndrome, its meaning and its course) is seen to reside not just in the sick person but also in the family and its members' networks. Their depleted *qi*, inefficacy, and possibly contagious bad fate constitute the illness experience as much as do the hallucinations, delusions, and other symptoms. The moral effects of chronic mental illness extend to the psychiatric hospital itself. "Walking through these gates," said the anguished father of a patient, "is like putting on a political cap." (During the Cultural Revolution, ceremonies of degradation were organized by the Red Guards for their victims in which so-called enemies of the people were shamed by being forced to wear dunce caps as visible stigmata of their bad political status.)

Recovery from schizophrenia in Chinese society, then, is as much a tale of revitalizing social networks as it is a story of the control of hallucinations, delusions, and other serious behavioral disturbances. Negative family responses intensify symptoms and increase relapse and rehospitalization. Family therapy for schizophrenia in China is successful in part because families are assisted in the practical task of relegitimating their local worlds and in the symbolic work of remoralizing their position in those worlds: acquiring face and gaining favor. (Xiong et al. 1994; see also Kleinman et al. 1995.)

Dissociation, Possession, and Healing: Transformation of the Embodied Processes of the Moral Order

In 95 percent of the world's cultures, trance and possession states are routine forms of experience (Bourguignon 1976). They may be normal or pathological (cf. Canquilhem 1989), but they are normative. Viewed from the perspective of contemporary neuropsychol-

ogy, such states are processes of dissociation in which the field of attention is greatly narrowed; perception, imagination, and memory
are absorbed into a particular focus; and as a result cognition is split
from affect so that the self may be experienced as divided or occu-
pied or lost. Among Chinese, these states are more common among
rural populations, who maintain a strong orientation to traditional
folk religion. Yet, even in urban Taiwan—one of the world's wealth-
iest and most technologically advanced societies—lower-middle-
class and even well-educated Chinese may participate in religious
ritual activities in which supplicants and healers experience possession by gods, ghosts, or ancestors (Davis 1992).

Trance and possession provide yet another angle from which to
view the interpersonal mediation and transformation of experience. I. M. Lewis (1971) was among the first to show, among
women who undergo possession in the Zar cult in Somalia, that
the possession is the appropriation, through an authorized trance
state, of a voice of criticism, which articulates a subaltern perspective on the power of patriarchy and other oppressive social institutions. The voice of a *jinn* spirit, or, for that matter, of a possessing
god or ghost among Chinese, not only expresses resentment but
demands retribution. Transformation in social space, though usually modest and transient, follows upon transformation of the
body-self (see Boddy 1989; also Comaroff 1985; Ong 1987). Case
examples of possession as social transformers come from a Taiwan
ethnography (Kleinman 1980, 210–43, 375–89) and could be described among patients in psychiatric facilities and folk healing settings in China. These patients quite frequently are women from
impoverished households who have been under great pressure and
have undergone deeply hurtful experiences of powerlessness in
family and work setting. The possessing god or ghost demands that
their grievances be heard and that they be compensated for them.
The presence of the possessing agent offers face, energizes experience, and demands favor from family and friends. Thereby, moral
experience is transformed. Illness through possession criticizes a local world; healing opens up a few more options in the social field.
The changes usually are modest in scope but often can be significant nonetheless.

If the mediation and transformation of possession involve the
embodiment of moral categories that have an effect within local
fields of power, how are we best to research these processes and
their effects? The chief methodological problem is set by the limits
imposed by the major disciplines that study trance and possession.

Cognitive neuroscientists and biological psychiatrists limit the object of enquiry to "central states," by which they mean the cognitive machinery involved in the processing of attention, perception, and memory. Their research studies take place in laboratories in which the vital context of action has been almost entirely removed. On the other hand, the ethnography of trance and possession often proceeds as if there were no person present, and when there is a self it is usually disembodied. Most anthropological studies emphasize the *representation* of dissociation, or its social effects, rather than the experiential phenomena of trance and possession.

A more adequate research frame would have to examine the microprocesses of interaction that transform person into god or ghost. From our own research experiences we would posit a model of the interpersonal flow of experience in which cognitive and affective processes aggregate, disaggregate, and reaggregate around different axes of experience from the deeply subjective through the dialogical to the communal, depending upon particular transactions in a local world (Kleinman and Kleinman 1991). Dissociation and association, in this framework, are to be conceived as processes that mediate that transpersonal field. Local worlds of demoralization, for example, may be mediated as embodied experiences of defeat.

In trance and possession states, the experiential flow is aggregated around an axis of self-body processes, associated linguistic and other symbolic forms, and social rituals that instantiate voices of gods, ghosts, and ancestors in the lived world in one cultural setting, and multiple personalities in another. Classical trance states may represent the aggregation in a moral world of exchange relations; multiple personality aggregation in a field of commodity relations (see Taylor 1992, 3–22). The *form* of dissociation is not limited to brain, mind, body, or person as discrete entities but is enacted as interconnected cognitive, affective, and transpersonal processes.

Trance and possession are transformations upon these axes of interpersonal experience such that local social psychological resonances and rhythms are altered, as are local physiologies. Seen from this perspective, the processes that mediate and transform routinized misery among the poor, bereavement and shamanistic trance, are of a piece; suffering cannot be regarded as logically separable into "natural" (that is, disease) and "social" states. The self is not the only locus of the mediation or the transformation; rather, it is only one of the axes of social experience. The object of medical and anthropological enquiry needs to be restructured to get at the constitution of axes of experience and their effects on society-mind-body states.

The problem of efficacy in healing requires the same restructuring of the object of research enquiry (Csordas and Kleinman 1990; Roseman 1991). Transformation in delegitimated local worlds is as central to therapeutic efficacy as is transformation of the alienated body-self in those worlds. What is transformed is the interpersonal moral order. This in turn transforms the moral physiology associated with one's position in the social field.

Certain of the models of traditional Chinese medicine (TCM), not surprisingly for reasons already reviewed, seem more adequate for appreciating these dialectical phenomena than are those of biomedical or psychological science. The categories of TCM can be used to complement or even substitute for analytic approaches. Efficacy in healing rituals, be they surgical or shamanistic, illustrates the point.

Efficacy, as the Chinese experience-near categories would suggest, involves the reaffirmation of face, the redistribution of favor, the reinterpretation of fate, and the reordering and reimagining of the lived experience of local worlds. Efficacy can involve an assemblage or only one of the areas of experience. "Relapse," "remission," "treatment failure or resistance," all technologize efficacy. There is no space in this biomedical construction of outcome for endurance as a valued experience, for remoralization, for transcendence. Eschewing teleology, just as it does such experiential states of the lived world as tragedy and courage, biomedicine, for all its technological power, misses the moral point of what is at stake in human conditions.

The Destruction of Local Moral Worlds: Social Suffering and Its Implications for Policy

The immense political and economic dislocations of recent times and their powerful effects on local worlds have created a pandemic of behavioral, social, and mental health problems that are affecting societies of the North and South alike (see Sugar, Kleinman, and Eisenberg 1991). Rates of alcohol and drug abuse and related violence, suicide, family breakdown with spouse and child abuse and abandonment, mental illnesses, sexually transmitted diseases, AIDS, trauma owing to forced uprooting secondary to ethnic conflict—all are high and most are rising rapidly (Sugar, Kleinman, and Heggenhougen 1991, 1992; Desjarlais et al. 1995). In Latin America, it has been estimated by the Pan American Health Organization, that these problems account for most adult mortality; in primary care settings, they are the most common cause for attendance.

Without invoking an exaggerated millenarian notion of apocalypse, it is important for the model we have advanced to examine the effects of certain large-scale political and economic transformations of the current era on local worlds. Routinized misery and contingent misfortunes are, of course, aspects of human conditions across historical epochs and cultural settings. The death of fifty million in the Second World War and the forced uprooting of hundreds of millions make even the worst contemporary tragedies seem manageable. What we wish to emphasize is not that societal developments are unprecedented but, rather, that our present period of social change is particularly destructive for local moral worlds and that situation holds special significance for social science and for social and health research and policy (cf. Kennedy 1993).

Lin Tsung-yi, Rin Hsien, Yeh Eng-kung, and their colleagues at National Taiwan University began a series of studies in the late 1940s, repeated in the 1960s and 1980s, that used the same diagnostic and assessment systems and even many of the same team of investigators to survey mental health problems in a Taiwanese village, a market town and a city (Lin et al. 1969; Yeh et al. 1987). These researchers found that rates of psychoses did not change much over the four decades of Taiwan's profound transformation from a poor, primarily agrarian society to a wealthy, high-technology-based urban country. However, rates of depressive and anxiety disorders increased several fold at each of the times of follow-up evaluation. The increase was greatest in the market town, which the researchers described as being under the most difficult pressures of urbanization. Taiwan as a whole has also experienced a tenfold increase in rates of serious alcohol abuse from the 1950s to the 1990s (Chang Ly-yun, personal communication). Rates of adolescent and adult crime and violence follow a similar trend.

Most such problems are initially interpreted and coped with not in the clinics and hospitals of the official system of mental health care but in family and folk-healing settings, where the language of distress and the methods of response are not those of psychiatry, psychology or social work but, rather, the everyday moral and religious languages of this still deeply familistic, ancestor-reverence-oriented, Confucian culture (Kleinman 1980; Davis 1992). These informal structures of response point to destructive changes in local worlds under the powerful pressure of societal transformation, such as the breakdown of the interpersonal code of behavior, the intensification of egocentric consumer practices, the worsening of class divisions, and escalating forms of violence, as the locus of responsibility for distress. It is a perspective worth considering.

In China, where the disintegration of the state's structures of diffused social control has brought with it not only diminished surveillance but also a return to rates of prostitution and sexually transmitted diseases, along with drug abuse and crime, that had not been seen since the social turmoil of the 1940s, there is a widespread fear of *luan* (chaos). That fear feeds on disturbing social memories of earlier periods of social disorder. Richard Marsden (1984), in his study of the effects of radical political movements since the 1950s on Chinese village structure, argues that these changes have broken the moral framework, yielding paralyzing bitterness and resentment, and destructive cynicism (see also Chang 1991). Other ethnographers, while charting the effects of equally profound change, describe much greater resilience and coping capacity (Huang 1989; Siu 1989; Yan 1992). Our own research in a large urban work-unit discloses that that local world is beset by an extraordinary disruption in the interpersonal processes delineated earlier in this chapter, including the unraveling of the fragile web of social obligation and responsibility. Members of the work-unit themselves see this development as a fracture of the moral order (cf. Liu 1990). It is visible at all levels of urban units in China. Hospital directors have competed for foreign exchange from wealthy overseas Chinese who receive the organs transplanted from newly executed criminals. Work-unit leaders cut off the life-sustaining medical insurance for severely ill members because it is perceived as too substantial a financial drain on the collective. Theft of collective and personal items, always a low-level concern, has become much more serious, as has open corruption. Our colleagues view these problems as the diminution of the virtues of communism, which has occurred along with the weakening of its oppressive features, and the rise of the problems of the "free market." A common local opinion is that because Chinese are both sociocentric *and* individualistic, a change in local values encourages the unfettered development of the latter at the expense of the former. Clearly, this viewpoint corresponds with a political line pressed by hard-liners within the government; nonetheless, it does pick up on a sea change in local conditions. Moreover, this is a change in local social patterns that ethnographers have noted in other parts of the world, where some have seen it as a transformation of local moral orders from ones based on gift-exchange relations to ones based on commodity exchange.

What are the implications for health, health care, and social welfare? Infant mortality rates are no longer improving in China; in the poorest villages, poverty and malnutrition have deepened. Perhaps 100 million Chinese are internally displaced for economic reasons from villages to shantytowns in and around cities. The once greatly impressive national system of public health services and health care has disintegrated. Infanticide of female newborns is once again a serious problem. There can be little doubt that with the economic reforms have come both substantial economic improvement for many and the worsening of health and social conditions for others. At the local level of the village and work-unit, the moral processes that we have detailed are undergoing profound change. It is our contention that to understand the problems that have resulted in order to fashion appropriate policy responses and preventive programs, research must focus on these transformations in local worlds.

Heretofore health and health care policy has used aggregated national indices to propose regional and national policy alternatives. Rarely have systematic efforts been made to ground these indices in local worlds. The key question is not whether to moralize or to demoralize health affairs, or whether the moral aspects of health are best configured as partisan ideology or universal ethical standards. Rather, we need to see health as inseparable from the local moral order of our everyday worlds (see Desjarlais et al. 1995; Chen, A. Kleinman, and Ware 1994). Those worlds are distinctive, plural, and changing. Hence, the study of the relationship of health and morality needs to accommodate variety, pluralism, local particularities, and local change based in history and culture.

References

Boddy, J. 1989. *Wombs and alien spirits*. Madison: University of Wisconsin Press.

Bourdieu, P. 1989. Social space and symbolic power. *Sociological Theory* 7(1): 14–24.

Bourguignon, E. 1976. *Possession*. San Francisco: Chandler & Sharp.

Canquilhem, G.1989. *The normal and the pathological.* New York: Zone Books.

Chang, J. 1991. *Wild swans: Three daughters of China.* New York: Simon & Schuster.

Chen, L., A. Kleinman, and N. Ware, eds. 1994. *Health and social change in international perspective.* Cambridge: Harvard University Press.

Chartier, R. 1988. Social figuration and habitus. In his *Cultural history.* Ithaca: Cornell University Press.

Comaroff, J. 1985. *Body of power, spirit of resistance.* Chicago: University of Chicago Press.

Connerton, P. 1989. *How societies remember.* New York: Cambridge University Press.

Csordas, T. 1990. Embodiment as a paradigm for anthropology. *Ethos* 18(1): 5–47.

Csordas, T., and A. Kleinman. 1990. The therapeutic process. In *Medical anthropology: Contemporary theory and method*, edited by T. Johnson and C. Sargent. New York: Praeger.

Davis, L. S. 1992. On the eccentric position of shamanism in Taiwan. Ph.D. diss., Harvard University.

Desjarlais, R., L. Eisenberg, B. Good, and A. Kleinman, eds. 1995. *World mental health: Problems and prospects in low-income countries.* New York: Oxford University Press.

Dewey, J. 1925/1989. *Experience and nature.* La Salle, Ill.: Open Court.

Dewey, J. 1922/1957. *Human nature and conduct.* New York: Modern Library.

Geertz, C. 1987. *Local knowledge.* New York: Basic Books.

Hallowell, A. I. 1955/1967. *Culture and experience.* Philadelphia: University of Pennsylvania Press.

Huang, S. M. 1989. *The spiral road: Change in a Chinese village through the eyes of a Communist Party leader.* Boulder: Westview Press.

Hwang, K. K. 1987. Face and favor: The Chinese power game. *American Journal of Sociology* 92(4): 944–74.

Jackson, M. 1989. *Paths toward a clearing.* Bloomington: Indiana University Press.

Kennedy, P. 1993. *Preparing for the twenty-first century.* New York: Random House.

King, A. Y. C. 1991. *Kuan-hsi* and network building: A sociological interpretation. *Daedalus* 120(2): 63–84.

Kleinman, A. 1980. *Patients and healers in the context of culture.* Berkeley: University of California Press.

————. 1986. *Social origins of distress and disease: Neurasthenia, depression and pain in China*. New Haven: Yale University Press.

————. 1992. Pain and resistance: The delegitimation and relegitimation of local worlds. In *Pain as human experience*, edited by M. J. D. Good, et al. Berkeley: University of California Press.

————. 1995. *Writing at the margin: Discourse between anthropology and medicine*. Berkeley: University of California Press.

Kleinman, A., and J. Kleinman. 1991. Suffering and its professional transformation. *Culture, medicine and psychiatry* 15(3): 275–301.

————. 1994. How bodies remember: Social memory and bodily experience of criticism, resistance, and delegitimation following China's cultural revolution. *New Literary History* 25(3): 707–723.

————. 1995. Remembering the Cultural Revolution. In *Mental health in Chinese culture*, edited by T. Y. Lin, W. S. Tseng, and E. K. Yeh. Hong Kong: Oxford University Press.

Kleinman, A., et al. 1995. Social course of epilepsy in interior China. *Social Science and Medicine* 40(10): 1319–30.

Kosslyn, S. 1992. *Wet brain*. New York: Oxford University Press.

Lewis, I. M. 1971. *Ecstatic religion*. London: Penguin.

Lin, T. Y., et al. 1969. Mental disorders in Taiwan 15 years later. In *Mental health in Asia and the Pacific*, edited by W. Caudill and T. Y. Lin. Honolulu: East West Center Press.

Liu, B. Y. 1990. *A higher kind of loyalty*. New York: Pantheon.

Marsden, R. 1984. *Morality and power in a Chinese village*. Berkeley: University of California Press.

Merleau-Ponty, M. 1962. *The phenomenology of perception*. London: Routledge & Kegan Paul.

Nakayama, S. 1984. *Academic and scientific traditions in China, Japan, and the West*. Tokyo: University of Tokyo Press.

Ong, A. 1987. *Spirits of resistance and capitalist discipline*. Albany: SUNY Press.

Phillips, M. 1993. Strategies used by Chinese families coping with schizophrenia. In *Chinese families in the post-Mao era*, edited by D. Davis and S. Harrell. Berkeley: University of California Press, 277–306.

Roseman, M. 1991. *Healing sounds from the Malaysian rain forest: Temiar music and medicine*. Berkeley: University of California Press.

Rosaldo, M. 1980. *Knowledge and passion*. Cambridge: Cambridge University Press.

Schieffelin, E. 1976. *The sorrow of the lonely and the burning of the dancers*. New York: St. Martin's.

Scott, J. C. 1990. *Domination and the arts of resistance: Hidden transcripts*. New Haven: Yale University Press.

Siu, H. 1989. *Agents and victims in South China: Accomplices in rural revolution*. New Haven: Yale University Press.

Sugar, J., A. Kleinman, and K. Heggenhougen. 1991. Development's "downside": Social and psychological pathology in countries undergoing social change. *Health Transition Review* 1(2).

Sugar, J., A. Kleinman, and L. Eisenberg. 1991. Psychiatric morbidity in developing countries and American psychiatry's role in international health. *Hospital and Community Psychiatry* 43(4): 355–61.

Taylor, C. 1992. *Milk, honey, and money: Changing concepts in Rwandan healing*. Washington, D.C.: Smithsonian Institution Press.

Tu, W. M. 1992. The exit from communism. *Daedalus* 121(2): 251–92.

Unschuld, P. 1985. *Medicine in China: A history of ideas*. Berkeley: University of California Press.

Ware, N., and A. Kleinman. 1992. Culture and symptoms. *Psychosomatic Medicine* 54:546–60.

Xiong, W., M. R. Phillips, X. Hu, R. Wang, Q. Dai, J. Kleinman, and A. Kleinman. 1994. Family-based intervention for schizophrenic patients in China: A randomised controlled trial. *British Journal of Psychiatry* 165:239–47.

Yan, Y. X. 1992. The impact of reform on economic and social stratification in a Chinese village. *Australian Journal of Chinese Affairs* 27:1–23.

Yang, K. S. 1987. *The Chinese people in change*. Vol. 3, *Collected works on the Chinese people* (in Chinese). Taipei: Kuei Kuan Book Company.

Yeh, E. K., et al. 1987. Social changes and prevalence of specific mental disorders in Taiwan. *Chinese Journal of Mental Health* 3(1): 31–42.

You, H. L. 1994. Defining rhythm: Aspects of an anthropology of rhythm. *Culture, Medicine, and Psychiatry* 18: 361–84.

The "Big Three" of Morality (Autonomy, Community, Divinity) and the "Big Three" Explanations of Suffering

Richard A. Shweder, Nancy C. Much, Manamohan Mahapatra, and Lawrence Park

A Discourse on Suffering: "Old Sins Cast Long Shadows"

Wherever one looks on the globe it appears that human beings want to be edified by their miseries. It is as if the desire to make suffering intelligible and to turn it to some advantage is one of those dignifying peculiarities of our species, like the ability to cook or conjugate verbs or conceive of the idea of justice. Human beings, unlike other living things, want to go to school when they are miserable. They want to make their suffering intelligible, even as it is unwanted, by answering one or more questions about the cause of their distress: What caused this to happen? Why did this happen to me? Am I responsible for this? What can I do about it? What does this imply about my social relationships? What does this suggest about my personal rectitude? In this chapter we explore some of the ways human beings understand suffering and turn suffering to advantage, by blaming themselves for illness, disaster, and distress.

The chapter explores the implications of imagining the world and the experience of suffering in terms of some of the moral metaphors of South Asia. (On the study of metaphors implicit in folk and scientific theories, see Lakoff and Johnson 1980, 1986; Johnson 1987; Lakoff 1987.) In South Asia, ideas about a sacred self, a sacred world, "karma" ("you reap what you sow; therefore suffering may be an index of moral failure") and what might be called "feudal ethics" exist both as "folk theories" and as highly developed "technical theories." In the United States, such ideas run counter to the official discourse of scientific explanation yet persist as "private" intuitions experienced as mysteries or with embarrassment or as personal or communal "counterdiscourses" to the official discourse of scientific explanation. Why do certain ideas, which are viewed as rational in South Asia and infused with publicly acknowledged social meaning, persist in our own culture despite the absence of a scientific ontology to support them and despite the preeminent prestige of a scientific-materialist discourse that disavows and disparages them?

It is our assumption that ideas about human experience that persist long, or are widespread, or become invested with social meaning and established as folk theories in a major region of the world are not likely to be merely "primitive" or "superstitious." It is our assumption that such ideas illuminate some aspect of mind, experience, or society and can be put to use not only to construct a valid "cultural psychology" (Much 1992, 1995; Shweder 1991; Shweder and Sullivan 1993) but to extend our "moral imagination" (Johnson 1993). We examine apparently "primitive" or superstitious" ideas, such as "old sins cast long shadows" and, relatedly, that illness is payment of or punishment for spiritual debts. This chapter spells out the wisdom that ideas about karma, the sacred self, the sacred world, and feudal ethics encode in their metaphors. It applies one of the central assumptions of cultural psychology: indigenous or folk theories (our own and others) should be taken seriously as cognitive objects and as potential sources of social scientific and practical knowledge (Much 1993, 6–7; Much and Harre 1994; Much and Mahapatra 1995; Shweder and Miller 1985; Shweder and Much 1987).

The Causal Ontologies of Suffering

A List of Ontologies

To suffer is to experience a disvalued and unwanted state of mind, body, or spirit. The experience might be an acute disease, a recurrent nightmare, an obsessive thought, an incapacitating sadness, a skin rash, a miscarriage, or a cancer. It might be the experience of chronic fatigue or pain or a prolonged decline in physical integrity and personal autonomy.

One way to render suffering meaningful is to trace its genesis to some "order of reality" where one may point the finger at events and processes that can be held responsible as suffering's cause. We shall use the expression "causal ontology" to refer to a person or people's ideas about the "orders of reality" responsible for suffering.

Although the varieties of suffering of soma, psyche, and spirit that have been experienced by human beings range widely over an indefinitely large territory of afflictions, symptoms, and complaints, the varieties of causal ontologies that have played a major part in explanations of suffering are in fact relatively few. On a worldwide scale, there seem to be at least seven kinds of causal ontologies (and associated therapeutic institutions) for comprehending and responding to suffering.

There is a biomedical causal ontology. That causal ontology is notable in its current official Western medical variety for its explanatory references to genetic defects, hormone imbalances, organ pathologies, and physiological impairments. It is notable in non-Western or unofficial Western varieties (for example, Hindu Ayurvedic medicine) for its explanatory references to humors, precious bodily fluids and juices (semen, blood, ascorbic acid), and felicitous ecological transactions that enhance feelings of strength and well-being. Biomedical therapy focuses on the ingestion of special substances, herbs and roots, vitamins, vegetable compounds, and chemical compounds, and on the direct or indirect mechanical repair (for example, through surgery, massage, or emetics) of damaged fibers and organs.

There is an interpersonal causal ontology. That causal ontology is notable in traditional societies for its references to sorcery, evil eye, black magic, spirit attack, poisoning, and bewitchment. We have our contemporary counterparts in harassment, abuse, exploitation, "codependencies" and "toxic relationships." It is associated with the idea that one can be made sick by the envy or ill-will of colleagues, neighbors, and associates who want you to die, suffer, fail, or fall under their control. Therapy focuses on talismans and other protective devices, strategies for avoidance or aggressive counterattack, and, quite crucially, on the repair of interpersonal relationships.

There is a sociopolitical causal ontology. That causal ontology is associated with the idea that suffering is the product of oppression, colonial (including ideological) domination, or adverse economic or family conditions. Therapy focuses on altering one's life circumstances through social reform or, more typically, on achieving some local or immediate successes or gains.

There is a psychological causal ontology. That causal ontology is associated with the idea that unfulfilled desires and frustrated intentions (for example, repressed wishes) or various forms of fear can make one suffer. Therapy focuses on a variety of intrapsychic and psychosocial interventions, including meditation, dialogue, therapeutic relationships, consciousness-raising, and realistic goal setting. Freud is a noteworthy contemporary Western variant of psychological explanation, much absorbed into North American folk theory, but non-Western cultures, including South Asia, use psychological theories of causality as well.

There is an astrophysical causal ontology. That causal ontology is notable for its references to malevolent arrangements of planets, moons, and stars, and to auspicious and inauspicious periods of time. Therapy emphasizes the theme that one should wait, with optimism, for some identifiable auspicious future time when recovery will occur spontaneously or remedial efforts can be effective. In the meantime certain protective or meliorative actions are often possible. This is a causal ontology that is foregrounded in many non-Western cultures. It is backgrounded or officially denied yet very much present in segments of the folk life of contemporary middle-class American culture (of European, African, or Asian origin).

There is an apparently emergent causal ontology rooted in the metaphors of external "stress," "pressure," and "environmental risk factors." This ontology seems contemporary in the forms of discourse with which we are all familiar. Along with CNN (cable television) and Visa (credit cards), the English word *stress* seems to have migrated to all parts of the world. It is possible, however, that this causal ontology has been around for a long time but in terms we have as yet failed to identify. For example, aspects of Ayurvedic medicine, South Asian home remedies, and Indo-Tibetan social theory contain "ecological" causal relationships perhaps not entirely dissimilar to the terminologies of this ontology, and recognize "destressing" tactics for remedial action. "Stressors" themselves may, of course, be of a social or a biochemical nature. Therapies emphasize the minimization of stress: relaxation; the creative use of leisure time; and the reduction of ambient "hazards" in one's environment through enlightenment, education, and foresight.

Finally, there is a moral causal ontology. That causal ontology is notable for its references to transgressions of obligation: omissions of duty, trespass of mandatory boundaries, and more generally any type of ethical failure at decision making or self-control. It is associated with the idea that suffering is the result of one's own actions or intentions, that a loss of moral fiber is a prelude to misfortune, that outcomes—good and bad—are proportionate to actions. Moral therapy focuses on unloading one's sin, confession, purification, reparation, moral education, and the adoption of "right practices" sanctioned by a sacred authority (from the pope to the surgeon general). Later in this essay we take as an example a South Asian conception of moral causation, the theory of karma, and explore its implications as a viable moral metaphor for rethinking the discourse of morality and suffering in our own contemporary society.

The Idea of Causation in Folk Psychology

Within the intellectual framework of folk psychology explanations of illness are instances of causal analysis. Although the idea of causation is an idea that all folk around the world seem to recognize, it is important for us to recognize that the idea of causation universally employed in folk psychology has several special characteristics that distinguish it from other uses of the idea of causation with which it should not be confused. The idea of causation in folk psychology deviates in significant ways from the logician's (for example, John Stuart Mill's) analysis of the idea of "causation" as all the necessary conditions that are jointly sufficient to produce an event. It deviates as well from the empiricist's (for example, Sir David Hume's) reduction of the idea of causation to directly observable events (e.g., one billiard ball making contact with another) that are immediately coincidental in time and locally proximate in space (see Collingwood 1938/1961; Hart and Honore 1956/1961). In folk psychology the idea of causation does not rule out the possibility of influence at a distance. It does not rule out influence by unobservable forces. It does not demand attention to all necessary conditions. It does not treat all necessary conditions as equally relevant or as of the same kind.

Quite crucially, the idea of causation in folk psychology is deeply shaped by human interests in assessing "normality," attributing responsibility or blame, and exercising control over future events. Thus, the numerous logically necessary conditions for the production of a given event do not all have equal status in the folk psychology of causation. Indeed, in folk psychology the elevation of this or that necessary condition to the intellectual status of an attributed "cause" is an act of selection and interpretation that can be understood only within the context of practices and institutions aimed at finding fault, righting wrongs, and gaining control over future events.

A classic account of the idea of causation in folk psychology can be found in Hart and Honore (1956/1961, 333, 335). As Hart and Honore note, distinctions are drawn in folk psychology (they call it "common sense" psychology) "between what is abnormal and what is normal in relation to any given subject-matter and between a free deliberate human action and all other conditions." For example, with regard to the distinction between "normal" conditions and "abnormal" conditions, the oxygen in the air is a necessary condition for the forest fire but it is a "normal" condition and is not viewed in folk psychology as a "cause" of the fire, while the lightning storm, although no more necessary than the oxygen, is an "abnormal" condition and hence is likely to be viewed as the "cause."

And as Hart and Honore point out with regard to the distinction between free deliberate human action and everything else, "We [folk psychologists] feel that it is not enough to be told that a man died from unusual quantities of arsenic in his body, and we press on for the more satisfactory explanation in terms of human agency." "Deliberate human action has a special status as a cause [in folk psychology] and is not regarded in its turn as something which is caused."

Collingwood (1938/1961, 303, 306) detects the following two basic senses in the folk concept of a "cause." In one sense, it is the idea of "a free and deliberate act of a conscious and responsible agent," which is best understood in terms of the ends the agent is trying to achieve and the means the agent believes is available for achieving them. For example, looking ahead to our discussion of the prevalence of interpersonal explanations of suffering within the intellectual framework of folk psychology, the cause of an event (for example, a miscarriage) might be treated as equivalent to someone's motives for acting (for example, a neighbor is envious, intends to subvert the childbirth, and employs the services of a sorcerer). Indeed, it is precisely by reference to the quality of those motives and intentions (are they good or bad?) that the agent who caused the event can be held responsible, or judged to be at fault, or even accused of being a witch.

In the second sense, "the cause of a given thing is that one of its [logically necessary] conditions which [one] is able to produce or prevent." Collingwood gives the following example:

> A car skids while cornering at a certain point, turns turtle, and bursts into flames. From the car-driver's point of view the cause of the accident was cornering too fast, and the lesson is that one must drive more carefully. From the county surveyor's point of view, the cause was a defective road surface, and the lesson is that one must make skid-proof roads. From the motor-manufacturer's point of view, the cause was defective design, and the lesson is that one must place the center of gravity lower.

Notice that in each case the selected necessary condition (the attributed "cause") is relative to the potential range of control of the attributer. Notice that the attributed "cause" (the selected necessary condition) is not everything that is logically relevant to a causal analysis but, rather, the one thing that is practically relevant because the attributer is in a position to set it right.

As we examine the causal ontologies of suffering available on a worldwide scale, it is helpful to keep in mind the true aims of causal analysis in folk psychology: to set abnormal outcomes right by gaining control over abnormal conditions that are within the range of one's expertise and power, and to attribute responsibility and to assign fault in a world of events presumed to be caused by "free and deliberate" acts by "conscious and responsible" agents.

The "Big Three" Explanations of Suffering: Interpersonal, Biomedical, and Moral

Among anthropologists the cross-cultural study of the types and distribution of explanations of suffering with special reference to illness has a distinguished history (see, for example, Whiting & Child 1953; Kleinman 1986; Wikan 1989), although interest in the topic has been erratic. In 1980 George Peter Murdock published a survey of explanations of illness in 139 societies, as recorded in extant ethnographies. Although the overall quality of that ethnographic data leaves much to be desired, the survey suggests that preferred or official causal ontologies for suffering are unequally distributed around the world and may cluster in broad geographically based "ideological regions."

In sub-Saharan Africa, Murdock discerns a preference for explanations by reference to moral transgression (for example, violation of sexual taboos). In East Asia, the folk seem inclined to the view that suffering is due to ancestral spirit attack and other interpersonal causes. In the circum-Mediterranean region (Europe and North Africa), it is witchcraft that is favored in accounts of the causes of misery and death. Explanations by reference to organ pathology, hormone imbalance, or physiological impairment were, among the societies surveyed by Murdock, never preferred.

A recent cross-cultural survey by Park (1992), reanalyzed some of Murdock's sources and recoded the data in several ways. Park's goals were threefold: (1) to arrive at an estimate of the relative worldwide prevalence of six of the seven causal ontologies mentioned above (the "stress" concept was not examined); (2) to assess the hypothesis that there is geographical clustering of different types of causal explanations of suffering into "ideological regions"; and (3) to examine the connection between specific illnesses and the particular types of explanations and therapies produced in response to illness.

In the present context we shall restrict our discussion to the question of the prevalence rates of various causal ontologies for suffering and parallel therapies, although the third issue—the connection between type of affliction and type of explanation—is relevant to our discussion as well. Thus, for example, on the basis of Murdock's and Park's surveys, it seems reasonable to imagine that particular afflictions (for example, a miscarriage, a rash, sterility) of particular parts of the body (say, the womb, the genitals, the mouth, a visible part of the skin) incline the mind in the direction of particular causal ontologies and not others. Witchcraft explanations, where and when they are adduced, seem to be associated with issues of generativity and fecundity (crop failure, miscarriage, infertility). Murdock himself suggested that agent-blaming moralistic explanations crop up when suffering is preceded by violations of sexual or food taboos or by acts of disrespect to figures in authority (parents or gods).

Indeed, it is tempting to speculate that sexual transgressions, dietary transgressions, and transgressions of the hierarchical ordering of things can at times have such a powerful influence on the way we think and reason that long-delayed misfortunes may be understood as punishments for prior sin, and as confirmation of the maxim "ultimately the past catches up." We return to this issue later, when we suggest that a transgression (for example, disregard for one's parents, incest) is most readily moralized if it is embedded in an intellectual framework such as an ethics of community and/or divinity, which carries with it the implication that the transgressor has violated the sacred order of things, as manifest in nature, society, or the self. The basic idea is that when things start to go bad in life (illness, misfortune) there is a special class of prior dreadful transgressions in one's life that are likely to leap out as suspiciously ill-begotten causes.

On the basis of Park's reading of ethnographic reports from 68 cultures, involving 752 illness episodes, it appears that on a worldwide scale, interpersonal, moral, and biomedical causal ontologies constitute something like the "big three" explanations of suffering. These explanations offer alternative accounts of the causes of misery.

According to the interpersonal mode of causal explanation suffering is an instance of victimization at the hands of, for example, witches, ancestral spirits, envious neighbors, or domineering relatives. The background assumption of an interpersonal explanation is that the ill-will of others is a force to be reckoned with and may have momentarily gained an upper hand. Interpersonal explanations of suffering externalize blame: others are held responsible for one's misery.

In contrast, according to the moral mode of causal explanation, suffering is a consequence of personal transgressions, misdemeanors, and spiritual debts. The background assumption is that we live in a world where one reaps what one sows. This mode of explanation is agent-blaming: agents bear the primary responsibility for their own miseries.

Finally, according to the biomedical mode of causal explanation, suffering is a by-product of events and circumstances that take place outside the realms of human action, responsibility, or control. Strictly speaking, within the terms of a biomedical explanation, suffering is a material event and should be understood in material terms. It should be controlled through material interventions. When it comes to the strict biomedical understanding and alleviation of illness, no further questions are asked about such ultimate issues as human society, social relationships, or personal rectitude. Pure biomedical explanations are by definition morally neutral and indifferent to the moral career of the sufferer or of others. Of course, biomedical explanations are not always practiced in their "pure form," and many medical practitioners in the United States, South

Asia, and East Asia appreciate a more ecological and interactive approach to medicine, lifestyle, and environment.

On a worldwide scale, interpersonal, moral, and biomedical explanations and therapies are overwhelmingly the most common. They seem to be the "big three" explanations of suffering, although the three causal ontologies seem to play a somewhat different role in explanation versus cure. On the basis of Park's findings the most frequent *explanations* for suffering are interpersonal (42 percent of all accounts), moral (15 percent) and biomedical (15 percent); the most frequent *therapies* are biomedical (35 percent of all accounts), interpersonal (29 percent), and moral (7 percent).

A second fascinating finding of Park's study is that sufferers are more likely to seek a biomedical therapy for a problem than to offer a biomedical explanation of it. This is not true of either of the other two modes of explanation and cure. Interpersonal therapies (repair of social relationships, countersorcery, exorcism) are less likely to be sought than interpersonal explanations of suffering are to be offered. Moral therapies (confession, sacrifice, austerities) are less likely to be sought than moral explanations of suffering are to be offered. Thus, although in general it is true that there is a rough parallelism between mode of explanation and mode of cure—a tendency for biomedical explanations to lead to biomedical therapies, interpersonal explanations to interpersonal therapies, and moral explanations to moral therapies—it is also true that when there is "misalignment" between explanatory ontology and therapeutic mode, the mismatch seems to be in the direction of using a biomedical therapy for an affliction believed to have an interpersonal or moral cause. This may have something to do with the perceived possibility for control. That is, when human beings suffer, an imperative may exist for direct, physical manipulation of the suffering body. Another reason for the slippage toward biomedical therapies may be the immediacy or relative efficacy of such cures. In any case, the drift toward biomedical therapies does not seem peculiar to our times or to our particular system of Western biomedicine.

The prevalence of interpersonal explanations of suffering suggests that the idea of "victimization" also is not peculiar to the contemporary United States with its particular social justice concerns. That prevalence of attributed interpersonal causes also may reflect an underinvestigated intuition of folk psychology, namely, that the attitudes and expressions of those around us, through various social-communicative and social-control processes, are effective in inducing psychosomatic stress, which can result in illness. Tibetan communities, for example, have the idea that the malicious or envious gossip of one's neighbors, without other intervening mechanisms such as sorcery or witchcraft, acts as a kind of force capable of wreaking havoc with one's life and health (Mumford 1989).

On a worldwide scale, then, moral explanations of suffering and moral therapies are among the three most salient forms of explanation and cure, although in Park's survey they rank third in prevalence behind interpersonal and biomedical modes of interpretation and response. It seems likely, however, that this kind of estimate of the prevalence of moral thinking in health practices underestimates the role and importance of moral agency in explanations of suffering.

For one thing, interpersonal explanations of suffering are often saturated with implicit secondary moral implications (for example, the ancestral spirit attack may have been related to an ethical failure to perform a ritual) that may not have been known to the ethnographer. Interpersonal causal explanations frequently involve moral features and moral offenses; there is some "quarrel" or bad feeling between the "victim" and the "aggressor." Repair of relationships and reestablishment of a just local order (for example, family) may be part of what sorcerers try to accomplish. Even in cases of pure victimization the very notion of "victimization" is inherently a moral idea, which may place the victimizer in jeopardy of becoming sick. Second, in some societies, such as eastern India, biomedical and interpersonal therapies do not necessarily occur in "pure" form. Such therapies are not isolated from religious elements, for example, something like "divine grace," which we would include in the discourses of morality, as we argue below. Ayurvedic doctors and sorcerers alike may call upon the power of God to accomplish their work and the act of healing may presuppose a moral relationship between the healer and the God (Much and Mahapatra, in preparation). Third, personal ruminations about moral reform may take place without being announced in public and without being made available to ethnographers. Finally, an examination of the use of moral explanations and therapies in the context of an existing illness (where it can be viewed only as a response to distress) does not take account of the role of morality as a form of "preventive medicine" upholding "right practices." It thus seems likely that moral explanations of suffering not only are part of the "big three" but are more prevalent than Park's data allowed him to estimate.

Perhaps the most noteworthy finding of Park's survey is the evidence that on a worldwide scale the biomedical causal ontology so prevalent in secular scientific subcultures in North America and Europe is only one of the "big three" explanations of suffering, and that it is probably the explanation least frequently employed (also see Murdock 1980). For example, when it comes to explaining afflictions such as insanity or death, the folk around the world almost never concern themselves with biomedical causes and almost always explain it in either other-blaming interpersonal terms or agent-blaming moral terms.

For most peoples of the world there are no faultless deaths. One is reminded of Hart and Honore's remark (1961, 333) that "it is not enough to be told that a man died from the presence of unusual quantities of arsenic in his body; and we press on for a more satisfying explanation in terms of human agency." In the minds of many peoples of the world, death would not take place without the push of human agency. On a worldwide scale it is as if any life-terminating biological happening (stroke, heart attack, and the like) is viewed the way we view the case of arsenic poisoning. Nature does not cause people to die without the assistance of human beings. We now turn to a more detailed account of the way faults are found and agents blamed within the framework of some South Asian discourses of morality and health.

The "Big Three" of Ethical Discourse: Autonomy, Community, and Divinity

An Analysis of Moral Discourse

Our analysis of the moral discourse of the residents of the city of Bhubaneswar, Orissa, India is derived from interviews with forty-seven informants (twenty-nine males and eighteen females, mostly adults and mostly Brahmans). The thirty-nine incidents shown in table 1 are brief descriptions of behavioral events representing actual or potential breaches of codes of conduct. They were developed over a period of several months on the basis of ethnographic knowledge of community and family life in Bhubaneswar. The moral discourse to be analyzed was elicited during a structured interview described in

TABLE 1

The 39 Incidents
and Their Loadings on Codes 1, 2 and 3

Incident Number	Code 1 Harm Rights Justice	Code 2 Duty Hierarchy Inter-dependency	Code 3 Sacred Order Natural Order Personal Sanctity
1. A woman cooked rice and wanted to eat with her husband and his elder brother. Then she ate with them. (the woman)	L	M	H
2. In a family, a twenty-five-year-old son addresses his father by his first name. (the son)	L	H	M
3. In a family, the first-born son slept with his mother or grandmother till he was ten years old. During these ten years he never slept in a separate bed. (the practice)	M	M	M
4. A woman is playing cards at home with her friends. Her husband is cooking rice for them. (the husband)	L	H	H
5. A beggar was begging from house to house with his wife and sick child. A home owner drove him away without giving anything. (the homeowner)	H	M	M
6. A man says to his brother, "Your daughter's skin is dark. No one will say she is beautiful. No one will wish to marry her." (the man)	M	M	M
7. The day after his father's death the eldest son had a haircut and ate chicken.	L	H	M
8. A father said to his son, "If you do well on the exam, I will buy you a pen." The son did well on the exam, but his father did not give him anything, spending the money on a carton of cigarettes. (the father)	L	M	L

L=Low   M=Medium   H=High

TABLE 1 *(continued)*

The 39 Incidents
and Their Loadings on Codes 1, 2 and 3

Incident Number	Code 1 Harm Rights Justice	Code 2 Duty Hierarchy Inter- dependency	Code 3 Sacred Order Natural Order Personal Sanctity
9. A young married woman went alone to see a movie without informing her husband. When she returned home her husband said, "If you do it again, I will beat you black and blue." She did it again; he beat her black and blue. (the husband)	L	M	H
10. A letter arrived addressed to a fourteen-year-old son. Before the boy returned home, his father opened the letter and read it.	L	H	L
11. A man had a married son and a married daughter. After his death his son claimed most of the property. His daughter got a little. (the son)	H	H	L
12. You went to a movie. There was a long line in front of the ticket-window. You broke into line and stood at the front.	M	L	L
13. Six months after the death of her husband the widow wore jewelry and bright-colored clothes. (the widow)	L	M	H
14. Immediately after marriage, a son was asked by his parents to live in the same house with them. The son said he wanted to live alone with his wife and that he and his wife had decided to live in another town and search for work there. (the son)	L	H	L
15. Once a doctor's daughter met a garbage man, fell in love with him and decided to marry him. The father of the girl opposed the marriage and tried to stop it, because the boy is a garbage man. In spite of the opposition from the father, the girl married the garbage man. (the daughter)	L	H	H

L=Low   M=Medium   H=High

TABLE 1 *(continued)*

The 39 Incidents
and Their Loadings on Codes 1, 2 and 3

Incident Number	Code 1 Harm Rights Justice	Code 2 Duty Hierarchy Inter- dependency	Code 3 Sacred Order Natural Order Personal Sanctity
16. There was a rule in a hote: Invalids and disfigured persons are not allowed in the dining hall.	H	M	H
17. A widow and an unmarried man loved each other. The widow asked him to marry her. (the widow)	L	M	M
18. A boy played hookey from school. The teacher told the boy's father and the father warned the boy not to do it again. But the boy did it again and the father beat him with a cane. (the father)	H	M	L
19. At night a wife asked her husband to massage her legs. (the wife)	L	M	M
20. A poor man went to the hospital after being seriously hurt in an accident. At the hospital they refused to treat him because he could not afford to pay. (the hospital)	H	M	L
21. A wife is waiting for her husband at the railway station. The train arrives. When the husband gets off, the wife goes and kisses him. (the wife)	L	L	M
22. In school a girl drew a picture. One of her classmates came, took it, and tore it up.	M	M	L
23. One of your family members eats beef regularly.	L	L	H
24. Two people applied for a job. One of them was a relative of the interviewer. Because they were relatives he was given the job although the other man did better on the exam.	H	L	L

L=Low   M=Medium   H=High

TABLE 1 *(continued)*

The 39 Incidents
and Their Loadings on Codes 1, 2 and 3

Incident Number	Code 1 Harm Rights Justice	Code 2 Duty Hierarchy Inter- dependency	Code 3 Sacred Order Natural Order Personal Sanctity
25. A man had a wife who was sterile. He wanted to have two wives. He asked his first wife and she said she did not mind. So he married a second woman and the three of them lived happily in the same house. (the man)	M	H	L
26. One of your family members eats a dog regularly for dinner.	L	L	H
27. While walking, a man saw a dog sleeping on a road. He walked up to it and kicked it. (the man)	H	L	M
28. After defecation (making a bowel movement) a woman did not change her clothes before cooking.	L	L	H
29. A man does not like to use a fork. Instead he always eats rice with his bare hand. He washes it before and after eating. He does this when he eats alone or with others.	L	L	H
30. A father told his son to steal flowers from his neighbor's garden. The boy did it. (the boy)	L	H	L
31. A brother and sister decide to get married and have children.	L	L	H
32. Two brothers ate at home together. After they ate, the wife of the younger brother washed the dishes. (the wife)	L	L	M
33. It was the king's order, if the villagers do not torture an innocent boy to death, twelve hundred people will be killed. The people killed the innocent boy. So the king spared the life of the twelve hundred people. (the people)	H	L	L

L=Low   M=Medium   H=High

TABLE 1 *(continued)*

The 39 Incidents
and Their Loadings on Codes 1, 2 and 3

Incident Number	Code 1 Harm Rights Justice	Code 2 Duty Hierarchy Inter- dependency	Code 3 Sacred Order Natural Order Personal Sanctity
34. A widow in your community eats fish two or three times a week.	L	H	H
35. You meet a foreigner. He is wearing a watch. You ask him how much it cost and whether he will give it to you.	L	M	L
36. Two men hold hand with each other while they wait for a bus.	L	H	M
37. A father, his eldest son and youngest daughter travelled in a boat. They had one life jacket. It could carry one person. The boat sank in the river. The father had to decide who should be saved. He decided to save his youngest daughter. The father and the eldest son drowned. (the father)	M	H	L
38. The day after the birth of his first child, a man entered his temple (church) and prayed to God.	L	L	H
39. A woman cooks food for her family members and sleeps in the same bed with her husband during her menstrual period, (the woman)	H	L	H

L=Low   M=Medium   H=High

Shweder, Mahapatra, and Miller (1987). All of the incidents listed are considered to be breaches or transgressions, with the exception of incident #3 (co-sleeping child and adult), #9 (beating the insubordinate wife), #18 (caning the errant schoolboy), #29 (eating with one's hands), and #36 (men holding hands with each other).

The basis for the analysis is the Oriya Moral Themes code (table 2), as described by Much. For the purpose of analysis, the rationales of all informants were pooled or grouped together to form collec-

TABLE 2

Oriya Moral Themes

1. **Virtue and Merit:** Acts that elevate and acts that degrade one's status as a human being, hence one's position in the social and cosmic (by karma) order. The development of a virtuous (elevated) nature.

2. **Social Order:** Effects of action in the social structure, within the family or community. Maintenance of patterns of social organization, harmony within the social structure, and one's own position within the social order.

3. **Souls and Sentiments:** Recognition of and respect for the non-material self of oneself and others. Regard for the feelings and the sensibilities of others and the well-being of their soul or non-material self. The goals and strivings of the spiritual self, hence individual will, desire and choice.

4. **Tradition, Custom, Culture, Relative Dharmas:** Hindu culture and traditional social law. The Hindu way of life. The relative Dharmas of different castes, religions, nations, ages, etc. The obligations one has by virtue of one's own particular social identity, place and time. Culture as an expression of the dharmic order; culture as an expression of natural law.

5. **Duty:** Role-based obligations within family and in society. The obligations that define one's particular role.

6. **Sacred Order:** The laws of God, the acts of gods, human actions that please and displease God. Worship, devotion, sacred scripture, scriptural and other religious authority.

7. **Interdependence, Relationship:** The interconnectedness of persons. One's own good as interdependent with the good of others. Asymmetrical reciprocity as bonding force at the social order.

8. **Hierarchy:** Respect for relative status within the family, in society or in the cosmic order (e.g., humans to gods). Patterns of behavior that signal acknowledgment of status differences.

9. **Nature, Biological Order:** Actions with intrinsic consequences for well being, based on a conception of the biological order.

10. **Justice, Fairness, Rights:** Distribution of rewards, privliges or punishments according to desert. One's rights and entitlements by various sources of entitlement.

11. **Purity, Sanctity, Pollution:** The maintenance of sanctity and purity of persons and environments. Actions, persons or animals, substances, or mental states that pollute sanctified persons or environments.

12. **Harm, Life, Well-Being:** Respect for life and material, biological well-being. Non-harming and protection of the life and well-being of others. Compassion.

TABLE 2 (continued)

Oriya Moral Themes

13. **Chastity:** Sexual conduct in keeping with social or religious norms of rightful sexual unions and sexual behavior. In particular, the conjugal faithfulness of women and actions that signal a chaste attitude vs. actions that signal an inclination to be unchaste.

14. **Respect for Possessions:** Respect for ownership and personal or private property.

15. **Truthfulness, Honesty, Trustworthiness:** Telling the truth, speaking honestly, honoring commitments and vows, being dependable and undeceitful in dealings with others.

16. **Transcendence:** Spiritual goals or spiritual realities that transcend material or social categories or concerns.

tive transcripts for each of the incidents. The collective transcripts for each incident ranged from three to twenty-five pages of single-spaced text. Much developed the code through inductive iterative reading and classification of transcript contents, first generating a set of categories sufficient to exhaustively catalog the content of the transcripts at a meaningful level of discrimination, and then combining categories where this seemed conceptually justifiable, to arrive at one parsimonious set. The purpose of the coding system was to identify the themes that occur in Oriya moral discourse and the ideas to which informants appeal when they give rationales for their moral judgments. The sixteen categories are not mutually exclusive.

A given stretch of text could instantiate more than one category. For example, if an informant expressed her moral condemnation of the events in incident #4 ("A women is playing cards at home with her friends. Her husband is cooking rice for them.") by stating, "The wife is the servant of the husband. The servant should do her work," the rationale would be coded as both "hierarchy" and "duty." After the texts were coded, a profile was calculated for each incident indicating the proportion of informants who had utilized each of the sixteen ideas listed in the Oriya Moral Themes code (table 2). In effect the degree of saturation was determined for each incident for moral ideas of particular kinds. For example, incident #2 ("In a family, a twenty-five-year-old son addresses his father by his first name") is highly saturated with ideas of "hierarchy" and "duty" but only moderately saturated with other ideas, and some ideas are entirely absent from the collective transcript on this incident. On the basis of the themes profiles for the thirty-nine incidents, Much utilized various statistical procedures, including cluster analysis and stepwise discriminant analysis, to distinguish three clusters of conceptually linked themes and to identify the degree of saturation of each incident by ideas from each cluster. The resulting three clusters are shown in figure 1.

The first cluster (Code 1: The Ethics of Autonomy) relies on regulative concepts such as harm, rights, and justice (see Oriya Moral Themes, table 2, items 10 and 12) and aims to protect the zone of discretionary choice of "individuals" and to promote the exercise of individual will in the pursuit of personal preferences. This is the kind of ethic that is usually the official ethic of societies where "individualism" is an ideal.

The second cluster (Code 2: The Ethics of Community) relies on regulative concepts such as duty, hierarchy, interdependency, and souls (table 2, items 3, 5, 7, and 8). It aims to protect the moral integrity of the various stations or roles that constitute a "society" or a "community," where a "society" or "community" is conceived of as a corporate entity with an identity, standing, history, and reputation of its own.

The third cluster (Code 3: The Ethics of Divinity) relies on regulative concepts such as sacred order, natural order, tradition, sanctity, sin, and pollution (table 2, items 4, 6, 9, and 11). It aims to protect the soul, the spirit, the spiritual aspects of the human agent and "nature" from degradation.

Presupposed by the "ethics of autonomy" is a conceptualization of the self as an individual preference structure, where the point of moral regulation is to increase choice and personal liberty. Presupposed by the "ethics of community" is a conceptualization of the self as an office holder. The basic idea is that one's role or station in life is intrinsic to one's identity and is part of a larger interdependent collective enterprise with a history and standing of its own. Presupposed by the "ethics of divinity" is a conceptualization of the self as a spiritual entity connected to some sacred or natural order of things and as a responsible bearer of a legacy that is elevated and divine. Those who regulate their lives within the terms of an "ethics of divinity" do not want to do anything, such as eating the flesh of a slaughtered animal, that is incommensurate with the

FIGURE 1

Society as Moral Order

Legitimate Regulation
Rational ⟶ External, Objective

Beast ⟶ Communitas ⟶ Angel

Autonomy	**Community**	**Divinity**
Code 1	*Code 2*	*Code 3*
Harm, Rights, Justice	Duty, Hierarchy, Interdependence, Souls	Sacred Order, Natural Order, Sanctity, Tradition
Individual as a Preference Structure	Actor in a Play	Way of Life
	Role-Based Social Status	Practice
		World-Soul
	Family	
obligations come from being a person	obligations come from being part of a community	displaying dignity by showing ultimate concerns
free agent	social, not just selfish	human, not beast
agency	community	heroic enchantment
appetites	holism	soul memory
free contact	sacrifice	angelic side of human nature
marketplace	membership	hermit-yogi

nature of the spirit that joins the self to the divine ground of all things.

Table 1 indicates the relative degree to which each of the thirty-nine incidents is saturated with ethical ideas from each of the "big three" types (autonomy, community, divinity) in the discourse of our Oriya informants. Table 1 shows, for example, that incident #4 (the wife who is playing cards with her friends while her husband cooks) is primarily conceptualized in terms of the "ethics of community" and the "ethics of divinity." In several cases where the reader might well reason in terms of harm, rights, and justice, our Oriya informants reason in terms of "duty," "sin," and "pollution." We now turn to a more direct and "thicker" discussion of the three Oriya discourses and the themes that play a central role in the cultural construction of ethics and well-being.

Our analysis of the rationales given by our Oriya informants suggests the existence of a "big three" domains of moral discourse, which we label "the ethics of autonomy," "the ethics of community," and "the ethics of divinity" (also see Shweder 1990, 1991; Shweder and Much 1987; Shweder and Haidt 1993; Haidt, Koller, and Dias 1993). We now elaborate on some of the "metaphors" that lend meaning to each of the domains.

Metaphors for the Moral Imagination: Multiplicity and Differential Saliency

The three thematic clusters introduced above may be thought of as culturally coexisting discourses of morality. Discourses are symbol systems for describing aspects of experience. More than one such symbol system may be applicable to any area of experience such as individual psychological development, ethics, health, or suffering.

There is no reason that one must select one and only one discourse to represent an area of experience. Indeed, there may be some advantage in possessing multiple discourses for covering the complexities of such an important area of human experience as ethics. No discourse corresponds so tightly to facticity that it cannot be separated from it. All discourses describe through interpretation and inference.

Experience is often so complex that its facticity is sometimes better described by one discourse and sometimes by another. Although different discourses in the social sciences and elsewhere—say, behaviorist, cognitivist, and object relations schools of psychological development—often seem to be in competition for definition of a realm of experience, this is usually a sociological effect more than a logical one. It is often advantageous to have more than one discourse for interpreting a situation or solving a problem. Not only alternative solutions but multidimensional ones addressing several "orders of reality" or "orders of experience" may be more practical for solving complex human problems. An anti-dogmatic casuistry with multiple (but rationally limited) discursive resources may be the most effective method to meet the vicissitudes of human ethical experience. It is useful to keep in mind the tenet that cognized reality is incomplete if described from any one point of view and incoherent if described from all points of view at once (Shweder 1993a, b).

The three ethical discourses of Orissa work together to promote three different types of "goods," which are meant to coexist in the Hindu social order. The Hindu ethical worldview is incomplete without any one of the three. All three goods are goods because they enhance human dignity and self-esteem. The rub, of course, is that the three goods are often in conflict. In the material world, the world of embodiment and constraint, there may never have been a place or time when all three goods have been or could have been simultaneously maximized. Although it is true that they often come into conflict with one another and create "moral dilemmas" (Much and Mahapatra 1993, in preparation), in India these conflicts are often opportunities for personal ethical discrimination and spiritual growth.

It seems to be the case that in direct contrast to secular society in the United States, the discourse of autonomy and individualism is backgrounded in Hindu society, whereas the discourses of community and divinity are foregrounded, made salient and institutionalized. That does not mean that there is no personal experience of autonomy and individuality in India or no personal concern with those goods as essential to well-being. The case is, rather, that the themes of personal autonomy are often absorbed into the discourses of community and divinity, in ways that we describe below.

Similarly, although ideas of community and, to an even greater extent, divinity have been backgrounded and left out of much of the world description produced and institutionalized by modernist Western social science, these communitarian concerns continue to live on, implicitly or explicitly, in the unofficial "folk culture" and its discourse.

Indeed, it appears that different cultural traditions try to promote human dignity by specializing in (and perhaps even exaggerating) different ratios of moral goods. Consequently, they moralize about the world in somewhat different ways and try to construct the social order as a moral order in somewhat different terms. Cultures differ in the degree to which one or another of the ethics and corresponding moral "goods" predominates in the development of social practices and institutions and in the elaboration of a moral ideology.

For example, in the United States today we are experts on the topic of the "ethics of autonomy." We have extended the idea of "rights" to different domains such as education and health care. We have extended the class of "rights" holders to include children and animals. We have expanded the idea of this worldly autonomy to such an extent that it has become imaginable that children should be free to choose the parents they want. We wish to be protected from every imaginable harm, protected from secondary cigarette smoke, protected from psychologically offensive work environments. We have enlarged the idea of harm to include such all-embracing notions as "harassment," "abuse," and "exploitation." We have stretched the notions of rights, autonomy, and harm, even as we wonder nostalgically how we lost our sense of community and divinity, and struggle to find a way to recover them. In rural India, on the other hand, the "ethics of autonomy" is much less salient, while the institutions and ideologies of community and divinity are highly elaborated and finely honed, which creates its own special distortions, of course.

One of the implications of this chapter is that there might be some advantages to expanding the moral discourse for health in Western scientific and popular culture. The potential for expanded discourse is latent in American folk culture. In this essay we bring the relevant discourses into relief by showing how they have become "official," locally rational, institutionalized discourses in a South Asian culture. We predict that some aspects of "traditional" thinking will appeal to many modern Americans.

Of course, it is not our goal to persuade North American science to adopt the metaphysics and metapsychologies of Indian Brahmans and yogins. Rather, we believe that by attending to explicit South Asian conceptions of the moral order, we will call attention to neglected ideas latent in our own cultural history and living contemporary culture. Ideas within one's own culture may be more easily seen by comparison with ideas from divergent cultures, which are the more "obvious" for the novelty of the ideational contexts in which they occur. We introduce in correspondence with our three domains of Oriya moral discourse (autonomy, community, divinity) three metaphors (the sacred self, feudal ethics, the sacred world) for the American moral imagination. Later we discuss a fourth overarching metaphor, the idea of "karma."

Autonomy and the Metaphor of the Sacred Self

The three discourse domains of Oriya ethics represent three goods, each related to well-being. It is good to have personal autonomy and control. It is good to be part of an organized community and to have an identity or place(s) within its social structure. It is good to experience communication and to be on speaking terms with the divine. These discourses seem to represent distinct but interrelated conceptual contexts for moral discourse. In the interview texts from which the Oriya Moral Themes were derived, we found that each could be used alone or in combination with any of the others in an informant's argument concerning a particular incident or event.

We focus first on the ethics of autonomy cluster that most closely resembles the harm-rights-and-justice code that is prevalent in American culture, with its emphasis on the individual's claim to self-interest and noninterference. The themes of this cluster (harm, rights, and justice) are by no means the most common discourse of Oriya moral argumentation. The discourse of cluster 1 represents the individual interests, desires, and preferences of the person. Although it resembles the harm-rights-and-justice code of North America, there are also differences in the way that Oriya Hindus talk about the interests of individuals.

In Orissa, the idea of the individual is linked to the idea of a "soul" and its particular dharma or obligation. This "soul" (what contemporary secular Western scholars might refer to as a "transcendental ego") is an entity identified with the realm of divinity. Embodied, it exists under many limitations and constraints. But peel away the gross layers of illusion and what is left is pure God-essence, capable of merging directly with the divine substrate of the phenomenal world. This ultimate (though not proximal) identity of the personal soul with God is what obligates respect for all living creatures, human and nonhuman, and what obligates tolerance of another person's free will. A concern for individual autonomy seems to act as a common denominator in the moral order and does not distinguish human beings from nonhuman animals, who are also regarded as having essentially the same soul and the same rights to protection from arbitrary harm or abuse and from interference with their natural needs and inclinations. Animal "souls" are not seen as particularly distinct from human ones, and souls may change places in transmigrations. The following didactic or "proverbial" narrative from Shweder's interview texts illustrates the point. Such narratives are one of the preferred methods of moral discourse and moral instruction in Orissa (see Shweder and Much 1987).

> There was a dog that always slept on the doorstep of the house of a certain Brahman. [Since dogs are polluted and polluting animals, this was problematic for the Brahman, who might have to bathe before entering the temple or his own house after accidental contact with a dog.] One day the Brahman threw cold water on the dog in order to drive it away. The dog went to God and complained. It said, "I am a dog. It is my nature to sleep on the road [or in doorsteps]. When the Brahman threw water on me, I shivered [that is, I suffered]. Let him take my sins and suffer as I suffer and let me take his merit." And God agreed. The Brahman became a dog. (From the Shweder interviews, Shweder, Mahapatra, and Miller 1987)

Any soul may be seen as having an individual dharma, designed for it either by God or by the precision of one's own karma (the fruits of one's work). One implication of this view of individuality is that there is a kind of specialness or even privilege to personal intuitions of right and wrong. Even odd and unconventional desires or overly adamant demands for normally forbidden things may be respected as possibly the "utterance of the soul." They are apt to be understood as a command of the deity within, pertaining to a person's particular course of spiritual development, something that no one else can fully know.

This highly particularistic individual dharma exists in addition to the dharma or obligation assigned to the person by virtue of features of social position such as gender, caste, age, family relationships, and so on. Hindu obligation structures are complex. The first metaphor for the moral imagination is the sacred self, whose obligation it is to know or discover its own individuated dharma.

Community and the Feudal Ethics Metaphor

The second thematic cluster, the ethics of community, pertains to the discourse of obligations engendered through participation in a particular community. It is a discourse of roles and statuses and obligations in relation to other members of the community. The themes associated with this cluster are duty, hierarchy, interdependence, and "souls" (selves). Notice that the theme of the individual soul or self is more closely connected in Oriya discourse to the role structure of a community than to the themes of this worldly self-sufficiency and individual freedom of choice. The identity of the person is defined in terms of community statuses. In Oriya Hindu discourse, personal identity is more closely associated with its statuses and relationships than with its individuality or distinctness.

Another reason for the association of "souls" or "selves" with relational concepts is that the protection and nurturance of the individual, and the satisfaction of individual desires are most often discussed as somebody else's responsibility. Persons rely on those to whom they are bound in institutionalized asymmetrical relationships to satisfy their needs. The person in the hierarchical position is obligated to protect and satisfy the wants of the subordinate person in specified ways. The subordinate person is also obligated to look after the interests and well-being of the superordinate person.

People often depend upon others to satisfy their needs and desires. Even when they are capable of looking after themselves, they may not think it appropriate to do so. The understood moral obligation of the interdependent "other" in such a relationship is sensitive responsiveness to the perceived or expressed needs of one's interdependent self. Sons and daughters should be obedient to their parents; parents should be sensitive and responsive to the wishes, feelings and inclinations of their children. Likewise, wives should be obedient to their husbands, and husbands should be sensitive and responsive to the needs, desires, and inclinations of their wives. That is why the theme of "selves" or "souls" clusters with the themes of duty, hierarchy, and interdependence.

One might (somewhat tongue-in-cheek) refer to this second metaphor for the moral imagination as the idea of "feudal ethics." It is a metaphor that is central to Oriya ethical argumentation in the context of communitarian concerns. What this discourse has to add to our own sense of community is the potential for rediscovery of some of the merits of the "feudal" mind.

Most Americans ideologically recoil at the idea of feudal ethics because a feudal ethic does not fit well with the philosophical underpinnings of our historically evolved political culture and our free-market mentality. We shall try to explicate a few major principles of feudal ethics in terms that Americans (who underplay this aspect of experience in their dealings with "persons") can understand. In true feudal systems, powerful persons take care of their "subjects": family members, employees, fellow caste members.

Along with hierarchy there is an obligatory responsibility for others. The less powerful respond with gratitude and loyalty that "sticks" when the chips are down. There are many specific principles for feudal leadership and feudal reciprocity, but these are beyond the scope of the present chapter. A cardinal principle, however, is "take care of one's own." Neither "networking," which is too market-oriented and ethically "thin," nor "social welfare," which is too impersonal and devoid of a sense of participation or alliance, are suitable substitutes for this concept.

A successful feudal "lord" or local "big man" (*bada loka*) uses his alliances sparingly; he does not exploit them unnecessarily. He tries to do more for others than they have done for him. That way he has a social "bank account" of debts due him when the really important issues arise. He cultivates alliances with those below him because they are the bedrock of his power. If he cultivates alliances only with superiors and equals, he will have no one to rule.

In a feudal social system, the "lord" (king, father, "godfather," or the like) knows that his well-being is closely entwined with the satisfaction of his "subjects." He knows that his understood obligation is to promote the satisfaction of those from whom he commands loyalty and that the obligation is proportional to his demands for allegiance and potential sacrifice. To do otherwise would be ultimately, if not immediately, self-destructive.

These policies are not necessarily easy for democratic-minded Americans to appreciate. The contemporary American mistrust of hierarchy and ready-made association of hierarchy with tyranny, exploitation, and overreaching entitlement seems to reflect what happens to hierarchy in a democratic market society, where "take care of one's own" is replaced by "survival of the fittest."

Nevertheless, in the cultural domain of health and well-being, the simple principle of "take care of one's own" might have far-reaching consequences if it were taken seriously as an ethical obligation. The principle has a direct bearing upon many social and psychological problems of the "postmodern" age, including community health problems such as "isolation" and "alienation," the problem of young and elderly persons without family members to take care of them in times of ill health, the problems arising from the national health insurance question, and related issues of what employers owe to their employees in the way of health benefits and health-protective working conditions.

The particular wisdom of the South Asian discourse of community is that the well-being of persons who live or work together or share other life projects is interdependent. If your actions weaken those you depend upon (whether in the upward or downward direction), they weaken you. This is true whether you are the "lord" or the "servant." Loyalties of this kind require continuous cultivation, which means caring about what happens to those with whom you live or work, caring about larger units of which you are a part, and being taken care of in return. Our second moral metaphor, then, from South Asia, is the feudal hierarchy, with its particular vision of allegiance, asymmetrical reciprocity, noblesse oblige, and ecological interdependence.

Divinity and the Metaphor of a Sacred World

The third thematic cluster, the ethics of divinity, expresses the Indian belief that a sacred order is immanent in the world, that godliness permeates or interpenetrates the human social order as well as the natural world and interacts with both, and that there are important communicative exchanges going on all of the time between persons and the realm of divinity. The basic idea is that matter (organic and inorganic) and all other forms—social hierarchies (parent, child, husband, wife), the tonal scales of music (raga), words (mantra)—are infused with spirit or divinity. This discourse is associated with the notion of a sacred tradition, the idea that a way of life—the Hindu dharma—is an earthly manifestation of divine design. Here there are partial (though not complete) correspondences with the Orthodox Judaic vision of society (Spero 1992). All things are encompassed within the sacred order, or one could say, divinity is immanent in all things. A view of this kind denies a radical separation between the secular and the sacred. Thus, even family life is a sacramental event, which is why the breach of a seemingly mundane domestic procedure can be rationally regarded as a kind of desecration.

The associated themes of the ethics of divinity are sacred order, sanctity, tradition, natural law. The cluster represents the idea that sacred law and natural law are the same thing. Both can be called "dharma." The sacred and the natural are not different orders of reality. The natural world with its shades of good and evil, merit and fault, dignity and degradation expresses the design of divinity. There is a corresponding idea that every entity in nature enjoys its particular right to exist and to be what it is according to its own nature, such that nothing is excluded from or contrasted to the moral order: everything is encompassed. This discourse ultimately brings one full circle, back to the origins of the sacredness of the individual, human or otherwise. The rights of human beings derive from and are protected under this same principle of a dharmic order in which every entity that exists is entitled to be what it is, and has its proper place in the order of things. That place is its protected realm.

Individuation also receives protection by this principle. Individual "souls" (selves) have desires that should be respected by others because those desires may be a form of wisdom that originates not in the discursive thoughts of the personal mind but ultimately in a kind of soul knowledge. Wishes and desires might be an indication from the divine order, which encompasses intimate knowledge of every individual soul. The wise sometimes feel it is better not to interfere with someone's wishes, especially if they are strong and persistent, even though wishes may seem irrational or maladaptive. After all, one never knows what the true source of the wish may be. The divine order interpenetrates matter, social form, and mind. And any apparent form, no matter how lowly (for example, a dog is lowly in India), is in essence, divine spirit. It may, in theory, "really be" a God, that is, manifest divinity in intensified form.

There are many such stories and myths. Lowly entities are always turning out to be something more than they appear. That is the classical test or trial of discrimination and genuine devotion that God imposes upon devotees. One kicks a dog. The dog turns out to be the Goddess in disguise and one is punished. One feeds a dog. The dog turns out to be the Goddess in disguise, and one is rewarded. A beggar or leper at one's doorstep turns out to be the Great God Siva in disguise, and so on. We are reminded of a similar idea expressed by the words of Jesus Christ, "As you did it to one of the least of these my brethren, you did it to me" (Matt. 25:31, 32).

The dignity of the individual person is also comprehended within the discourse of this ethics of divinity. It is represented in part by the idea of sanctity. This conception of sanctity is the basis of traditional social rank in Hindu society. It relates to one's ability to approach and communicate with the divinity, which in turn relates to social rank and personal fulfillment in the traditional Hindu social order. Individual dignity is also represented as the obligation to uphold the practices of a way of life (tradition) felt to originate in the design of a divine order. It is further represented by the possibilities for heroic expression of godlike personhood through concern with the ultimate aims of human existence and the disengagement from moment-to-moment temptations and sufferings of life.

It is worth noting that the idea of divinity has begun to reenter the discourse of psychiatry and psychology, though at present it is still on the fringes. Spero (1992) has recently made an argument for considering personal relationship to divinity as an important psychological reality without reducing divinity to a psychological structure. Spero also argues that a personal relationship with divinity is a primary psychological good and a fundamental aspect of psychological development. The experience of divinity may or may not be theistic. It may or may not involve a personified God or Goddess. Mystical-aesthetic experiences of a more diffuse kind are also communications with divinity.

A particular feature of the Hindu worldview is the disposition to make connections between all aspects of secular, domestic, and psychological life and a sacred order that is the ultimate reference point for all sources of obligation. One might speak of a Hindu sense of "sacred world" (Much and Mahapatra 1993, in preparation). Thus, the third moral metaphor we invoke is the sacred-world metaphor, the idea that persons communicate with the divine and the divine communicates with persons through actions in the world, whether special rituals, work, or ordinary domestic activities.

The relevance of a discourse of divinity for considerations of health and well-being in the contemporary United States rests upon the way it functions as a ground or foundation for obligations and boundaries, as an existential support for personal identity, and as a source of personal meaning and satisfaction. In the most abstract and secularized form, which some people prefer, "divinity" still has meaning as the forms through which personal life and social life are cultivated and given excellence (Sapir 1986). If divinity reveals itself through the forms of the world, there is no necessary contradiction between theistic and nontheistic senses of the sacred. The idea of the sacred does not demand that one separate out a personified or transcendent God-concept. The central theme is reverence for the forms of the world, the realization that pleasure and pain, right and wrong, are communicated through those forms and that the world communicates its message in accordance with the way one acts toward its forms. Reverence motivates taking seriously the obligations inherent in autonomy and community. It motivates as well a suspension of ultimate judgment and an antidogmatic attitude toward the "letter of the law." A reverential attitude places responsibility

...oral discrimination with personal intentionality, intellect, and

The three ethics (autonomy, community, divinity) and the three metaphors for the moral imagination (sacred self, feudal ethics, sacred world) represent an expanded repertoire of discourse for construing the grounds of obligation, the nature of particular obligations, and the consequences of remissiveness in matters of obligation. They represent an expanded discourse for considering the social, psychological, and behavioral context of health maintenance because they all relate to the kinds of responsibilities persons have to take care of themselves and others, and to treat the environment, the ecological matrix of personal life, with respect. We suspect that the development of similar discourses, in ways consistent with the beliefs, traditions, and roots of Western culture, would be a contribution to a postmodern resolution of contemporary problems of personal well-being and social responsibility. We conclude our chapter with a brief discussion of a fourth overarching moral metaphor, the Hindu idea of karma, which is at its core a theory of personal responsibility.

An Overarching Moral Metaphor: Karma and the Laws of Personal Responsibility

In India the human tendency to interpret fortune and misfortune in terms of spiritual or moral merit and debt is institutionalized in the widespread cultural doctrine of karma. Karma, which is the idea that actions have "inherent" consequences, has been a topic for reflection and debate for many centuries (see, for example, Babb 1983; Daniel 1983; O'Flaherty 1980; Kakar 1981, 1982; Keyes and Daniel 1983; Mahapatra, Much, and Shweder 1991; Obeyesekere 1980; Shweder and Miller 1985). In what follows we examine the way the connection between morality and health is represented in the discourse of karma that is found in and around Bhubaneswar.

The South Asian theory of karma exists indigenously as a complex and technical subject matter. Karma is not, as Westerners sometimes suppose, a naive or primitive theory of immanent justice, and in South Asian theories about karma there are specific mechanisms postulated to account for its operation. These theories depend upon a metaphysical ontology quite different from either the classical traditional Judeo-Christian one or the materialist metaphysics of modern science (Much and Mahapatra 1993, in preparation). That metaphysical ontology includes for example, the idea of a transmigrating soul, a mental self that goes on from one birth to another, taking with it its past deeds and the latent results of its actions. Karma pertains to several "orders of reality," although most of this complexity is beyond the scope of the present discussion.

Just like scientific Western biomedical theories, karma is part of an esoteric knowledge of indigenous experts yet also has its counterpart in widely disseminated folk knowledge that is closely but unevenly related to the expert's knowledge system. We will be concerned here with the form karmic discourse takes in folk theory.

Despite the metaphysical mismatch, certain aspects of karmic conceptions translate well into ideas present in Western thought. The "folk" discourse of karma is probably closer to Western discourses of moral responsibility, cause and effect, efficacy and control, than are the technical versions. As several ethnographers have observed (Babb 1983; Mahapatra, Much and Shweder 1991; Much and Mahapatra 1993, in preparation; Wadley and Derr 1990), karma has an operational quality of transference. That is, a person's karma affects not only the person's self but also others who have relationships or transactions with that person.

Generally, the closer the relationship or transaction, or the greater the degree of "participation" in the sin or merit, the stronger the effect of one person's karma upon another. There are subtle qualifications for all these rules of thumb. We give here only the most general outlines of the folk theory. The more general we are in our formulation, the more potential there is for a convincing correspondence between karmic and Western traditional socio-psycho-somatic moral causal thinking. For example, Western biomedical knowledge postulates that children of alcohol-addicted parents are a relatively "high-risk" population for alcohol dependency and other socio-psycho-somatic problems. The risk is created not only by genetic inheritance but by the behavioral patterns of alcohol-addicted parents and the participation of children in those patterns. Karma is not so different from our understanding of these kinds of complex causal relationships. It is only broader, including a more expansive discourse of obligation and encompassing more extended domains of cause and effect. Some ethnographers (Babb 1983; Daniel 1983; Keyes 1983; Wadley and Derr 1990) have noted that not all Indian conceptions of karma depend upon a theory of transmigration. A certain part of the population appears to believe that karmic results come within the life span. Even those who believe that karma operates across lives, such as our Oriya informants, also believe that it operates within lives, and they are able to narrate many local "case histories" of karmic cause and effect.

We focus our interest here on karma as a theory of personal responsibility and its close connection to the idea of dharma (objective obligation or duty). This close connection, which has been noted by Wadley and Derr (1990) and others, denotes simultaneously natural law as well as a divine or sacred order to things.

The conception of karma as a law of personal responsibility may surprise many Westerners who are vaguely familiar with the construal of "karma" as a theory of moral "determinism" (see Babb 1983). It is a great irony of Western understanding that karma is often misinterpreted as a description of how Indians excuse themselves from responsibility by describing themselves as passive objects of the force of their past actions. Babb attributes this bias to the historical fact that karma was first studied intensively by Western scholars in the context of development economics, where it acquired the interpretation of a "passive" and "fatalistic" life view, which encouraged acceptance of the status quo (for example, Kapp 1963, Myrdal 1968). What was missed was the powerful potential of karmic theory to generate prescriptions for agency and control.

It is apparently true that some Indians do use this kind of reasoning to account for their failures or abnegations of responsibility, and others criticize them for this very attitude (Daniel 1983). But it is not the case that this is how South Asian folk theories of karma (much less the technical versions) typically work in the narration and construction of the meaning of life events. A more accurate interpretation is that the idea of karma creates a feeling of inevitability that one's actions will have proportionate consequences for the self, which lends a motivational force to the felt obligatoriness of the many demanding practices in Indian domestic, social, and ritual life. It is ironic that the idea of karma is often given a fatalistic interpretation in the West because the theory of karma contains not only many mechanisms for the remedy of situations but also numerous preventive procedures for exercising a willful control over one's life.

At the level of social thought, karma is a theory of responsibility (Mahapatra, Much, and Shweder 1991; Much and Mahapatra 1993, in preparation). Karma means "action" or "work" (the same word is used in modern Oriya for any task or work one does). Along with the notion of work or action, karma implies the natural result or "fruition" of action. Generally speaking, the "fruits" (*phala*) of actions are proportionate to the action in quality and magnitude. The quality (for example, whether good or evil—finer distinctions exist but are not relevant here) relates closely to the three types of ethical obligations discussed above.

The "teachings" of karma are disseminated in part through local narrative gossip. Narratives about the karmic events in the lives of other persons or in one's own life are locally circulated, told to intimates and friends, and commented upon. The principles of karma are also amply illustrated in mythology and in "proverbial" tales. Several examples follow:

> There was an old Bauri woman (the highest of the local formerly "untouchable," now "scheduled" or "Harijan," castes) who was suffering a painful and lingering death. She suffered for a long time but she could not die. Finally, her relatives asked her to remember if there was any sin that she had committed in her lifetime, and to confess. She confessed that she had once accepted boiled food (boiled food is more readily polluted than fried food) from a Kachara (Bangle-Seller). [Though the Bauris are an "untouchable" caste, they regard the Kachara as inferior to themselves in purity; and so the Bauri caste prohibits accepting boiled food from the Kachara.] She also confessed that on one occasion she had bound a cow in the cow shed and [as a result of the way she had tied it and left it unattended] the cow had died during the night. After the woman had confessed these sins, she died peacefully. (Local neighborhood narrative; Mahapatra, Much, and Shweder 1991, 13)

The Bauri woman had breached the ethics of autonomy and of divinity by "polluting" herself with food offered by a person considered more impure than she. She had breached the second and third codes by carelessly binding the cow (a sacred animal in India) and then neglecting to look after it. She had allowed it to die during the night, unnoticed, while she was responsible for it.

> There was a married woman in Old Town, who treated her mother-in-law cruelly. The mother-in-law was a widow, and her son took no interest in her well-being, so there was no one to protect her. Her daughter-in-law [who lived in the same house] tormented the old woman without pity. Having to bear this, the old woman cursed her daughter-in-law to have the same fate in

her old age. As soon as the son's children were grown, the daughter-in-law became a widow. She is still living in the same sahi (ward) in Old Town. Now her children care nothing for her, but rather torment her just as she had tormented her mother-in-law. (Local neighborhood narrative; Mahapatra, Much, and Shweder 1991, 13)

The daughter-in-law breached the ethics of autonomy and community. She treated another person with cruelty. Worse yet, the person she treated with cruelty was her mother-in-law, a person whom she is obligated to respect and care for.

A man and his wife lived with the husband's elderly father. The daughter-in-law was always thinking of how they could get rid of the old man. One day she had an idea. She told her husband, let us carry Father to Puri [a place of pilgrimage] in a basket. There we will leave him on the Great Road in front of the Temple of Jaganath. [This road is a gathering place for the homeless and destitute. In those days there were no trains or buses, nor any other easy means of transport, so the old man would never be able to return on his own but would have to remain where he was left.] The husband agreed to this plan. But their son had overheard everything. He first warned his grandfather of the plot. Then he went to his father and said, "Father, you leave Grandfather at Puri just as you have said. But please do not leave the basket. Bring the basket back. Otherwise, what shall I use to carry you to Puri when you become old?" Then the husband understood. He confessed everything to his father and begged his father's forgiveness. (Proverbial narrative from the Shweder interviews, Shweder, Mahapatra, & Miller 1987)

In each case, the wrongful treatment of others, the breach or neglect of some obligatory action covered by one or more of the three ethical codes (autonomy, community, divinity), predicts future suffering, including physical illness or pain, psychological suffering, and social disharmony. Many other narratives of this kind are to be heard in rural India.

As Babb (1983), O'Flaherty (1976), and Wadley and Derr (1990) point out, the karmic theory of causality entails indeterminacy, uncertainty, and unpredictability. In Orissa, persons who are suffering from an illness or misfortune may consult sacred specialists, holy persons, or oracles to ascertain the karmic causes of their suffering.

Sacred healers, such as various oracles, may not only diagnose karmic problems but also prescribe remedial actions. This is especially true for illnesses or misfortunes that are not amenable to "immediate" or proximal remedial interventions (medicine, magic, or astrology).

> A man was blind in one eye. He consulted the oracle concerning this defect. The oracle told him that during his last life he had propitiated a certain Goddess. But, failing to obtain what he desired, he had spoken to her abusively, calling her "widow" [implying inauspiciousness and accursedness] and had torn out one eye from her image. Because of that, he now suffered blindness in one eye. The oracle advised him to bathe seven images of the Goddess [a ritual bathing performed by a qualified temple priest] on seven Thursdays [the day sacred to the Goddess Laxmi]. Then he should prostrate flat on the floor before the [image of the] Goddess and beg her forgiveness. Calling her "Mother," he should remind her that he himself is her own son, so that she might be moved to forgive his error. After this, he should return to the oracle for further instructions. (Mahapatra, Much, and Shweder 1991, 16)

Karma can be viewed as a kind of economic account of accumulated ethical merit and demerit. Metaphorically speaking, one's karmic bank account affects one's overall circumstances and provides opportunities for improvement, as well as constraints upon improvement. When the accumulated demerit is great, meritorious action also becomes more difficult. Through immoral, adharmic actions, obstructions are accumulated.

The teleological presupposition of the doctrine of karma is that the natural aim of the soul is to recognize its own divine nature and so liberate itself from entrapment in the illusion that causes inappropriate impulse and action with its consequent suffering. In Western parlance, this could (roughly, and with some loss of meaning) be called a state of flourishing or optimal well-being. Adharmic acts create obstacles to this achievement.

Whatever one's present status in life it is always possible to improve it by doing the dharma specific to one's existing capabilities and potentialities. A person's individual dharma is whatever is morally obligatory for the person, given his or her particular situation. This notion takes account of two things: (1) what it is possible for a particular individual to do in the particular case, and (2) the ideal conduct that is in accord with the three discourses of moral obligation. When the discourses of obligation come into conflict in specific situations, features of context plus the resources and constraints of the agent enter into casuistic consideration of the principles that govern the case in point. Morality, therefore, is not simply a matter of following rules (see Shweder and Much 1987). It involves personal effort of discrimination and judgment. This is something that must be cultivated. It is a personal responsibility to cultivate this kind of knowledge and intelligence.

There are certain classes of action that are not obligatory but are meritorious by nature. One can perform these actions and so gain or accumulate merit in order to better one's position in the future. These can be done as a kind of investment in one's future welfare.

Many of these measures involve either charity or the support of religious institutions. Sacrifice often enters into meritorious activity, and in some cases personal austerities are prescribed or considered efficacious. Acts of worship in themselves, as well as reading, reciting, and contemplating the scriptures, are meritorious. Many people in India do these things routinely. At the level of personal hygiene there are many ways to maintain or enhance personal "sanctity." One may follow certain laws of purity, avoid polluting places or substances, and seek out those with beneficial effects.

Merit-producing actions exist for each of the three codes of ethical discourse. The effects of these actions (for example, going on pilgrimage, performing rituals) promote personal hygiene and dignity, contribute to social welfare, and enhance one's sense of spiritual inspiration.

"Karma yoga" (liberation by means of meritorious action) is, of course, a very long-term project. The classical karmic worldview of South Asia envisions many lifetimes for the development of the soul. At the same time, certain known wrongs may be expiated in part or in whole by duly prescribed meritorious action. Local folk healers, especially sacred healers and ritual specialists, may prescribe meritorious actions that will benefit people who are suffering (Mahapatra, Much, and Shweder 1991).

Thus our final and overarching "metaphor" for the "moral imagination" is the metaphor of karma. The significance of karmic discourse for our present argument lies in the way it rationally motivates responsible action for those who comprehend and internalize it. The fundamental presupposition is that traditional codes of ethics are part of the divine and natural order of the universe and are established for the purpose of enhancing the well-being of persons in their worldly existence as well as the "afterlife." In this view morality and obedience to the obligations and limits of the three ethical discourses directly affect physical and mental health, social harmony, status, and well-being. Spero (1992) finds the same kind of reasoning in traditional Judaic Halakhic metapsychology. We note in passing that the classical Hindu conception of the worthy and obligatory goals in life include artha, dharma, moksha, and kama (roughly, wealth, duty, liberation, and pleasure; see Kakar 1981, chap. 1, for a highly readable account). We believe the three moral discourse realms of autonomy, community, and divinity are related to the classical concepts of artha, dharma, and moksha, although we cannot expound upon these connections in this chapter.

According to the theory of karma, intended immoral action, careless action, or even ignorant and misguided action is certain to lead to personal suffering unless some intervening correction can be made. For those who appraise the world in karmic terms, effects are not conceptualized as risk factors represented as aggregated population level odds, ratios, or probabilities, where one is at liberty to perceive oneself individually and as an exception. To conceive of the world in karmic terms is to know with certainty that the transgression of obligations will catch up with the transgressor sooner or later unless he or she does something to reverse the situation insofar as possible. Intervening corrections sometimes can be made if the sufferer has the insight to ask for help. But the interventions are costly to the sufferer and require great investments of effort and will. The results of corrective efforts may be incomplete. The full results may be a long time in coming. Therefore, it is better to avoid the problem in the first place if one can. The karmic metaphor emphasizes personal responsibility in regulating behavior and wise investment in actions that accrue benefits to oneself in the long run.

Theodicy and Public Health

In this chapter we have examined some ethical discourse realms and moral metaphors that are customary in many corners of South Asia with an eye toward enhancing the conceptual resources of our own culture for thinking about the connection between action, personal responsibility, and public health. We have assumed that one way to extend our own discourses for causation and morality is take account of the relevant indigenous theories of another complex culture that institutionalizes and supports intuitions that are suppressed or peripheralized by our own "official" scientific culture. To do this, it has been necessary to explicate certain beliefs that do not fit standard Western conceptions of reality. At the end, however, we believe it is possible to show the relevance or partial translatability of these metaphors to our own ways of life and to raise some questions about how South Asian ideas about autonomy, community, divinity, and karma might change our outlook on existential issues of universal importance: suffering, responsibility, and remedial change. In a sense, we have asked the reader to rethink the contemporary secular theodicy of Western biomedical beliefs and acknowledge both its limitations as well as its strengths.

Theodicy is the philosophical inquiry into the question of how the presence of evil in the world is to be explained. The presupposition of such an inquiry is that evil exists in the world, that it is distinguishable from good, and that the fact of its existence presents us with a problem. The prototypical problem formulated in terms of Judeo-Christian metaphysics is this: If God is good and omnipotent, then why does evil, which is antithetical to good, exist in the world (O'Flaherty 1976)?

There are variations of possible answers to this question. The philosophical possibilities include the conclusion that so far as "God" or "nature" are concerned, there is no distinction between good and evil, that there is no reason to consider suffering as evil. This theodicy is a relatively counterintuitive view of reality. It does appear in certain arcane philosophies (and sciences) but rarely as an ordinary folk intuition derived from the experience of an embodied human self. It is counterintuitive because suffering is organismically "felt" as a disvalued state, quite distinct from other "felt" valued states (well-being, happiness, pleasure). The intuitive distinction between good and bad, felt in the body as well as the consciousness, seems to be a difficult distinction to dispel.

Another possible theodicy is that suffering, although painful, is not really or ultimately evil because it results in an end state that is good. People are known to interpret narratively the benefits of their own suffering in a variety of ways. They may interpret suffering as a discipline through which human selves become wiser and stronger; or as a path of learning and personal growth; or as an experience that brings human beings closer to God, and so on. This is not necessarily a counterintuitive idea. Some persons do seem to feel empowered by and/or benefit from their suffering. They experience themselves as stronger, wiser, better protected, and more morally fit than they were before. Some develop exceptional skills because they suffer.

The South Asian causal ontology has an explanatory advantage with respect to supporting this type of interpretation of suffering. It postulates a soul that continues its "life" through countless births until conditions are ultimately worked out for the good. The metaphor is the arduousness of acquiring wisdom and skillfulness and the sense of empowerment that comes from working off spiritual debts. Of course, in any society although some people will manage to transform suffering into growth, others will suffer and remain miserable.

A quite different interpretation of suffering is favored by much of the contemporary Western scientific community, at least in its official canons. That theodicy involves the disjunction of moral good and evil from large areas of the experience of suffering, including illness, adverse living situations, and "behavior problems" of various types. According to this theodicy, although suffering is real, it is outside the domain of good and evil. It is outside the domain of the intentional agency of the sufferer.

One reigning metaphor of this contemporary official secular theodicy is "victimization." The sufferer is a victim, under "attack" from natural forces devoid of intentionality. Suffering is decontextualized and separated from the narrative structure of human life. It is viewed as a kind of "noise," an accidental interference with the life drama of the sufferer. It is as though suffering had no intelligible relation to any plot, except as a chaotic interruption. This image of suffering is most congruent with a theodicy that asserts that suffering is and must remain a mystery because it has no existential meaning or purpose. A metaphorical image associated with this view is suffering as an accident, as an event governed by chance.

Under this interpretation, suffering is to be treated by the intervention of second- or third-party agents who possess expert skills of some kind relevant to treating the problem. The solution is sought at the proximal level of alleviating and curing a condition and not at any more fundamental level in which ultimate questions about "who is responsible for this" and "who is to be blamed" get asked. Under this interpretation, the way to deal with suffering is to treat it, not to ask where it came from or why someone in particular is suffering. This type of secular theodicy is pragmatic and in keeping with (at least parts of) the known observable facts of many mishaps, injuries, or illnesses, and in line with some of our powers to remedy them. It is well to keep in mind, however, that nothing is really "by accident" in a true sense and that "chance" is an illusory explanation, a distortion of a far more complex determinism. What "by accident" really means is that we do not and cannot know all of the specific events that have converged to create a causal chain.

If a person is hit by a motor vehicle while crossing the street, there is in fact a complex chain of events that led to that convergence. Our discourse of chance says these are irrelevant. The South Asian discourse of karmic causality, which we explored above, says that each link in the chain is meaningful and related to responsible or irresponsible actions.

Even within the discourse of our own scientific causal discourse the illness-as-accident metaphor is sometimes shown to be mistaken. For example, only several decades ago it was not known that cigarette smoking put some people at high risk for very serious illnesses or was dangerous to the fetus of a pregnant woman. A genuine behavioral cause of suffering was missed because the linkage of action to outcome was not yet recognized by the scientific-medical community. At the same time there was a folk discourse that saw excessive smoking as an unsavory practice. It was said to be a "dirty" or "filthy" habit. There was a folk idea that women in particular ought not to smoke and there was a common discourse among smokers about "smoker's cough" and about addiction and other effects viewed explicitly as unhealthy and undignified by those who smoked and suffered. The respect for scientific authority and the absence at that time of a solid "scientific" linkage between cigarette smoking and serious health conditions enabled many people to ignore their own or others' experiential intuitions that excessive smoking was an unhealthy habit and damaging to the body. Although the "chance" view of suffering may sometimes be the best available representation, we suspect there may be many more linkages between behavior and suffering or well-being than are yet recognized by mainstream medical science.

From the sufferer's point of view the "random catastrophe" explanation is not especially appealing. It is about as appealing as is the invocation of "chance" as an explanation for a striking and world-altering series of "coincidental" events. Even with scientific sanction plus reasoned evaluation of known proximal causal factors the idea of "chance" misfortune may not be felt by the sufferer to have much experiential validity. The "chance" explanation does not help the sufferer make sense of an experience so intense that it feels as though it should be meaningful. This is especially the case for major or catastrophic illnesses. Yet even people who contract common colds and brief viral infections are often heard to say things such as "I guess I was supposed to slow down" or "I just wasn't supposed to go on that trip." Intuitively, human beings often feel as though their illness was a meaningful intervention in an intended course of action.

It is increasingly recognized among health scientists in our culture that the "chance" account of suffering is consistent with the facts of only a limited set of known conditions. Many forms of suffering today are known to have multiple determinants, and at least some of those determinants (sexual behavior, food consumption, and so on) are under the control of the agent. In matters of health, it is no longer news that suffering is caused or mediated by one's own behavior: by ingesting dubious substances (smoke, alcohol, fatty foods); by engaging in sexual acts and other actions that bring you in contact with hazardous body fluids (semen, saliva, blood) or airborne viruses; by embarking on adventures that place you at risk (driving a car, entering a hospital). Given the connections between personal behavior and health outcomes, it is not surprising that human beings should be willing to accept personal responsibility for their suffering and pain. In many cases, blaming yourself when you get sick can be the rational thing to do.

Not surprisingly, there are major theodicies that locate the origin of evil in the realm of human action. Some theodicies hold that God created both evil and its antidotes as a challenge to humankind (Spero 1992) to develop the character and will to choose good over evil. Other theodicies hold that suffering is evil and it is the human community, not God, that created it. A shared focus of these theodicies is the idea that God gave humankind free will (agency and intentionality) and the ability to choose good or evil.

This belief has had a long and fluctuating history in our own culture's ideologies and the discourses of suffering. At various times we have gone from one extreme to another in presuming or rejecting this kind of explanation. At one pole is the idea that every sufferer is at fault because of flaws of moral character and that those who suffer have engaged in unwholesome practices that have led to the dissolution of personal integrity. At the other extreme is the discourse wherein virtually every sufferer is a victim and no one is at fault for his or her suffering. At that extreme, it becomes unethical to suggest that someone who suffers may be to blame for that suffering, although he or she may be represented as the victim of the evil actions of others or of unjust social environments. It is a bit paradoxical to think that a person can be the victim of others' evil actions but not of his or her own. This is an issue not well worked out by that position.

Currently in the United States there is a mixed and perhaps changing discourse for talking about suffering and fault. In many scientific circles, the most widespread discourse depersonalizes as many kinds of suffering as possible. It removes the idea of the agency of the sufferer as a relevant contributory factor. Attributions of "fault" to suffering persons are disparaged as "blaming the victim."

There is some wisdom in this, of course. We are only imperfectly capable of judging others, particularly little-known others, and it is presumptuous at best to infer moral defect from the fact of suffering. Perhaps our depersonalization of suffering is in part a form of self-criticism for any tendency in us moralistically to cast blame on people less fortunate than ourselves, persons from whom we would like to distance ourselves, persons whose fates we fear.

There is a problem, however, when "victimization" becomes the dominant account of suffering and when it becomes "politically incorrect" ever to hold people responsible for their misery. The problem is that descriptions of agents as "victims" ironically depersonalize the sufferer. The sufferer is described (and encouraged to envision himself or herself) as a passive "victim," which is hardly a more health-inducing description than "villain." If the "victim" has no fault, neither has he or she any control over or responsibility for remedial action. The "victim's" only recourse is reliance on the intervention of "experts" and on people with resources of power and knowledge that constitute the means for remedial action. The sufferer is seen as possessing no resources and capabilities of his or her own that could ameliorate present conditions and future prospects.

Of course, there are illnesses and other conditions of suffering for which the sufferer is not "at fault." Some of these conditions are extremely serious, and as far as we know some of them may be entirely biologically predetermined. There are also social or ecological environments where only those who are endowed with unusual psychosomatic gifts could flourish or survive. But the cases are far more frequent in which biological predispositions and events, social-environmental conditions, and a person's actions all contribute to the state of suffering or well-being. If we seem to suggest that some "blame" be given back to sufferers, the critical point is not to say that they "deserve punishment" but, rather, that they deserve to be made aware of whatever degree of personal control they may have over their own conditions. They deserve the acknowledgment that there may be something that the sufferer can and should do to change his or her state of being.

What is ironic about the rhetoric of (not) "blaming the victim" is how often the "victim" is the most difficult person to convince of this position. "Therapy" may be necessary to provide the intensive persuasion needed to make sufferers agree that they are not to blame. The "no-blame" position seems, in fact, to be somewhat counterintuitive to sufferers. After all, suffering feels like "punishment." There are deep intuitions linking suffering to emotions such as guilt and shame, which are emotions that presuppose that one has done something wrong. It is not unheard of for highly educated scientifically trained women to be shocked and overwhelmed by the unbidden and unwanted feeling that their own miscarriage must be an indication that they have done something "bad" or that they are being punished for being a "bad person." Such intuitions are real experiences for sufferers in the contemporary Western world, where those intuitions are judged irrational by the sufferers themselves, as they are for sufferers in other societies, where those intuitions make rational sense within the terms of an official karmic worldview.

In a sense there is nothing surprising about the tendency of human beings narratively to link misfortune to personal agency and to blame or accept responsibility themselves when things go wrong. The experience of guilt and regret when things go wrong may be the affective side of a universal (and generally correct) human intuition that (in the aggregate and in the long run) outcomes tend to be proportionate to actions. The experience of guilt and regret may be merely the phenomenological corollary of the universal (and correct) intuition that personal effort deserves to be exercised in life precisely because it tends to be efficacious. When things go wrong human beings acknowledge their sense of agency and power by wondering how they are at fault. What is surprising is the insistence with which so many secular-scientific scholars in the West choose to analyze that commonplace mental association as some kind of "problem" or "pathology" or "primitivism" rather than asking what kind of wisdom might be expressed by such recalcitrant human thoughts and attitudes. What is surprising is the way those intuitions are summarily disparaged in modernist discourse as "blaming the victim." Such a doctrine ought to seem surprising because it violates the common-sense or folk psychology of most peoples of the world.

It is noteworthy that recent policy-making and economic concerns over public health issues have double-edged implications for questions of personal control over health-related behavior. Risky behavior once was assumed to be the private concern of the individual, and it was thought to be nobody's business but one's own. It was relatively easy to remain ignorant about or willfully ignore the consequences of high-risk behaviors like cigarette smoking. At present individual health behaviors are increasingly discussed in the context of community concerns. There is renewed attention to the economic and social problems of high-risk behaviors and how they affect others. There is a communitarian discourse that has reemerged and is expressed in terms of insurance rates, treatment facilities, family responsibilities, care for the uninsured, and the distribution of risk (for example, the effects of secondary cigarette smoke, sexually transmitted diseases, and so on). There has been a concurrent trend to regard personal health behaviors in a community context. With increasing social pressures, say, in the family and workplace, people might be expected increasingly to develop feelings of community responsibility concerning their own health-related practices.

One possible outcome of this renewed communitarian discourse is that collective concerns will proceed in the direction of a form of "neo-puritanism" (Shweder 1993b), with escalating state controls over increasingly medicalized life practices. That is to say, more and more of personal behavior will fall within the domain of the medical, and medical issues will be subject to centralized control. The weaker the responsibility given to potential "victims" of suffering, the more sweeping may be the control taken by "protective" centralized social control agencies.

A more promising trend in the discourse of American medicine, which is of course a complex culture in and of itself, is the movement toward preventive medicine with its encouragement to participate in the responsibility for personal health. The rising public concern over how individual health practices affect groups and communities suggests that it would be advantageous for individuals and communities alike to cultivate a discourse of informed personal responsibility toward health-related behaviors. Informed by the moral metaphors of South Asia, we would prefer a future scenario in which individual persons adopt a discourse in which their own health was considered a "life goal," a personal duty, and a "good" to be achieved, like a satisfying career, economic security, or a satisfying network of community relationships. We would much prefer this to the horrific alternative of a centralized medical hegemony in which individuals and even local communities lose the capacity to define the limits of a moral way of life.

It should be obvious to the reader that the linkage of health and personal integrity, as we construe it, is not a simple one. We do not intend to say that healthy people are dignified and sick people are not. We acknowledge that the experience of illness can in some cases contribute to a sense of personal dignity. We are aware that suffering may be represented narratively or biographically as "trials" of moral strength, or as periods of personal growth, as an expansion of awareness and understanding, and even as a condition for the development of exceptional skills.

As we engage the public health issues of the day it is probably advisable to avoid a dogmatic preference for any one discourse of health, suffering, and well-being. It may be desirable to cultivate a casuistic flexibility in applying the appropriate moral discourse and theodicy to particular cases or situations, but in order to do this, there must be a general awareness of possibilities for expanding our discourses of health and responsibility. For this reason, one of our aims in this chapter has been to call attention to some alternative discourse possibilities for considering questions of suffering and well-being on the one hand, and questions of personal obligation and responsibility on the other. These possibilities already exist within various enclaves of our own contemporary culture, even though they have not been well represented as part of the official, institutionalized scientific model. Though they exist in our culture, they most often are "not heard" by social scientists or by medical practitioners functioning in their "official" roles. Yet there are signs that this is changing. At the very least, there is growing reemergence of interest among social scientists and clinical theorists in folk wisdom and traditional world conceptions (for example, see Rozin and Nemeroff 1990; Sabini and Silver 1982; Spero 1992) and in the role these play in psychological life and health-related behaviors. We have attempted to bring forward what is culturally backgrounded in contemporary North America by looking at how it is culturally foregrounded in contemporary South Asia and in the sensibilities of many premodern peoples in various regions of the world.

A Parting Prophetic Remark

An ethics of community and an ethics of divinity still flourish in South Asian villages and towns such as Bhubaneswar. The doctrine of karmic consequences and the idea that "old sins cast long shadows" flourish there as well. To some readers these ethics, doctrines, and ideas may seem antiquated. Nevertheless, as the United States enters a new phase in public health policy, we are likely to witness an increase in agent-blaming moralistic explanations of illness not unlike those discussed in this essay. The connection between action and outcome (health behavior and illness) is going to be advertised, regulated, and evaluated in terms of social or community costs, and the idea of a "sin tax" is going to enter collective consciousness and be enforced by the state. Whether our highly individualistic ethics of autonomy will give way to an ethics of community or divinity in a world full of anxieties about illness and contagious disease remains to be seen. Yet, as we search for "postmodern" ways to rethink our responsibilities to society and nature, it would not be too surprising if we began to acknowledge the intuitive appeal of ideas such as "sacred self," "sacred world," "karma," "duty," "pollution," and "sin." It would not be surprising if we began to worry a lot about how those ideas are to be reconciled with the individualism that we value as well.

Note

We gratefully acknowledge the support we received for research on moral reasoning and explanations of suffering from several sources: The National Institute of Child Health and Human Development, the MacArthur Foundation Health and Behavior Research Network, the MacArthur Foundation Research Network on Successful Midlife Development (MIDMAC), and a research grant (to Nancy Much) from Georgetown University.

References

Babb, L. 1983. Destiny and responsibility: Karma in popular Hinduism. In *Karma: An anthropological inquiry*, edited by C. F. Keyes and E. V. Daniel. Berkeley: University of California Press.

Collingwood, R. G. 1961. On the so-called idea of causation. In *Freedom and responsibility: Readings in philosophy and law*, edited by H. Morris. Stanford: Stanford University Press.

Daniel, S. B. 1983. The tool box approach of the Tamil to the issues of moral responsibility and human destiny. In *Karma: An anthropological inquiry*, edited by C. F. Keyes and E. V. Daniel. Berkeley: University of California Press.

Haidt, J., S. H. Koller, and M. G. Dias. 1993. Affect, culture, and morality, or, is it wrong to eat your dog? *Journal of Personality and Social Psychology* 65:613–29.

Hart, H. L. A., and A. M. Honore. 1956/1961. Causation in the law. In *Freedom and responsibility: Readings in philosophy and law*, edited by H. Morris. Stanford: Stanford University Press.

Johnson, Mark. 1987. *The body in the mind*. Chicago: University of Chicago Press.

Johnson, M. 1993. *Moral imagination: Implications of cognitive science for ethics*. Chicago: University of Chicago Press.

Kakar, S. 1981. *The inner world: A psycho-analytic study of childhood and society in India*. Oxford: Oxford University Press.

———. 1982. *Shamans, mystics and doctors*. Boston: Beacon Press.

Kapp, W. 1963. *Hindu culture, economic development and economic planning in India*. New York: Asia.

Keyes, C. F. 1983. The study of popular ideas of karma. In *Karma: An anthropological inquiry*, edited by C. F. Keyes and E. V. Daniel. Berkeley: University of California Press.

Keyes, C. F. and E. V. Daniel. 1983. *Karma: An anthropological inquiry*. Berkeley: University of California Press.

Kleinman, A. 1986. *Social origins of distress and disease*. New Haven: Yale University Press.

Lakoff, G. 1987. *Women, fire and dangerous things*. Chicago: University of Chicago Press.

Lakoff, G., and M. Johnson. 1980. The metaphorical structure of the human conceptual system. *Cognitive Science* 4:195–208.

———. 1986. *Metaphors we live by*. Chicago: University of Chicago Press.

Mahapatra, M. 1981. *Traditional structure and change in an Orissan temple*. Calcutta: Punthi Pustak.

Mahapatra, M., N. C. Much, and R. A. Shweder. (1991). Sin and suffering in a sacred city: Oriya ideas about spiritual debt and moral cause and effect. Working paper.

Much, N. C. (1992). The analysis of discourse as methodology for a semiotic psychology. *American Behavioral Scientist* 36(1): 52–72.

———. 1995. Cultural psychology. In *Rethinking psychology*, edited by J. Smith, R. Harré, and L. van Langenhove. London: Sage.

Much, N. C., and R. Harré. 1994. How psychologies "secrete" moralities. *New Ideas in Psychology* 12:291–321.

Much, N. C., and M. Mahapatra. 1993, in preparation. *Karma as theory and experience: Symbolic contexts and the construction of meaning.*

Mumford, S. R. 1989. *Himalayan dialogue: Tibetan lamas and Gurung shamans in Nepal.* Madison: University of Wisconsin Press.

Murdock, G. P. 1980. *Theories of illness: A world survey.* Pittsburgh: University of Pittsburgh Press.

Myrdal, G. 1968. *Asian drama: An inquiry into the poverty of nations.* New York: Pantheon.

Obeyesekere, G. 1980. The rebirth eschatology and its transformations: A contribution to the sociology of early Buddhism. In *Karma and rebirth in classical Indian traditions*, edited by W. D. O'Flaherty. Berkeley: University of California Press.

O'Flaherty, W. D. 1976. *The origins of evil in Hindu mythology.* Berkeley: University of California Press.

———. 1980. *Karma and rebirth in classical Indian traditions.* Berkeley: University of California Press.

Park, L. 1992. Crosscultural explanations of illness: Murdock revisited. Available from Lawrence Park, Committee on Human Development, University of Chicago, Chicago, IL 60637.

Rozin, P., and C. Nemeroff. 1990. The laws of sympathetic magic: A psychological analysis of similarity and contagion. In *Cultural psychology: Essays on comparative human development*, edited by J. W. Stigler, R. A. Shweder, and G. Herdt. New York: Cambridge University Press.

Sabini, J., and M. Silver. 1982. *Moralities of everyday life.* Oxford: Oxford University Press.

Sapir, E. 1986. Culture, genuine and spurious. In Sapir's *Selected writings in language, culture and personality.* Berkeley: University of California Press.

Shweder, R. A. 1990. In defense of moral realism: Reply to Gabennesch. *Child Development* 61:2060–67.

———. 1991. *Thinking through cultures.* Cambridge: Harvard University Press.

———. 1993a. Fundamentalism for highbrows. *University of Chicago Record* 28 (October 14): 2–5.

———. 1993b. "Why do men barbecue?" and other postmodern ironies of growing up in the decade of ethnicity. *Daedalus* special issue "Children in America: Three to eleven" 122(1):279–308.

Shweder, R. A., and J. Haidt. 1993. The future of moral psychology: Truth, intuition and the pluralist way. *Psychological Science*, November.

Shweder, R. A., M. Mahapatra, and J. G. Miller. 1987. Culture and moral development. In *The emergence of morality in young children*, edited by J. Kagan and S. Lamb. Chicago: University of Chicago Press. Reprinted in *Cultural psychology: Essays on comparative human development*, edited by J. Stigler, R. A. Shweder, and G. Herdt. New York: Cambridge University Press.

Shweder, R. A., and J. G. Miller. 1985. The social construction of the person: How is it possible? In *The social construction of the person*, edited by K. G. Gergen and K. E. Davis. New York: Springer-Verlag. Reprinted in 1991 in R. A. Shweder, R. A. *Thinking through cultures*. Cambridge: Harvard University Press.

Shweder, R. A., and N. C. Much. 1987. Determinations of meaning: Discourse and moral socialization. In *Moral development through social interaction*, edited by W. Kurtines and G. Gewirtz. New York: Wiley. Reprinted in 1991 in R. A. Shweder. *Thinking through cultures*. Cambridge: Harvard University Press.

Shweder, R. A., and M. Sullivan. 1993. Cultural psychology: Who needs it?. *Annual Review of Psychology* 44: 497–523.

Spero, M. H. 1992. *Religious objects as psychological structures*. Chicago: University of Chicago Press.

Wadley, S. S., and B. W. Derr. 1990. Eating sins in Karimpur. In *India through Hindu categories*, edited by M. Marriott. New Delhi: Sage.

Whiting, J. W. M., and I. L. Child. 1953. *Child training and personality*. New Haven: Yale University Press.

Wikan, U. 1989. Illness from fright or soul loss: A North Balinese culture-bound syndrome? *Culture, Medicine and Psychiatry* 13:25–50.

Morality and Behavior
in Historical Context

Sugar and Morality

Sidney Mintz

From the mid-seventeenth century onward, the consumption of sugar in the West was colored by moral judgments, positive and negative. Much the same is true now. This essay considers why the use of sugar may have given rise to moral issues, and why it still may.

In any society, the act of eating can be encumbered with moral overtones—as can the act of not eating when others eat. Such acts take on their power as means of scoring moral points in contrast to their opposite: either of eating some things and not eating others; or of eating or not eating at all. Needless to say, to redefine ingestion as an arena for the acting out of moral principles is a distinctively human achievement. It operates according to rules that are by their nature culturally specific, socially and historically derived, not common to all members of the species.

The English literary critic Edmund Gosse (1907) provides a touching example of the symbolic power of food, both eaten and abjured. His book *Father and Son* is an autobiography, from his first memories to the end of his youth, entangled within a biography of his father, Philip Gosse, the anti-Darwinian naturalist. Philip Gosse was a founding member of the Plymouth Brethren, an ascetic Calvinist sect. For him, food—like all else—was a moral instrument. As leader of a small band of the faithful, Philip Gosse decided on one occasion at the end of his sermon to arrest the backsliding among his parishioners by announcing, without warning, a one-day, bread-and-water fast of contrition. To his nine-year-old son Edmund's amazement, the congregation took this stern admonition wholly to heart. Edmund describes in chilling detail the day he spent, hungering and praying, with his father and the congregation,

The memory of this miserable little boy stays with the reader, for Edmund shows us how deeply he experienced (and suffered from) his father's moral rigor and irresistible power.

Though eating is essential to continued life, both the use of food and intentional abstention from it are cultural practices that express deep emotions. Food habits serve as vehicles of such emotion. They are normally learned early and well, and are mostly inculcated by affectively significant adults; hence they acquire enduring sentimental power. One does not become an adult in the abstract; it must happen in terms of a particular substantive body of cultural materials. Food and eating are positioned near the core of such materials exactly because of their life-giving and essential (though usually routine and spuriously perfunctory) nature. Children are trained in eating according to their social group's values. Such things as the learning of manual skills, personal fastidiousness, cooperation and sharing, restraint and reciprocity are commonly linked to the consumption of food by children. Indeed, in some cultures getting to eat with the adults as an adult, rather than as a child, is a major hurdle when growing up.

Perhaps moral conviction commonly attaches to this sphere of human activity not only because it is frequently practiced, regular, and necessary but also because it is a sphere in which *some* choice is usually possible. For each individual, eating is a basis for linking the world of things to the world of ideas through one's acts, and thus also a basis for relating oneself to the rest of the world. The intuition that one is somehow substantiated out of the food one ingests can be said to carry some kind of moral charge. Because we are "manufactured," as it were, out of what we consume, must there not be a bad and a good to the choices we make? It would probably be more surprising if, as symbol-using creatures, we did *not* somehow burden ingestion with a moral onus.

Among foods, processed sugar, or sucrose, is a latecomer with a special status. A granular sucrose, extracted in liquid form from the grass called sugarcane, is about two thousand years old in the Middle East. Sugar was scarcely known in the West before the eighth century; its introduction there dates mostly from the Crusades. After reaching Europe, and until it became a sweetener for more and more Europeans around the start of the eighteenth century, sugar was subject to powerful social, economic, and political forces that, among other things, transformed it from luxury and rarity into prosaic necessity.

Yet, throughout this time it remained a much-prized and affect-ridden treat, even if not always for the same classes of consumers. Though used at first as medicine and spice, sugar's distinctive taste became known widely in the West particularly in association with the bitter stimulant beverages, all of them exotic and novel in the seventeenth century: coffee, tea, and chocolate.

The popularity of sugar in most western European countries continued to grow during the eighteenth and nineteenth centuries. Northern Europe and much of middle Europe changed into heavy-sugar-eating regions between 1750 and 1900, partly owing to the addition of beet sugar production in the temperate zone after 1830. The sugar-eating habit then spread outward, especially to major overseas anglophone areas (the United States, Canada, Australia, New Zealand, and others).

Questions about the suitability of sugar as food had been raised early in its history in the West. For example, Hart (1633) recognized that "immoderate" use of sugar could rot the teeth. But matters of health of this kind lacked any specifically moral dimension. In fact, the moral issues that were connected to sugar during its early history in the West did not have to do so much with sugar itself as with related matters. For example, we find the moral place of sugar tested in relation to fasting. Thomas Aquinas found for it, in this case. Aquinas was asked whether the eating of spiced sugars constituted a violation of the religious (Catholic) fast. He concluded that such sugars were medicines, not foods: "Though nutritious in themselves, sugared spices are nonetheless not eaten with the end in mind of nourishment, but rather for ease in digestion; accordingly, they do not break the fast any more than the taking of any other medicine" (cited in Lippmann 1970 [1929]:368).

Another more compelling linkage of sugar to morality marked events in the North European country that had first proved itself most hospitable to it. In the early years of the final decade of the eighteenth century, British abolitionists who had hoped to abolish the slave trade came to realize they had lost that fight, at least for the moment. Parliamentary defeats of the special measures they had struggled to secure in 1791–1792 led them to call for a new strategy. The decision was made to pursue the same goal, this time through economic pressure rather than legislative action. In pamphlets and broadsides the abolitionists told their readers that the consumption of West Indian produce was tantamount to the commission of murder.

As with all such political events, cartoonists found a funny side.

In one cartoon dating from 1792, George III, his wife, and their reluctant daughters are depicted, about to drink their sugarless tea. The daughters display varying degrees of disdain or disgust, while their parents urge them on. The queen beseeches them to drink bitter tea: "Consider how much work you'll save the poor blackamoors." The young ladies are unmoved. But the abolitionists themselves were deadly serious about finding sugar eaters guilty for the sins of slavery: "[S]o necessarily connected are our consumption of the commodity, and the misery resulting from it, that in every pound of sugar used (the product of the slaves imported from Africa) we may be considered as consuming two ounces of human blood."[1]

Ragatz (1928) writes:

> All Christians were called upon to give a practical demonstration of the principles of their faith by refusing to use products defiled with blood; children were asked to forgo accustomed sweets and thus prevent the selling of their little black brothers into bondage; royalty was urged to set an example of abstinence which must needs be followed by all persons of importance in the country.[2] (262)

The end of the trade in slaves came soon after the turn of the century; and the end of British slavery itself finally arrived, less than three decades later.

Some critics thought sugar itself morally questionable. In an anonymous essay (probably written by the reformer Jonas Hanway), the reader is first harangued about the evils of tea, and then:

> To these we may add another pernicious Foreigner, called *Sugar*,—which not only inflames the poor man's expences, but his blood and vitals also. If you please, then, join them all together, and compute the expence, the loss of time taken in breaking and washing the dishes, sweetening the tea, spreading the bread and butter, the necessary pause which defamation and malicious tea-table chat afford, and they will largely account for half a day in winter, spent in doing that which is worse, very much worse than doing nothing. (Anonymous 1777, 13)

Hanway's tirades against tea and sugar criticize this use of the laborer's income, the time wasted in consumption, and the effects of tea. Hanway does not criticize sugar so much; he even concedes later that it may be beneficial in some ways. Yet his argument has moral implications: luxury and excess (sweets included) are corrosive of the will; wasting time and wealth are equally intolerable morally.

Another, quite different case bears mention. A provocative paper on the history of ice cream in Scotland by McKee documents the early inclination of Glaswegians to associate ice cream with immorality, particularly (it seems) because the pioneers of ice cream retailing in Glasgow were Italians (McKee 1991). McKee's argument is provocative because the role of sugar (here, in the form of ice cream) is given a sexual cast, as others have done with alcohol, for example. Thus, testimony before a joint parliamentary committee is reported in the *Glasgow Herald* of June 7, 1906, as follows:

> Cross examined, witness added that he had seen the boys and girls kissing and smoking and cuddling away at each other. . . . Detective Young, Northern Division, stated that he had known many little girls when about twelve or thirteen years of age who had since been before Magistrates, and were now prostitutes. The boys who had accompanied them as girls were now living off them, and were going out acting as their bullies at night. Q. Do you ask us to believe that the downfall of these women was due to ice-cream shops? A. I believe it is. (McKee 1991, 203)

The association of sweet things with luxury and excess, and hence with issues of morality, is clear.

McKee descries a link between sugar and vice. As we have seen, the abolitionists boycotted sugar to help to free the slaves. Here is an example of a religious boycott of sugar, though unrelated to any intrinsic quality of the sugar itself.

Redcliffe Salaman (1949), author of *The History and Social Influence of the Potato*, observed that the Old Believers, who broke away from the Russian Orthodox Church after Patriarch Nikon's reforms, defined certain foods and other substances as abominations:

> Chief amongst these were sugar, tobacco and potatoes, none of which, it will be noted, are mentioned in the Bible. Cane-sugar, a luxury in England, must have been a great rarity in Russia of those days; tobacco and potatoes, both new arrivals, were not only rarities but, sharing the primal curse of the *Solanums*, were

considered to be generated by some peculiar botanical form of incest. (Salaman 1949, 116)

The creation of a new taboo by a religious sect has many parallels; it is of interest here only because one of the tabooed foods is sugar. Collective repudiation of practically anything can figure importantly in the stimulation of positive in-group feelings, for those who share in the act ideationally. In the case Salaman describes, the *Bozpopovschini* ("priestless ones") were showing themselves to be purer than the priestist (*popovets*) church they had abandoned because its priests and members had not renounced such foods. The forswearing of foods is a feature of religious change, and seems always to be invested with moral weight.

The historical examples that have been provided up to this point suggest that sugar has been forgone for the good of others, as in the case of the antislavery antisaccharites; and for the sake of God, as in the case of the *Bozpopovschini* and the Plymouth Brethren. But what about repudiating sugar for one's own personal, moral reasons? Surely, that sort of repudiation must figure in any contemporary reflection on sugar and morality. Paul Rozin (1987) has suggested three reasons that today's sugar eaters may consider sugar consumption morally dubious or sinful: First is its association with "sinful" substances (such as coffee); second, he posits an asceticism that views all pleasurable sensations as inherently questionable morally; third, there is the possible link between sugar and obesity, since obesity itself can be perceived as sinful. That eating should be subject to such strong moral overtones Rozin attributes to the intimacy of ingestion. I share this view. But such association is highly variable cross-culturally; people in different societies perceive such connections very differently. Moreover, although obesity may be seen as unfortunate (or even sinful) by people in some cultures, others draw no such conclusions.[3] I propose to try a somewhat different route toward understanding the abnegation of sugar and other substances as immoral, by suggesting that we use feelings about obesity as a clue. Moral feelings about the body deeply affect how foods are perceived in the West today and, I think, in a manner markedly different from that which was true three centuries ago.

The modern individual, of whose body and needs we now speak, is the product of the Industrial Revolution and the rise of an economic system given over more and more to the gratification of individual consumption. That system has distinguished itself by its success not only in producing the consumables but also in specifying and defining the needs. Such processes of production and need definition have stretched over nearly three centuries, and continue still, ever stronger. They began to take on a modern form, I suspect, when the first commodities changed from being luxuries into daily needs, including such things as tea, tobacco, and sugar, soon to be followed by clothing, china, and much else.

This is not to assert that ordinary working people in late-eighteenth-century Britain became totally different sorts of human beings simply by becoming consumers of such substances. Nonetheless, consuming what were at first new and often exotic products bought with their own labor—which allowed them to see themselves as *being* different because they were able to choose to consume differently—surely helped to *make* them different. In the new scheme of things, what one consumed became a changing measure of what (and of who) one was. Status no longer so much defined what one could consume; what one consumed helped to define one's status. The individual producer as consumer has desires that must now be continuously remodeled. Collective (social) needs take on a different form, altered by the expansion of individual needs, as these became more immediate, more apparent, and more widely justified in the press, by the political organs of the state, and even from the pulpit.

To link morality to sugar for the modern individual, we must see needs as *changing morally* over time. The relationship between work and ensuing satisfactions becomes more intimate. Specifying the nature of satisfaction becomes a more individual and personal matter. For this new individuality to take shape, society had to succeed in shifting people's perceptions of where the locus of desire lies. That desire, now defined in terms of the individual, is relocated, so to speak. It acquires a voice of its own, a voice I believe to be conditioned in part by society's new ways for publicizing and elaborating what is desirable. The motor of desire, now speaking in what is perceived as being its own voice, becomes one of the most powerful of all signals attesting to the *existence* of the individual. This highly divisible, modern self is now a "bundle of desires," elements of which come together and express themselves unitarily at certain moments, probably with special clarity at moments of deciding (choosing) to consume.

This conception of the individual can be aligned with the issue of food and morality, and, more specifically, with the issue of sugar and morality. Then it becomes a *refusal to consume* that needs examination from a moral standpoint. But this construction is qualitatively different from what precedes it. It has to do with the forgoing of sucrose in the consecration of the self. One "cuts out," "gives up," "swears off," "does without" sugar, in order to live longer, be healthier, prettier, shapelier, more competitive. But it also means to consume even more of a different kind, according to one's personal conceptions of what one can become.

Such forswearing can be done without apparent commitment to other humans, to other species, to one's own society, to other societies, or to the world—without any commitment at all, in fact, except to a newer, lovelier you. But it should be apparent that the "you" in this instance is far more frequently female than male; and that the newer, lovelier you may be forged with others very much in mind. Any discussion of dieting in American society must take account of maleness and femaleness, and of its clearly gendered rendering of the female body image. Women who diet may do so primarily to please themselves, but they do so also to make themselves members of a gender-defined group of abnegators, self-defining and self-fulfilling. By doing so successfully, they also define themselves as *outside*—indeed, above—another, larger female group. Their highly individualized sacrifices validate their membership. Such sacrifices are often meant to please males as well, either in the abstract or specifically. The encouragement to consume; to consume various goods and services simultaneously; to use consumption as an index of one's status; to show no interest in ceilings for consumption or, for that matter, floors for consumption, either—all militate against conceptions of the human body as a *satiable* entity. The material world, which is (and is envisioned as being) unimaginably rich in both goods and services for those with the means to pay, is refashioned to yield infinite, not finite, satisfactions. One simultaneously consumes less of some things and more of others—exercise costumes, special shoes, fitness magazines, sports equipment, special videotapes, exertion weekends, new foods and food-preparation instruments, new clothes, and so on. Such a reconstruction of needs and their satisfaction developed in particular during the past century, and had the important subsidiary effect of changing the ways in which the individual is definable in relation to others. The acceleration of such consumption and the multiplication of its objects in the past decade or two is particularly obvious.

The link between morality and sugar in the modern world must be descried against the background of an army of consumers prepared to consume messages about health, love, and beauty on the one hand; and, on the other, to repudiate large quantities of sucrose, prepared in an infinite number of ways—particularly in pruriently labeled desserts but also in everything from bread and salt to salad dressing and catsup. To those who reject sucrose, the only immediately visible moral principle in this picture is that of self-discipline. It involves responsiveness to definitions of the self that may seem for the most part to omit society at large—and, for that matter, the needs of other societies or of other life forms. It is as if the reason that individuals should forgo the consumption of sucrose is solely for their individual improvement: no reward but self-defined virtue.

But the self is rarely disengaged wholly from its social context. Judith Goldstein (1993) writes of a "female aesthetic community," precisely because appeals to a gendered self in modern life are based on social connections, real or imagined. It is the intent of health and beauty advertising to accentuate simultaneously the appeal of intensely self-oriented improvement by self-denial *and* the appeal of membership thereby in some imagined group that shares elite consumerist interests.

The renunciation of certain consumables—sugar, for instance—is often accompanied by alternate or increased consumption of other things. Such renunciation generally proceeds because of self-referential (that is, individual) decisions about behavior. Also commonly involved are ideas about the ordering of lifestyle—of blazing behavioral trails to a new personality. These claims fit well with positions advanced by Jonathan Friedman (1989), who argues that consumption under capitalism simultaneously involves individualism, consumerism, and romanticism. Friedman declares that before the rise of modern consumerism, the individual was embedded in networks of dependency that defined his or her identity in relation to others in the same social system: "All relations, from those within family networks, to the class structure were defined in terms of established forms of interaction and etiquette. Who one was and how one was to act were related as essence to appearance" (125). To replace the older, more fixed system, capitalism breaks down the socially defined meaning that system provided individuals, depersonalizes the public sphere, and increases people's feelings of anonymity, of not belonging. The public and the private become acutely different. As an older social system becomes dilapidated, one's individual identity is called into question more. The use of consumption as a means to define oneself becomes commoner; the market emerges as a mirror of what is, and of what can become. The romantic ethic, which enables the individual to pursue some different lifestyle, comes into its own by means of the market. This new sort of individual is truly different; the market has created her, by encouraging her to buy her new self.

"In order to be a romantic," Friedman writes, "one must endure the experience of alterity, of otherness. One must, thus, be formally alienated from any specific social reality in order to seek new realities. One must be an individual whose essence is independent of all specific social and cultural attributes" (127) The individual as a consumer who creates cultural forms by which to live and then discards them in order to create new ones, accords with the repudiation of particular practices or objects (including of course certain foods) as a means of enhancing and intensifying individuality and distinctiveness. Such creativity does not mean reducing consumption but molding it to accommodate changing needs and images, which are enhanced exactly because they are changing. Its romantic aspect is clear: the consumer arranges her desires in a coherent manner, both for self-definition and for novelty. Without addressing directly the estimates accorded obesity in such individual schemes, we see that consumption forgone can satisfy differing ends simultaneously.

The triad of individualism, romanticism, and consumerism fits well with the picture of a new self. The repudiation of a desired good bestows virtue, while opening the door to additional consumption of different kinds. Exercise of choice heightens the illusion of individuality. The utilization of choices of consumption to create an effect of changing form (in this instance, quite literally, changing form) fits with the romantic conception of the self. In these ways, the rejection of sugar—tobacco, drugs, coffee, television, cholesterol, unfiltered water, synthetic fiber, irradiated fruit, red meat, whatever—enables one to march to the beat of a different drummer, made more attractive because one can also believe one is among the first to hear its tattoo. But this individuality is conditioned by the postulation of a "group," membership in which is attainable among other things by certain consumptions of sacrifice, based on inner will—on difficult choices, freely made, to validate one's fitness for belonging. Such a "group" consists not of one's family or alumni association but of an abstraction from the pages of certain magazines and from television, generated by the best salespersons in world history. An imaginary group of this kind corresponds well with Friedman's idea of "an individual subject with no necessary socially established essence." Using the products (or, in the case of sugar, not using them) is how the imagined group is joined. By such urgings to "moral" performance, individuals learn to consume with more discipline; morality, detached from society itself, thus becomes a new consumable.

Notes

1. My colleague Gillian Feeley-Harnik wonders whether such imagery may have arisen within a particular religious tradition, in view of the anti-communionist overtones. The question is a good one. Many of the abolitionists were Quakers; other religious groups in Britain also struggled against the slave trade and slavery. But the stress upon what might be called the "cannibalistic" aspects of sugar eating also deserves notice.

2. The proslavery faction was quick to respond to such politics with arguments of its own. Its own propaganda apparatus was brought actively into play. An example turns up in the *European Magazine* for March 1792. There, a writer who dubs himself "Consistency" submits a purportedly authentic letter from a five-year-old, reasoning against the moral petition to abstain from sugar in order to save the lives of the slaves.

> Dear Lady L_____:
>
> Forgive me for applying to you to release me from my promise not to drink anything that has Sugar in it. To be sure, I would not wish to have my promise back again, if I was convinced of the truth of what you told me, that every lump of Sugar I put in my mouth, consumed some of the flesh of a poor dead Negro Slave.

The letter continues; the little boy complains of the ridicule to which he was subjected by grownups for persisting in his sacrifice,

> and while they are laughing at me, I see them eating such nice tarts, and cakes, and sweetmeats. . . . Some of the gentlemen told me they had been to the country where the Negroes make Sugar; and that they are never so fat and so happy as when they are making Sugar; and they eat and drink as much as they can; and they love it as much as we do.

Among those who ridiculed him, he says, were those who said that the Negroes are engaged in many other activities, such as mining gold and silver, dyeing cloth, cutting trees, and so on. Hence, he reasons, all of the objects produced through their labor are similarly contaminated by slavery. Those who forswear sugar while using mahogany tables and sterling flatware must be hypocrites:

> I cannot think, dear Lady L———, how anybody who will not eat Sugar because it is eating Negro flesh, can handle gold or silver, or feed themselves with silver spoons or forks; for if eating sugar is eating Negroes flesh, sure every time anybody puts a fork or spoon in their mouths, it is putting a poor dead Negro's finger or toe there. (185).

But the planters' spin doctors labored in vain. The end of the trade came soon after the turn of the century; the end of slavery itself finally arrived, less than three decades later.

3. Contributors to the recently published volume edited by De Garine and Pollack (1995) provide some extremely interesting examples of socially induced and approved obesity in non-Western cultures.

References

Anonymous. 1777. *An essay on tea, sugar, white bread . . . and other modern luxuries*. Salisbury, Eng.: J. Hodson.

De Garine, I., N. J. Pollock, eds. (1995). Social aspects of obesity. In *Culture and ecology of food and nutrition*, vol. 1. Sydney, Australia: Gordon & Breach.

Friedman, J. 1989. The consumption of modernity. *Culture and History* 4:117–30.

Goldstein, Judith. 1993. The female aesthetic community. *Poetics Today* 14(1): 143–63.

Gosse, Edmund. 1907. *Father and son*. New York: Scribner's Sons.

Hart, J. 1633. *Klinike or the diet of the diseased*. London: John Beale.

Lippmann, E. von. 1970 [1929]. *Geschichte des Zuckers*. Niederwalluf bei Wiesbaden: Dr. Martin Sandig.

McKee, Francis. 1991. Ice cream and immorality. In *Public eating: Proceedings of the Oxford symposium on food and cookery*, edited by Harlan Walker. London: Prospect Books.

Ragatz, Lowell J. 1928. *The fall of the planter class in the British Caribbean, 1763–1833*. New York: Appleton-Century.

Rozin, Paul. 1987. Sweetness, sensuality, sin, safety, and socialization: Some speculations. In *Sweetness*, edited by J. Dobbing. London: Springer Verlag.

Salaman, Redcliffe N. 1949. *The history and social influence of the potato*. Cambridge: Cambridge University Press.

Food, Morality, and Social Reform

Warren Belasco

In a September 1990 column titled "Restaurant Industry Moved by New Moral Fervor," the editor of *Nation's Restaurant News* observed that successful food service operators would have to be more "ethically sensitive." Hungry customers wanted more than tasty dishes, comfortable settings, and fair prices; they were "shopping for a better world." Good food had become "a moral imperative." But simply switching to vegetable oils to whip Mr. Cholesterol would not be quite enough to satisfy the "new righteousness." The current food worries went beyond obesity and coronary health to encompass "environmental disasters, the savings-and-loan failures, insider trading, and corporate mergers," not to mention "declining voter turnouts [and] the nuking of the nuclear family." Catering to the emerging "high-visibility social consciousness" would challenge even the most politically correct chef. "Today's consumers are demanding safe and nourishing food that is served with personal integrity in an environmentally responsible manner. They want something to believe in" (Telberg 1990, 22).

The busy editor of a restaurant trade newspaper did not often have an opportunity to ponder the modern crisis of faith, so it was probably inevitable that the "moral fervor" of affluent food shoppers would seem unprecedented. As I will argue, however, there was nothing new about the tendency to link private food choices to broad moral issues and social problems.

To those of us who have studied the social, ecological, and historical dimensions of eating, it comes as no surprise that food has ethical implications. Obviously, the way we dine has enormous impact not only on our personal health but also on nature, animals, other people, and the distribution of power. In eating even the simplest dish we join a chain of events linking people and places across the globe—past, present, and future. Yet, the very complexity of our modern food delivery system tends to hide those ties. However cheap a fast-food burger may seem, few of us can see the "external" costs—for example, the impact on Corn Belt groundwater, overgrazed grasslands, rain forests, energy reserves, or our children's welfare.

If eating ethically means taking a degree of responsibility for the wider impact of our diet, then modern dining tends to be fundamentally *amoral*. I doubt that many consumers *want* to do harm—that would be *immoral*—but few want to hear about the problems either. Such obliviousness has long benefited the food mass marketers, who have been able to work their wonders largely unimpeded by public concern for the "externalities." Thus, in his recent environmental history of Chicago, William Cronon writes that the turn-of-the-century meat industry thrived on "forgetfulness." "In the packers' world it was easy not to remember that eating was a moral act inexorably bound to killing" (Cronon 1991, 256). But now it is hard to consider meatpacking without also recalling Upton Sinclair. It has long been the job of food moralists like Sinclair to *insist* that we remember the wide social consequences of what and how we eat.

To be sure, such moral fervor was not new even at the time of *The Jungle* (Sinclair 1906/1981). Rather, Sinclair had inherited a tradition of dietary radicalism that went back at least seventy years—to the heyday of Sylvester Graham—and that continued for another seventy or eighty years, to its recent rediscovery and rejuvenation by the environmentalist wing of the counterculture. This chapter examines that critical tradition, both for its long-term continuities and for the variations in three particularly contentious periods: the mid-nineteenth century (Graham), the Progressive Era (Sinclair), and the 1970s (the countercuisine). In addition, I will look at the interaction between the moral radical reformers and the dietary mainstream: which moral appeals worked to spur changes in the production and consumption of food and which did not?

Continuities

Although academic historians often resist long-term generalization, there *are* some common themes in 150 years of food protest. Most obvious, food moralists share the belief that there is a connection between eating and social problems, digestion and corruption: bad diets produce bad societies, and vice versa. If there is a common social context spanning almost two centuries, it is the rise and consolidation of an urban-industrial civilization, and with that, a growing distance from the sources of our food. Sylvester Graham and Upton Sinclair would have recognized Wendell Berry's (1989) description of "the industrial eater [as] one who does not know that eating is an agriculture act, who no longer knows or imagines the connections between eating and the land, and who is therefore necessarily passive and uncritical—in short, a victim" (126). And what exactly is the modern eater a victim of? Four concerns recur—all addressing the crisis of moral accountability in a complex mass society.

Adulteration. Given the increasing distance between producer and consumer, it is all too easy for commercial food to be poisoned by hidden contaminants, some the inadvertent by-product of modern processing, some the deliberate result of marketers' greed. The anonymity of the modern market encourages (or at least allows) food sellers to act less responsibly toward buyers.

Short-term versus long-term efficiency. Modern society prizes efficiency, which means getting the most output from the least input. In criticizing this conventional calculus of efficiency, food moralists call for an extended time frame for assessing costs and benefits. When viewed from an elongated time perspective, the modern diet is both ecologically and medically wasteful, that is, inefficient.

Hubris. The classical Greeks believed that the gods would punish those who overstepped natural limits. Similarly, food moralists fear the catastrophic results of the unnatural way that we produce and consume foods.

Alienation. Modern food consumption isolates us from nature and from other people. Conversely, as one of my countercultural sources put it, joining others in seeking radical dietary change becomes an "edible dynamic"—a way to find personal wholeness (health) and to restore an "organic" community of mutual responsibility.

In exposing and decrying these persistent problems, food radicals advocate solutions that are ascetic (you are what you don't eat), nostalgic (back to nature and imagined folk tradition), decentralist (anticorporate, antiurban), egalitarian (antiprofessional), and, as the "edible dynamic" suggests, communitarian.

Radical reformers are not the only people who worry about the food supply or about the larger social dimensions of eating. Because food is so important not only as a biological necessity but also as an economic resource, political tool, and moralistic metaphor, dietary issues are hotly contested. In each historical period of heightened concern there are conservative reform alternatives to the more radical critique. More compatible with a *slowly* evolving status quo, conservative reform delegates the responsibility for finding solutions to advanced technology and centralizing institutions.

Lest all this become too abstract, it is now time to examine the three historical variations on these overall themes.

The Jacksonian Variation: Sylvester Graham

A passionate advocate of home-baked whole wheat bread and vegetarianism, Sylvester Graham is still best (or worst) remembered as the first great American "food nut," but recent reappraisals have suggested that Graham had a much broader agenda. Although his scientific rationale for giving up "bolted" (refined) flour and meat now seems hopelessly arcane, his social vision is still compelling. For Graham, a diet based on white bread and red meat reflected and reinforced the more vicious and self-destructive tendencies in Jacksonian America (Green 1986; Nissenbaum 1988; Walters 1978, 145–72; Whorton 1982).

Adulteration. Adulteration was a particularly powerful image in the vocabulary of the mid-nineteenth-century food reformers because it embraced many threats—from the literal poisoning of commercial foods to the seductive tastes of corrupting modern culture. Fear of adulteration reflected the acute crisis of confidence at a time of rapid, unregulated urbanization and unbridled commercial hucksterism. Beset by crooks, con men, and conspiracies, Jacksonians could trust no one—not even the local baker, who if Graham was right, routinely extended inferior flours with copper, alum, clay, and chalk.

Long-term inefficiency. Urban consumers bought commercial bread because it saved time, labor, and space, but Graham doubted that convenience was such a bargain in the long run. "Bolted" white flour was too easy to eat, thereby depriving the teeth and digestive system of the exercise necessary for long-term health. Afflicted with a "lazy colon," sedentary city dwellers sought harmful stimulants, especially alcohol, meat, and spices—along with corrupting commercial amusements. Moreover, the lucrative market for commercial bread was encouraging wheat farmers to overproduce, thereby "debauching" their soil (and robbing future generations) for the sake of instant profits (Nissenbaum 1988, 6).

Hubris. The "debauchery" was not only agricultural. Graham's belief that excessive excitement unleashed powerfully destructive forces struck a chord in the early Victorian culture. Graham first rose to prominence during the 1832 cholera epidemic, which he attributed to the irritating effect of modern foods on the stomach. Metaphorically, the mass epidemic could be interpreted as a sign that Jacksonian Americans were going too far in allowing their "animalistic" appetites (both dietary and sexual) to run amok (Nissenbaum 1988, 88–101).

Alienation. If there was a root cause of modern disease, Graham suggested, it was the disintegration of "organic" connections to the body, the family, the land, and other people. Graham suggested several ways to reestablish such links. First, monitor the body closely and rein in its self-indulgent impulses by eating simple pure foods (and by curbing sexual activity). Wheat should be bought personally from local farmers and then ground at home. Home-baked bread not only disciplined the colon but also bolstered family ties. As Nissenbaum writes, Graham was acutely nostalgic for an idyllic self-sufficient peasant household run by a dutifully nurturing (and bread-baking) mother—a home he never experienced personally. But Graham went beyond the sentimentalized nuclear family when he inspired the establishment of boardinghouses for unrelated single followers. Many of the alternative communities of the mid-nineteenth century did attempt to follow versions of the Graham diet (Nissenbaum 1988, 140–73).

Graham's radicalism also stimulated a full-scale backlash. Adopting the now-familiar tone of bemused disdain, journalists sided with the doctors in ridiculing the claims of food faddists. "What can surpass that which finds long life in starvation, sees 'moral reform' in bran and cabbage, and promises to revolutionize the world with john-cake and boiled beans?" quipped the *Boston Courier* in 1838 (Green 1986, 50). And he was physically attacked by obviously threatened butchers and bakers. Yet, Graham's fears about the direction of modern society *were* widely shared, and following the dialectic on conservative reform, the mainstream did respond to those worries—but without threatening the status quo.

Perhaps the most important adaption was the cult of the separate spheres, which delegated responsibility for humanizing a brutal economic order to the wife and mother. In her dedication to home cooking and moral uplift, the Victorian housewife roughly resembled Graham's vision of the bread-baking colonial mother—but with important exceptions. For one thing, the lady was urban, middle-class, and, baking aside, an avid consumer—certainly no self-sufficient preindustrial peasant. The control of atavistic appetites was confined largely to the private sphere, where women avoided meat (and sometimes all food) and children learned the rules of etiquette (Brumberg 1989; Kasson 1987). Meanwhile, men were left free to indulge their cravings in the public economic sphere. Another irony was that whereas Graham was more worried about the health of the bread-buying working class, it was the middle class that took up, in piecemeal fashion, Graham's therapeutic prescriptions—especially bran bread, more vegetables, exercise, fasting, temperance, and hydropathy (Green 1986).

The Progressive Variation: Upton Sinclair

Needless to say the middle-class codes of domesticity and gentility were unable to curb the voracious hunger of U.S. business leaders, whose ample bellies and Roman-scale banquets were widely caricatured in the popular press. But the outrageous gluttony of the plutocrats was not just symbolic, for some of the most sensational scandals at the turn of the century involved the food industry: for example, the deaths of children from drinking contaminated milk; and the "embalmed beef" that killed more American soldiers in Cuba than the Spanish army. Measured against the widespread price fixing, fraudulent advertising, and blatant poisoning of processed meats and packaged foods by the cynically named "trust," the flour-adulterating techniques of Sylvester Graham's local bakers seemed almost innocuous, even quaint (Cummings 1940; Levenstein 1988; Whorton 1982). Inevitably these abuses provoked a full-scale elaboration of both radical and conservative-reform themes.

Adulteration. The *adulteration* of basic foodstuffs with traditional extenders and new chemicals was clearly the most spectacular theme in muckraking. No one exposed that muck more literally than Upton Sinclair, with his graphic descriptions of the offal on the killing-room floor, the consumptive women wading through murky pools in the pickling shop, or the ingenious recycling of odd materials into sausage. The inability to trust what went into something so basic as meat suggested a fundamental crisis of confidence. Like Graham, Sinclair suggested that the anonymity of food production fostered irresponsibility—but on a much grander scale than anything imaginable seventy years earlier.

Hubris. Indeed, the managers and owners of the slaughterhouses were *so* anonymous that they hardly even appeared in the novel. What was most frightening in *The Jungle* was that the system seemed to operate on its own, without apparent direction. "It was like some horrible crime committed in a dungeon, all unseen and unheeded, buried out of sight and of memory" (Sinclair 1906/1981, 35). If Mary Shelley's *Frankenstein*, an 1818 work, was the archetypal story of scientific hubris, then the slaughterhouse was the industrial variant—a headless monster running amok, routinely killing thousands of animals (and, ultimately, humans) without much thought or remorse. Worse, as the prototype of mass production, the animal disassembly line served as a harbinger of more technological horrors to come (Bloodworth 1979).

Inefficiency. Like Graham, Sinclair believed that there were major long-run costs in modern convenience foods—in *The Jungle*'s case, precooked canned meats. Although the mass production system was scrupulously efficient in using "everything about the hog except the squeal"—it was enormously wasteful in its abuse of workers, who were routinely discarded after just a few years of service. Noting that many workers and fellow activists were often too ill to fight for social justice, Sinclair advocated a simple diet as the best preparation for the long struggle.

Alienation. By exposing slaughterhouse brutality Sinclair hoped to bridge the growing gap between middle-class consumers and the people who fed them. Perhaps workers and consumers could join forces against the businessmen who victimized them both—one step toward Sinclair's socialist utopia (Bloodworth 1979; Dickstein 1981). Moreover, in suggesting that pigs and cattle had feelings, integrity, and rights, too, Sinclair attacked the ethical myopia that tolerates killing on such an unprecedented scale.

Although Sinclair may have cared most about overcoming bourgeois alienation from production and nature, it was the adulteration angle that moved the mainstream. ("I aimed at the public's heart, but hit its stomach," he supposedly lamented [Levenstein 1988, 39].) The strong but narrowly focused political reaction to *The Jungle* typified the dynamics of conservative reform. For Sinclair, adulteration was an inevitable by-product of corporate size and anonymity; for the wider public, food contamination resulted from the greed of individual businessmen, not from the business system itself. Thus, rather than openly confronting the "trusts," Congress passed a few inspection, labeling, and worker-safety laws that curtailed the worst abuses of the greediest individuals but also helped, in the long run, to legitimize those large firms most able to afford compliance. As Susan Strasser (1989) shows in *Satisfaction Guaranteed*, mass marketers were quite successful in convincing consumers that only nationally branded processed foods could be trusted. Progressive Era worries about food safety and accountability actually accelerated centralization—the very opposite of Sinclair's intent.

Food manufacturers also profited from the Progressive Era concern about efficiency. Sinclair (like Graham before him) suggested that ascetic self-control enhanced personal and social vitality, but marketers obviously favored more consumption. In this they were aided by the period's growing faith in statistics-wielding professionals. Thus, nutritional scientists used unimpressive-sounding food-composition tables and weight/height charts to argue that Americans were not getting enough protein—a clear boon to the milk and meat industry. The discovery of vitamins would soon bolster sales of citrus, breakfast cereals, and "enriched" versions of Graham's nemesis, white bread (Levenstein 1988). Purveyors of consumer goods also got help from another emerging profession: home economics. Inheriting the Victorian lady's faith that enlightened domesticity could tame a brutal world, leading home economists used time-study jargon in recommending appliances, canned soups, Jell-o, and other convenience foods. And through their recipes, school classes, and cafeteria menus, home economists spearheaded the drive to modernize (and homogenize) the American diet (Strasser 1982).

The Countercuisine

By the late 1940s the battle was largely over. Harvey Levenstein (1988) characterizes the victory of the Americanizers, nutrition professionals, and corporate caterers as a "revolution at the table," but given the professional-managerial status of the victors, it might more accurately be called a "coup." Supported by the moral power of the statistics and biochemical analysis, the emerging nutrition consensus had several basic articles of faith:

- When judging whether a diet is "adequate," the whole is less than its parts. That is, as long as you can get the right biochemical nutrients—amino acids, vitamins, minerals, and so on—it really does not matter what final form they take.

- A healthy diet is a well-balanced one, composed of lots of animal protein—whether in the Basic 7 or, after 1955, Basic 4—and consumed in three square meals.

- Thanks largely to advanced technology (farm machinery, agrichemicals, mass production) the United States has the safest, cheapest, most varied food supply in the world.

Enter the counterculture, which questioned every axiom. Motivated partly by generational revolt, partly by genuine fear of environmental apocalypse, and partly by sheer boredom with the Basic 4s/3 Squares, hippies discovered the health-food underground. Creating what I have dubbed a "countercuisine," they revived and updated the moralistic critique of Sylvester Graham and Upton Sinclair. Like earlier dietary missionaries, they believed that the battle for the stomach would determine the fate of the world (Belasco 1993).

The word *adulteration* was rarely used, perhaps because its sexual connotations were now outdated. But the more popular epithets, *poison, plastic, junk, pig food*, and *artificial*, suggested the same thing: the commercial food supply was hopelessly polluted—thanks, again, to corporate anonymity and irresponsibility, now symbolized by the faceless "conglomerates" and impersonal suburban supermarket. (The Orwellian-sounding Safeway seemed about as safe as the old trusts were trustworthy.)

Concerns about *efficiency* were both personal and planetary. A diet full of poisons obviously sapped energy from the daily struggle for "survival" and "the revolution." But for youthful "health food nuts" the main threat was more ecological than medical. Through their intensive use of petrochemicals for fuel, fertilizers, and pesticides, modern farmers were poisoning the water, land, and wildlife. Thus, just as Graham's Ohio wheat farmers had "debauched" their land, "agribusiness" was sacrificing for the sake of present greed.

Frances Moore Lappé (1982) made a similar case against the "Great American Steak Religion" in *Diet for a Small Planet*, the bible of the countercuisine: converting feed grains to animal protein was sinfully wasteful and *unsustainable*—the environmentalists' synonym for long-run inefficiency. And giving up meat did not necessarily mean sacrificing freedom—indeed, quite the reverse: freedom was the capacity to make intelligent choices "based upon awareness of the consequences of those choices" (1982 ed., 26, 52).

Fear of an impending eco-catastrophe was reflected in the recurrent theme of technological *hubris*. A generation reared on science fiction and grade-B horror flicks had little trouble envisioning an agricultural hybrid of *Brave New World* and *Godzilla*. Mixing strange white powders in their secret labs, white-coated food engineers seemed embarked on a mad, Faustian defiance of mortality and natural law. Indeed, in their enthusiastic embrace of Pop Tarts, Tang, and other artificial wonders, Americans were thoughtlessly participating in a gigantic experiment (a common image in muckraker exposes and the guinea pig books of the 1920s and 1930s).

The solution for all this was a drastic decentralization of the food system: organic revolution. Regional, nonchemical agriculture would revitalize family-based farming and rural communities, reduce energy use, save the soil, and produce healthier food, too. To counter anonymity and return responsibility to the market, the countercuisine looked to revive the face-to-face contacts of the farmers' market and the mom-and-pop grocery (or co-op). Growing at least some of your own food—preferably in community gardens—would restore contact with nature and neighbors. And eating "lightly"—especially by shifting protein sources from meat to grain—would free up resources to feed the hungry elsewhere. A holistic cure for modern fragmentation and *alienation*, whole foods would heal the whole earth (Belasco 1993).

Considering the long history of dietary radicalism—with its links to agrarian and ascetic traditions—none of this was really new, and neither was the strong counterreaction it provoked. As I have argued elsewhere (Belasco 1993), the food establishment—comprising mostly people who had won Levenstein's (1988) "revolution" thirty years before—led a "moral panic" in the early 1970s that ridiculed every radical claim and proposal. When the dust had settled (by around 1980), the more far-reaching aspects were largely marginalized—especially organic agriculture, which the public came to associate with drugs, granola, and dirty hippies rather than with its squarely agrarian roots.

But, in the familiar pattern of conservative reform, the mainstream absorbed fragments—particularly those of the most interest to affluent people and the marketers who catered to them. Responding to concerns about poisons, federal agencies banned a handful of pesticides and additives, and marketers rolled out a few premium-priced "natural" foods. Ethnic, gourmet, and regional foods boomed in response to widely shared boredom with homogenized American cuisine, but these, too, tended to become stereotyped and predictable with mass exposure. "Lite" foods were probably a more lasting innovation because they addressed long-standing female concerns about fat and fatness. Nightmares of technological hubris apparently made little impact, for corporate research in biotechnology—the next frontier in the food engineers' war against nature—went on largely unimpeded. Indeed, the food industry of the 1990s was more consolidated and high-tech oriented than ever.

True, the research literature on sustainable alternatives was now vast and impressive, and some highly successful chefs were making noises about going "green." The upper half of the population probably did eat a bit *better* (in cardiovascular terms) than before (Food Marketing Institute 1992a, 1992b; Rich 1992). But it was hard to detect much consumer interest in eating more *responsibly*. Indeed, by mid-1992—just two years after Earth Day revivals—market research seemed to show that consumers and marketers alike were highly cynical about products that claimed to be environmentally safe. "Green" was no more credible than "brown" (natural) (Chase and Smith 1992).

What Works? What Doesn't?

Stepping back from this historical overview, is it possible to generalize about the effectiveness of dietary moralization? Which ethical appeals are most likely to have some impact on mainstream diet, and which appeals are likely to fail? To get at this I first want to introduce a very rudimentary model of food selection that I find useful when I teach about the American food system: normally, people decide what to eat based on a rough negotiation between the dictates of *convenience* and *identity*. "Convenience" encompasses such variables as price, availability, and ease of preparation (which is related to the requirements of energy, time, and skill). "Identity" is a hybrid of personal and cultural influences. The "personal" components include taste, family context, and individual memories. The "cultural" aspects of identity include widely shared values and ideas, extravagant notions about the good life, as well as the community's particular food habits and practices. Deeply rooted in childhood and tradition, the culinary dictates of identity are hard to change.

The challenge for food moralists is to introduce a third set of considerations into the decision-making process: a sense of *responsibility* for the more distant consequences of one's actions. Such consequences encompass not only the effect on one's personal health thirty years down the road but also the impact on other people and places, both today and tomorrow. In effect, the reformer tries to turn the bipolar struggle between convenience and identity into a triangle. Looking back over our history, is it possible to generalize about the American moralist's chances of substantial successes?

First some impressions about the moral appeals that do not work very well. Clearly doomed are reforms that seem excessively *inconvenient*: Sylvester Graham did not make much headway against store-bought bread; the Progressive Era crusader Horace Fletcher was unable to get many people to chew slowly, and few people in our day are willing to spend the time or money to find fresh organic lettuce. Perceptions of cost remain a major obstacle to eating responsibly. Marketers have recently discovered that more affluent shoppers will pay a bit more to save their arteries and reduce waistlines, but few seemed ready to pay a substantially higher price to save the planet—pieties about "green marketing" notwithstanding.

Personal identity also gets in the way, especially strong childhood associations with a particular dish. As marketers know well, consumers consistently resist "healthy" foods that do not "taste good." Although some of this disdain is culturally determined, it is also true that fat, sugar, and salt have inherent taste appeal.

As for *cultural* parameters of identity, it is clear that Americans consistently resist ethical vegetarianism, not just because it seems inconvenient but also because of strongly held moral arguments *for* meat eating: for example, the Bible (man's "dominion" over animals), natural law ("the food chain," "the struggle for survival"), and custom ("we've always eaten meat"). On the other hand, some Americans—particularly middle-class women—have been willing to change the type of meat (beef to chicken) if that seemingly produces tangible and quantifiable benefits (say, a thinner waist.) Perhaps in a culture so enamored of consumption, reforms are more likely to succeed if they entail product *substitutions* rather than overall *reductions*. Although few Victorians accepted the abstinence strategies of Graham and Kellogg, they were willing to replace traditional breakfast meats with whole-grain cold cereals. Upton Sinclair's arduous fasting went largely unnoticed, but many shoppers did switch to seemingly safer branded goods. Eco-poet Gary Snyder's injunction "to live lightly on the earth . . . clad in the sky with the earth for a pillow" is a beautiful countercultural dream, but the reality in the supermarket is the proliferation of "lite" frozen dinners.

There are other cultural determinants. Adulteration exposés have the most impact if they involve wrongdoing in the factory rather than on the farm (or the dump *after* the meal). The public's much-invoked "right to know" rarely extends to the more remote links in the food chain. Scares involving "innocent" children (for example, poisoned milk, Alar) have a great weight, but threats to children who are already born are more worrisome than threats to unborn future generations. Wartime injunctions to conserve and abstain work well, but only until the cease-fire. Appeals with a nostalgic tone (for example, neoethnic, folk, pastoral) may have some force— say, the populist critique of monopolies, the hippie's invocation of natural virtues—but not if they would mean forgoing the low cost and wide accessibility offered by mass production. And, finally, given the cultural "bias of the center," moral appeals must seem moderate, not extreme, made with good humor and good sense; they can't appear humorless or "moralistic."

In short, the food moralist has a very tough row to hoe. It is hard to get adults to think beyond the already-complex dictates of *convenience* and *identity*. Indeed, changing adults may well be a lost cause. Rather than imposing a sense of *responsibility* as an artificial and unloved intruder, reformers need to work on making ethical considerations an inherent part of a child's cultural upbringing. This may be why the more long-lasting dietary transformations have occurred within self-reproducing alternative communities (examples: the Adventists or The Farm). It may also account for Deep Ecology's fascination with the Iroquois Confederacy, whose Great Law equated cultural identity with ethical foresight. "In our every deliberation we must consider the impact of our decisions on the next seven generations." Considering seven generations might be too much to expect of anybody—even the Iroquois—but even one or two would be a good start.

References

Belasco, W. J. 1993. *Appetite for change: How the counterculture took on the food industry*. Ithaca: Cornell University Press.

Berry, W. 1989. The pleasures of eating. *Journal of Gastronomy* 5:125–31.

Bloodworth, W. 1979. From *The Jungle* to *The Fasting Cure*: Upton Sinclair on American food. *Journal of American Culture* 2:444–53.

Brumberg, J. J. 1989. *Fasting girls: The history of Anorexia Nervosa*. Cambridge: Harvard University Press.

Burros, M. 1992. Environmental politics is making the kitchen hotter. *New York Times*, September 30, C1, C6.

Chase, D., and T. K. Smith. 1992. Consumers keen on green but marketers don't deliver. *Advertising Age*. June 29, S2.

Cronon, W. 1991. *Nature's metropolis: Chicago and the Great West*. New York: Norton.

Cummings, R. O. 1940. *The American and his food*. Chicago: University of Chicago Press.

Dickstein, M. 1981. Introduction to *The Jungle*. New York: Bantam.

Food Marketing Institute. 1992a. *Trends 92: Consumer attitudes and the supermarket, 1992*. Washington, D.C.: Food Marketing Institute.

———. 1992b. *Shopping for Health*. Washington, D.C.: Food Marketing Institute.

Green, H. 1986. *Fit for America: Health, fitness, sport and American society*. New York: Pantheon.

Kasson, J. 1987. Rituals of dining: Table manners in Victorian America. In *Dining in America, 1850–1900*, edited by K. Glover. Amherst: University of Massachusetts Press.

Lappé, F. M. 1982. *Diet for a small planet*. New York: Ballantine.

Levenstein, H. 1988. *Revolution at the table: The transformation of the American diet*. New York: Oxford University Press.

Nissenbaum, S. 1988. *Sex, diet, and debility in Jacksonian America: Sylvester Graham and health reform*. Chicago: Dorsey Press.

Rich, S. 1992. Healthful habits of the 1980s may go way of the hula hoop. *Washington Post*, March 12, A2.

Sinclair, U. 1906/1981. *The jungle*. New York: Bantam.

Strasser, S. 1982. *Never done: A history of American housework*. New York: Pantheon.

———. 1989. *Satisfaction guaranteed: The making of the American mass market*. New York: Pantheon.

Telberg, R. 1990. Restaurant industry moved by new moral fervor. *Nation's Restaurant News*, September 3, 22.

Walters, R. 1978. *American reformers, 1815–1860*. New York: Hill & Wang.

Whorton, J. C. 1982. *Crusaders for fitness: The history of American health reformers*. Princeton: Princeton University Press.

The Culture of Public Problems: Drinking–Driving and the Symbolic Order

Joseph R. Gusfield

In 1945 the Yale Summer School of Alcohol Studies published the landmark *Alcohol, Science, and Society*, a collection of the twenty-nine lectures used in its classes (Yale University Center of Alcohol Studies 1945). In his introduction to the book, E. M. Jellinek, the director of the school, wrote that in the past scientists had remained aloof from public issues. The Yale School of Alcohol Studies, of which he was a member and which presented the Summer School, represented for him a redressing of this tendency in science. "In a sense this [Summer] School will be a test of the applicability of scientific thought to the problems of alcohol."

The post-Repeal era of the 1930s and the 1940s was dominated by the ghost of Prohibition and the political conflicts between Wets and Drys (Roizen 1991). The Yale School of Alcohol Studies, founded in 1940, represented the first major effort of an academic research university to address the problems of alcohol from the impartial and factually grounded approach of empirical science. It was an effort to take the issues of alcohol out of politics, morals, and religion; to scientize and depoliticize a public conflict. Mark Keller, one of the original members of the Yale School of Alcohol Studies, describes the mood that inspired him and his colleagues at the time. "Were we not in the age of science? Could not the power of science be brought to bear on these problems?" (Keller 1974, 20).

In the discourse of modern medical science, morality and health seem to represent contrasting ways of thinking about the use of alcoholic beverages. Concern for morality suggests the image of Prohibition, of a religiously motivated criticism of seemingly innocent pleasures. It blurs the distinction between drinking that creates harm and drinking that is part of enjoyment. Concern for health suggests a very different attitude: one that treats conditions that are creating harm without any judgment of sin or virtue. The attitude of morality judges drinking as inherently good or bad, innocent or evil. It mutes the distinction between the uses of drinking and its abuses.

In the contemporary United States alcohol is talked about in the arenas of public health in the language of ethical, moral, and religious neutrality; the language of medical science and social research. Such ways of speaking and writing are presented as a clear contrast to the nineteenth- and early-twentieth-century eras of Temperance and Prohibition in which drinking was seen as inherently sinful and harmful by the movement's partisans.

Despite the seeming break with the ethos of the Temperance and Prohibition eras, a moral paradigm has remained and, even within the scientific modes of discourse, continues to be mixed with the conceptions of health implicit in the scientific perspective. A latent "Puritanism" persists and accentuates the conflicts over the regulation and control of alcohol in the United States and over the designation of health and illness connected with the use of alcohol. The frames of health and morals remain intertwined.

The Frames of Health and Morality

The Social Construction of Reality

In much of human action the real, everyday world in which we act is not the objective, unmediated world of a pristine, self-contained reality. It is infused with meanings and connotations in interaction with those who observe it. It is a product of that interaction constructed within the context of historical, institutional, and cultural elements (Berger and Luckmann 1967).

The term *frame* applied to everyday conduct is a means of defining situations and objects. As Erving Goffman (1974) wrote, "There is a sense in which what is play for the golfer is work for the caddy" (8).

So too in the case of *health*. A condition of the body can be viewed from different points of view or from several at the same time by the same person. What constitutes "health" and "illness" can be perceived within different frames, which permit some conditions to be "in" the frame and others "outside" (Tesh 1988). Pre-existent conditions that might be unnoticed may become noticed. They may be viewed as matters of health and open to treatment, as aspects of inevitable and irremediable human conditions, as matters of political or religious concern. They may be seen as illness in one historical period; as moral dereliction in another; as normal, "healthy" behavior in another.

A good illustration of how the meanings of conditions can change is the phenomenon of pregnancy in industrialized societies. Prior to the late nineteenth century pregnancy and the delivery of babies was not viewed as a condition that normally required the services of physicians (Wertz and Wertz 1989; Arney 1982). The transformation of homosexuality from immorality to emotional disorder to alternative sexual style is an instance of movement out of psychiatric, medical categories into the frame of cultural difference.

Medicalization and Moralization

During World War II an American soldier treated for a venereal disease would lose salary for the time spent in being cured. Though it was seen as disease—a medical condition—there was also a moral judgment that differentiated venereal disease from the common cold or kidney failure. In the decades since World War II venereal diseases have been increasingly viewed in public discussions as medical conditions akin to cancer, pneumonia, or broken bones. The transformation from venereal disease to sexually-transmitted disease has by no means been a complete one. A moral meaning is still attached to sexually transmitted diseases. The patient confronts a world of shame and opprobrium unlike that visited on the victim of heart trouble, cancer, or multiple sclerosis (Brandt 1985).

In recent years a wide number of conditions have been transformed or are in process of transformation from matters of moral judgment into matters of health and medicine. Among these are habitual drunkenness, smoking, opiate addiction, child abuse, gambling, and wildness in children (Conrad 1992; Conrad and Schneider 1980). A striking example is the history of "insanity and hysteria," which has become "mental illness and neurosis" (Foucault 1965; Scull 1979; Rosen 1968).

Sociologists and historians have utilized the concept of "medicalization" to describe the process by which phenomena become perceived as matters of health or illness and thus amenable to understanding and to practical action as medical conditions (Conrad 1992; Conrad and Schneider 1980; Goffman 1961, 321–86; Szaz 1961).

Two dimensions of the medicalization process need to be distinguished. One is the cultural dimension, which refers to how we think about and understand a condition. The concept of "mental illness" is such. A second dimension is the institutional dimension, which refers to the institution and personnel responsible for ameliorating the condition. The transformation of pregnancy into a condition to be treated by physicians is an example.

The Mix of Health and Morality

The cultural and institutional dimensions interact with each other. A consequence of the cultural process of medicalizing is to bring the condition into the agendas of the medical institutions: doctors, nurses, clinics, and so on. In the quest for power and influence, groups and occupations seek to establish the validity of their conceptions of reality and sometimes refashion them as well. Throughout the nineteenth century allopathic medicine sought to establish a dominant role in U.S. medicine and had succeeded by the twentieth (Starr 1982).

Elsewhere I have used the concept of the "ownership of public problems" (Gusfield 1981, 10–11). This phrase describes the group or groups that have legitimacy as the definers and claimants to authority over a public problem. In medicalization, the medical institutions become the "owners"—the legitimate authorities and controllers of the condition. The condition is thought about and described in medical language and imagery, in the culture of medicine.

A condition is moralized, in the context of this paper, when its possessor is perceived and described in terms that define him or her as good or bad, evil or righteous. Institutionally, the immoral person can be treated as a criminal, a sinner, or a villain. Shame and guilt attend the immoral; honor and applause attend the moral. Cigarette smoking in the United States has been moving toward an immoral, deviant status since the initial surgeon general's report of 1964 (Gusfield 1993).

These distinctions between the medical and the moral constitute a necessary background to understanding the place of alcohol and drinking in American life across the past two centuries. The two cultural perspectives—the moral and the medical—are linked in American life, with resultant consequences for social and medical policy.

The differentiation, between the moral and medical, is perhaps more a characteristic of public discourse in American life since World War II than in earlier periods. The cholera epidemic of the 1830s was seen as a visitation of God's wrath by many, retribution for the sinful character of American life. By some others, it was seen as the result of an unjust social system (Rosenberg 1962). The ways in which alcohol is talked about and written about in the United States have usually involved both discourses but in varying degrees and with varying degrees of dominance and marginality. The very problem of this chapter and this volume—the relation of morality and health—is perhaps more salient in the contemporary medical culture because it presupposes the segregation or desegregation of these two arenas of discourse as a problem for understanding and analysis.

Morality and Health in Temperance History, 1800–1933

Drinking has been a political issue in the United States for more than 150 years, sometimes treated as an issue of public morals, sometimes as an issue of public health, sometimes as an issue of public order, often as all of these. The history of drinking in this country is the history of its definition and redefinition (Room 1974).

In a great many societies and in most historical periods the drinking of alcoholic beverages has been viewed as dangerous and risk-producing, as well as pleasurable and even healthful (Heath 1976; Keller 1976; MacAndrews and Edgerton 1969). An illustration of the continuity of fearful concern is found in the British Act of 1606 regulating the operation of alehouses. That legislation described drunkenness as the cause of "Bloodshed, Stabbings, Murder, Swearing, Fornication, Adultery and such like" (Wrightson 1981, 12). Drinking per se was not condemned, but its perceived consequences were feared.

However, although drinking and drunkenness are matters of comment and concern in many places, the circumstances under which that concern is manifest and the beliefs about the role of drinking and its consequences vary considerably. Harry G. Levine (1978) has shown that colonial America recognized a relationship between drunkenness and physical incapacity but did not use the chemical effects of drunkenness as an explanation of accidents or socially disapproved behavior. Alcohol was "the goodly creature of God" and as such not a source of evil. During the nineteenth century this attitude was reversed; many people came to believe that drinking and drunkenness did result in physical harm and social vice. It was also during the nineteenth century that the concept of alcohol as addictive began to emerge (Levine 1978). Alcohol became "Demon Rum."

It was also during the late eighteenth century and early nineteenth that alcohol was claimed by some to be associated with ill health. In the late eighteenth century the physician Benjamin Rush described the consequences of alcohol use in medical terms. Throughout much of the nineteenth century, a conception of the addictive qualities of alcohol was prevalent, even though in a muted form.

Although the harmful effects of alcohol were proclaimed, it was not until the twentieth century that the physiochemical consequences of drinking loomed significantly in condemnation of alcohol use. In the 1940s habitual drunkenness began to be viewed as a medical condition and to be called alcoholism. The consequences of that change and the apparent closing of that era in recent years form an essential part of the story related here.

Colonial America: "The Goodly Creature of God"

One historian has described the drinking habits of colonial America: "Virtually everyone drank virtually all the time" (Blocker 1989, 3). Quite probably this is an exaggeration, but it serves as an apt contrast to later periods. Alcoholic beverages, chiefly hard liquor, were used in many social and work contexts. They were an ubiquitous accompaniment to work, public and familial ceremonies, and entertainments, and of home hospitality, of diet, even of ministerial ordinations (for accounts of drinking in colonial America, see Blocker 1989; Gusfield 1963b; Levine 1978;

Rorabaugh 1979). It was an accepted part of everyday life, useful to health, to social order, and to personal happiness. It was, as the Puritan divine Increase Mather called it, "the goodly creature of God."

Drunkenness was far from uncommon but did not appear to create a problem that led to public action. Taverns were licensed, but there is little evidence of community problems created by drinking. The habitual drunkard was recognized as a distinct social type whose condition was a matter of choice.

Such acceptance of alcohol and drunkenness was not universally applauded. Drunkenness that led to social disorder was a matter of condemnation from some Puritan ministers including Cotton Mather, who distinguished between acceptable use and unacceptable abuse. What elicited much of their criticism was drunkenness among the upper classes and the public disorder that ensued rather than the use of alcohol per se (Rorabaugh 1979, 30–31).

Self-Control and Self-Transformation: The Antebellum Period

The emergence of the Temperance movement in the 1820s occurred under the leadership of evangelical Protestant Christianity. It was a response to a cluster of changes occurring in American society. For the old elite of Federalists, drunkenness was associated with the fear of a popular electorate whose power spelled the demise of the colonial hierarchy (Gusfield 1963b, chap. 2). For employers in a newly developing economy, it was part of a quest for a more disciplined labor force (Tyrell 1979). For the church leadership, drunkenness threatened its vision of purity and the moral man. Urbanization, geographical and social mobility, and familial disorganization had lessened the authoritative controls of earlier periods. The problem of social disorder was on the public agenda, as was an increasing revival of religious sensibilities (Rothman 1971; Boyer 1978).

In the early nineteenth century the weakening of the web of communal, familial, and religious institutions meant that the external, institutional authorities could no longer be depended upon to insure social order (Boyer 1978; Levine 1978; Nissenbaum 1980; Rothman 1971). In colonial America the capacity for self-control as distinct from the controls of external authority was deemed rare (Gusfield

1992; Levine 1978). The appeal to develop self-control and self-transformation was a major part of the Temperance movement. Drinking and drunkenness had been seen as inevitable in colonial America; in the nineteenth century they came to be condemned as deviations from a now-expected capacity for self-control.

This period is marked by the growing role of Temperance organizations. Sobriety was becoming a mark of moral character and a sign of dependable workers. Although the leadership of the early Temperance societies was in the hands of clergy and business or professional elites, in small towns and in other organizations, such as Sons of Temperance, artisans, skilled workers, and farmers were important parts of the membership (Blumin 1989, chap. 6; Gusfield 1963; Ryan 1981, 132–42). In 1848 the Washingtonians, the movement among self-labeled "drunkards" represented still another strand in the efforts to achieve sobriety.

Whether these movements are seen as modes of self-transformation among drinkers or as forms of validating self-identification among upright elites, a common theme of self-control and a fear of its loss are as deeply embedded in Temperance appeals as in evangelical Protestantism. In colonial America the evangelical temperament saw the undisciplined impulses of the self as threats to internal and public order that had to be rooted out through stern external authority (Greven 1977). Temperance preached that self-denial was possible through individual control, through control by the individual (Levine 1978, 1983).

The Moral Character of Health

In the early nineteenth century health and morality were not clearly distinct. Healthy living included abstinence from alcohol, and health was a sign that the person had led a good and moral life. The self-control of a healthy life was also a sign of character, of moral purity (Gusfield 1993). Despite Rush's 1784 essay, a conception of addiction and illness does not appear to dominate the understanding and evaluation of chronic drunkenness in colonial America.[1]

A prevalent view in the antebellum United States often linked health with moral character, and social disorder with epidemics (Fellman and Fellman 1981; Gusfield 1992; Rosenberg 1962; Whorton,1982). Temperance, as well as moderation in diet and other aspects of virtuous habits, showed adherence to God's laws of nature and were ways of achieving good health. Illness was a sign of moral dereliction and a flawed character. In this sense, the conception of the moral man was linked to the conception of the healthy man. For example, Sylvester Graham, the founder of the "natural foods" health movement in the 1830s, described alcohol use as inherently dangerous to human physiology and its use a deviation from God's natural laws (Gusfield 1993).

Nevertheless, to understand how many nineteenth-century Americans perceived issues of health, the general medical culture of the times needs to be understood. The early decades of the 1800s were characterized by the dominance of a view of illness that emphasized the idea of a balance between mind and body. Diseases were not specific but were attributes of a general dysfunction of the body and its relation to the environment. As Charles Rosenberg (1979) has described it:

> The model of the body, and of health and disease, . . . was all-inclusive, antireductionist, capable of incorporating every aspect of man's life in explaining his physical condition. Just as man's body interacted continuously with his environment, so did his mind with his body, his morals with his health. (10)

Although this medical culture was under attack during much of the nineteenth century, especially from elite physicians and science, it persisted among many laypeople and in the practice of many physicians. The medical literature of the late nineteenth century still contained much evidence of a view that health depended on a harmony between nature and the life of the individual (Fellman and Fellman 1981). In this fashion, the social and moral behavior of people was perceived to relate to their health.

By the Civil War, drinking had lost its acceptance throughout society. This is not to say that few people drank or that drunkenness had disappeared but that drinking was now a point of public conflict. It differentiated persons and groups in American life and its public appreciation had lessened. For the churchgoing Protestant middle class, the problem of drinking was preeminently a moral question. The chronic drunkard was a symbol of degradation; the middle-class drunkard a symbol of what could happen through self-indulgence; and lower-class drinking was the source of economic ruin. The tavern, later the saloon, was seen as a site of immorality and political corruption.

From Temperance to Prohibition:
The Quest for Cultural Supremacy

The long movement culminating in Prohibition was composed of several highly organized movements in localities, in states, and ultimately in the nation. These movements were marked by the quest for legal controls on the sale and use of alcoholic beverages. Although this had been a facet of the earlier movements, it was balanced by the self-transformative character of much of the antebellum actions. What stands out in the activities of organizations like the Woman's Christian Temperance Union, the Prohibitionist Party, and, especially, the Anti-Saloon League is the advocacy of the coercive controls of law to restrict the abused substance of alcohol. It is this direction that aroused the conflicts that marked alcohol as a political issue. Whatever its sources, the Temperance movement was not conducted in the spirit or under the auspices of public health. It was a religious and social conflict that marked drinking and abstinence as political symbols.

The battles over legislative acts to restrict or permit the use of wine, beer, and liquor were part of the conflicts over social and political power in American life. Catholics, urban dwellers, and European immigrants were much more accepting of drink as part of everyday life than were Protestants (especially evangelical denominations), native Americans, and rural or rural-origin people. The reform of drinking habits through political action was also a defense of a culture, a style of life in which drinking was a sin. It also informed the efforts to assimilate alien cultures into American life (Gusfield 1963b).

Drinking was also viewed as a threat to the middle-class drinker (Levine 1979, 1983). The saga of the "Face on the Barroom Floor" was the image of the once-established man whose drinking cost him all that was dear: his work, his family, his good reputation. An alternative saga was that of the workman who, by his patronage of the saloon, squandered his salary (Gusfield 1991). The debility of the body was a natural accompaniment to the social and moral downfall of the drinker. Addiction was constantly portrayed as a fear of the middle-class drinker. Temperance literature portrayed the fear of physiological as well as social degradation, but social descent and the loss of good reputation were fears with much greater intensity.

The saloon was also an important focus for movements of the late-nineteenth and early twentieth century. "The working man's club" was seen as a source of crime, prostitution, and the power of the political machine (Duis 1983; Rosen,1982).

In the Temperance and Prohibition movements of the time what role was played by considerations of health? Certainly, the issue of drinking was not approached as a medical one—one in which medical institutions had a special claim to ownership. Nor was the treatment of the chronic inebriate well developed as a specialty of medical institutions. In the last quarter of the nineteenth century, institutions to cure chronic inebriety did appear and were separate from insane asylums as places for the treatment of habitual drunkards. Some physicians began to specialize in the treatment of habitual inebriates and to perceive addiction as a psychological disorder (Baumol 1990). The *Journal of Inebriety* was begun in 1870 and lasted several decades.

We cannot speak of the medicalization of alcohol abuse, however, before the repeal of the Prohibition amendment in 1933. Although all drinking might be viewed as leading to habitual inebriety, individual or public problems of alcohol were neither understood as problems of health nor seen as responsibilities of the medical profession.

The Temperance Ethic and the Ethic of Drinking

In analyzing the history of public actions toward alcohol, it is necessary to keep in mind the diversity of a heterogeneous society and always ask: Whose morals? Whose health? Whose sense of social order? A sense of excessive drinking was common to the nineteenth century in the United States as well (Levine 1978). Despite the dominant role of Protestant churches in the movement for abstinence and the political drive toward Prohibition, there was unease about excessive drinking among Catholics and others in the society. The Catholic Temperance Union was concerned about drinking, but its focus was on excessive drinking and the habitual drunkard; it did not support Prohibition (Bland 1951). It is the distinction between alcohol use and alcohol abuse that is at question. It is the disposition to define all alcohol use as abuse that is the focal point of the Temperance ethic.

A culture that prizes the joys of drinking sustains its detrimental consequences without demanding its eradication. For some, there is a definite yet vague line that separates alcohol abuse from all alcohol use; for others, most use is abuse. This distinction is deep and essential to an understanding of the cultural bases of political and social conflict over the uses of alcohol.

In his history of early modern popular culture (1500–1800) Peter Burke describes how drinking and drunkenness were a source of conflict between elite and popular culture in much of the Europe of that period (Burke 1978, chap. 8; also Clark 1983). Even though any simple thesis of similarity between sixteenth-century Europe and the United States in the nineteenth century is highly misleading, the ethical diversities Burke relates share much with later conflicts in American life and politics.

> In short, we find in this period two rival ethics or ways of life in open conflict. The ethic of the reformers was one of decency, diligence, gravity, modesty, orderliness, prudence, reason, self-control, sobriety, and thrift. . . . The ethic of the reformers was in conflict with a traditional ethic . . . which involved more stress on the values of generosity and spontaneity and a greater tolerance for disorder. (Burke 1978, 213)

The culture of temperance and its ethic of self-control never quite achieved the dominance that the Temperance and Prohibition movements sought. Whether the opposition is within one's own social group or possessors of an alternative culture, an ethic of drinking, as well as an ethic of temperance, is a constant part of American life. While alcohol became the icon of evil for some, it remained the symbol of joyous release from repressive social control for others. A more common attitude unites the two attitudes ambivalently.

From the standpoint of the temperance ethic, the drinker is sinful and in his sinfulness creates trouble for himself and trouble for others. The emphasis is on rowdiness, on violence, on crime, on sexual "misconduct," on accidents involving others, on political protest and riot, on sickness and debility. It is the impact of alcohol on immorality that is the focus. The vision of a harmonious, peaceful, and sedate society without intoxicating beverages is contrasted to the society in which drink is a part of life. Here is the appreciative description by a Fall River textile manufacturer of 1871 of the Fourth of July, usually a rowdy affair among workers for whom it was a joyous holiday: "I have boasted a good deal about them [the workers] since our last Fourth of July celebration, when all were clean, well-dressed and orderly; when everything was quiet; when there was a smile on the face of everyone, and no one was in liquor" (Rosenzweig 1983, 65).

Public Health and the Post-Repeal Era

The Alcoholism Movement: The Deviant Drinker and Health

Dominating the temperance ethic through much of the nineteenth and early twentieth century was a belief in the sinfulness and degradation of drinking per se. Use of spirits, beer, and wine was inherently threatening to the self-control that marked the moral and potentially successful person. Use endangered reputation, social standing, and income, and inevitably brought chronic inebriety and all its attendant harms. The doctrine of abstinence had no place for a distinction between alcohol use as the "goodly creature of God" and alcohol abuse as "Demon Rum." Anything short of abstinence threatened to become addiction and endangered the drinker and those around him.

With the repeal of the Eighteenth Amendment in 1933 the distinction between use and abuse emerged and came to dominate the meanings of alcohol in American life. Alcohol continued to be viewed as a "dangerous commodity" whose sale in most states and localities was limited as to hours, places, and age of customer, and was prohibited in many communities and several states. Nevertheless, the attention of organizations to abstinence disappeared and the focus swung toward a minority of drinkers for whom alcohol was particularly associated with trouble: the alcoholic. The problems of drinking came to be perceived as the problems of some deviant drinkers—of alcoholics and alcoholism.

In several respects the focus on the problem drinker was congruent with the paradigms of modern medicine and its inclusion of emotional disorders into the subject matter of physicians. Here it broke sharply with the religious and medical frameworks that had been part of the pre-Repeal culture. It reflected also the greatly expanded role of medical science and federal government health agencies in defining and publicizing medical science and its advice.

It is of crucial significance to my thesis to recognize that the transformations in the context of alcohol and drinking were also deeply affected by shifts in the society and in medical institutions

occurring in the late nineteenth century and well into the mid-twentieth century. It is these five changes that work to separate the discourses of morality and health.

1. The disease concept of alcoholism. The word *alcoholism* was
   itself relatively new to Americans. It pointed to a specific disease rather than a general condition of the body. To see the alcoholic as suffering from a disease was a clue to alcoholism's
   reception as a problem of medicine, akin to other diseases such
   as cancer, diabetes, or mental illness. The alcoholic was not to
   be classified in religious categories. Even Alcoholics Anonymous, sometimes seen as religiously oriented, shared the view
   that the alcoholic was afflicted with a specific disease. In this
   fashion alcohol addiction was brought into the paradigm of
   disease and therapy that had by now assumed dominance in
   medical culture (Rosenberg 1979).

2. The medicalization of deviant behavior. This was a period in
   American history and in medicine when many emotional states
   were coming into the ambit of medical discussion (Conrad and
   Schneider 1980). The very concept of "mental illness" suggests
   how conditions once experienced as nonmedical were being
   made part of medical institutions.

3. The idea of treatment. If problem drinkers suffered from a disease, then treatment should be possible. An industry of medical, psychiatric, and quasi-medical personnel developed to
   attempt the cure of alcoholism (Fingarette 1988, 23–24; Cahn
   1970, chap. 6). Research in the biological and social sciences
   could address the conditions of the alcoholic.

4. The alcoholic could be seen as a patient rather than a sinner.
   Modern medicine has been distinguished from earlier paradigms
   by its scientific attitude. Alcoholism and the alcoholic were not
   to be blamed for a condition that afflicted them but not other
   drinkers. Taking the onus of moral dereliction from the alcoholic was an almost explicit element in the promulgation of the
   term and in its medicalization (Jellinek 1960, chap. 1).

5. Shift from institutional to personal change. In Roizen's (1991)
   term, alcohol as a substance was "devilified." A consequence
   of the changed perspective was that drinking was a problem
   for only the deviant drinker. As the alcohol industry expressed
   it, "The problem is in the man and not in the bottle." An in-

ference could be drawn from the discourse and logic of the health perspective: if drinking had no unhealthy or pathological consequences, there should be no objection to it.

Prevention and Public Health: The Continuance of Moral Stigma

Although the disease concept helped support governmental aid for treatment, it is doubtful that it was ever widely accepted by most Americans. Surveys indicated that many respondents agreed that it was a disease, but they also deemed the alcoholic responsible for his condition (Moore 1972; Mulford 1964; Rodin,1981; Room 1983a).

Nevertheless, facilities and personnel for treatment of the alcoholic grew considerably during the sixties and seventies. Not only psychiatrists but other physicians were drawn into provision of treatment services, and insurance companies began to consider alcoholism a medical condition warranting health insurance payments for treatment. Roizen's (1991) conclusion that after Repeal alcohol was devilified should be tempered by the realization that its status as a dangerous commodity remained. The moral condemnation of all but abstinence remained an active force in American life, though weakened by the retreat of active religion from the field of battle. If Prohibition was dead, its ghost still hovered in the wings, whether in new or old clothes. As Room (1983b) has put it: "Whatever one may think about the wisdom of the provision, a society which does not allow children into pubs with their parents is not a society which is treating alcohol like any other commodity" (266).

The Public Health Movement in Alcohol

By the early 1970s the alcoholism perspective began to lose its dominance in public arenas and policy areas. The line between the deviant drinker, the alcoholic, and the population of other drinkers became blurred. In the concept of "problem drinker" the object of concern was broadened (Cahalan, Cisin, and Crossley 1969). The issue of drinking and driving, involving harm to others, was the focus of much public attention to alcohol issues in the late 1970s. In keeping with the general movement toward prevention of illness in many areas of medicine, attention turned toward the drinking habits of the general population: alcoholics, problem drinkers, nonproblem drinkers. It became an issue of public health (Bruun et al. 1975).

In practice the prevention movement in alcohol has been largely associated with attempts to diminish the total consumption of alcohol through measures such as increased taxation and laws that mandate signs or education about such issues as the fetal alcohol syndrome and the dangers of drinking and driving. This point of view reintroduces the vilification of alcohol. Analogous to the Temperance movement, it places attention on the institutional aspects of market and legal controls that affect the availability of alcohol for the total population. Although the cultural sources of this public health framework are very different from the older Temperance movement, the object, total consumption, is similar.

But drinking has become an object of public health and medicine from another standpoint, widening the spectrum of people who are seen as at risk in drinking. The healthful lifestyle or health-fitness movement provides another source for the revilification of alcohol based on medical science and carrying the legitimation of governmental medical agencies.

Alcohol and the Health-Fitness Movement

The conception of health is itself undergoing a shift away from the view of illness as an agent of external factors such as bacteria and viruses. For a variety of reasons beyond the scope of this chapter, the habits of patients have come to be seen as instrumental in preventing or creating illness. The promotion of health through changes in lifestyle is today a significant part of public health promotion (Goldstein 1991).

Rather than perceiving illness as a condition divorced from personal character or lifestyle, to see cancer or heart trouble as consequences of personal habits is to shift, to some degree, the nature of the disease and responsibility for its occurrence onto the person (Crawford 1979). In this fashion, medicine comes to emphasize prevention of diseases by proper living.

Who, then, is the healthful person? What is the lifestyle enjoined by the transformation of health from the treatment domain of the medical institution to the domain of the individual? The healthful person incorporates the pursuit of good health into his or her daily life, at work and at leisure. He or she eats nutritiously, exercises, has only "safe sex," doesn't smoke and avoids smoke, limits or eliminates drinking, watches caloric intake, and aims at reducing weight (Goldstein 1991). Health is not the absence of illness but something pursued in the very way we behave (Stone 1986; Zola 1978; Gusfield 1992). The healthful person is also a person of moral character, of self-control.

The Changing Medical Paradigm

The healthy-lifestyle movement, whatever its sources in institutional and economic concerns, presents a framework of meanings analogous to the older frameworks of nineteenth-century thought. It places the causes of disease and pathology, in part, in the behavioral conduct of the individual. "Immoderate drinking" is part of the complex of pathogenic behaviors. Illness is neither random nor external to the conduct of the person. Alcohol, like tobacco, is seen as increasing the risks of a variety of illnesses, including accidents, heart troubles, kidney distress, fetal deformities, and other ailments, as well as those mostly specific to it, such as cirrhosis of the liver. Such risks are not confined to people labeled "alcoholic." The advice is generalized to the total population of possible drinkers (U.S. Department of Health, Education, and Welfare 1979).

It is in this sense that both the alcohol-prevention movement, with its emphasis on total consumption, and the healthy-lifestyle movement return to a position that blurs the differences between use and abuse so that most use is abusive.

Criminalization of Drunkenness

In one area of alcohol control there has been a distinct move toward substituting a medical for a legal, quasi-criminal attitude toward drunkenness. This is the movement toward placing public drunks in the hands of detoxification centers rather than jails (Pittman 1991); of defining public drunkenness as a health problem rather than a law-enforcement problem. However, in the past two decades there has also been a decided move toward more severe punishment for drinking drivers, lowered minimum ages for buying alcohol, and harsher punishment of drinkers involved in accidents harming others (Gusfield 1988; Reinarman 1988). The "new Temperance movement" has involved a sharper, more condemnatory approach to drinking than marked the period of focus on alcoholism. These changes in public attitudes have occurred with little, if any, evidence that alcohol problems connected with them had increased.

This should not be understood to mean that I am describing a total return to the moral condemnation of alcohol that inspired the Temperance and Prohibition movements of the nineteenth century. The public health perspectives, both the total consumption and the disease preventions, are products of academic, scientific, and public health institutions. They are presented in the discourse and style of amoral medical and social science. Yet the break with the nineteenth century and the religious-moral basis of judgment is not as sharp nor as deep as meets the casual eye.

The Pathological Framework: Alcohol in Law and Research

The ubiquitousness of the mind-altering usage for alcohol suggests that it is a persistent and very widespread part of human leisure.[2] Studies abound of how drunkenness results in dangerous behavior or in detrimental results, such as injury, death, or addiction. Studies of drunkenness that does not have such results are absent from the literature. Drunkenness is not studied as "normal" or "natural" behavior. Nor are the pleasurable aspects of tavern life (Oldenburg 1989).

The "Malevolence Assumption"

Where drinking is associated with a detrimental or disapproved condition, it is usually assumed that alcohol was the cause. In a review and assessment of the impact of alcohol on wife beating and child abuse, Claire Hamilton and James Collins, Jr. (1981) have coined the useful phrase "the malevolence assumption" to describe this significant element in much current alcohol research (261).

The assumption persists that if alcohol is present in any incident of accident, crime, or other "trouble," it is the causal factor responsible for the action. In cases of felony drunken driving where an injury has occurred, the presence of a blood alcohol count above the legal limit is sufficient to prove guilt. A relation between the condition of the driver and the accident need not be shown. The act of drinking cannot be beneficial. Its appearance displays the malevolent character of the drinker.

It is rare to find studies of the exact relation between accidents and alcohol. Social research into drinking and driving generally also presumes that the existence of alcohol in association with an accident implies a causal relationship. Similarly, most research on alcohol concentrates on the pathology, the evil consequences, and ignores whatever may be the beneficial or pleasurable but nonpathological consequences. It is symbolic of the perspective toward drinking that underlies its meaning in relation to illness that proposed increases in taxes on alcohol and cigarettes are called "sin taxes."

There is a continuity between these views of the assumed evil of drinking and the place of alcohol in the health-fitness movement described above. What is prized is the person able to control himself or herself, to resist temptations of food or sex or cigarettes or alcohol. Those who cannot resist are the fools and villains of this drama. The movement reintroduces a moral element in the characterization of health and illness. What is prized is a person who possesses capacities for self-control and self-denial. As one student of the movement has put it in a paper on jogging: "But the enduring interest in fitness reflects a profound conviction on the part of the educated, affluent segment of America that clean, good living is at the heart of good individual and societal health" (Gillick 1984, 383).

All of these elements—the assumed malevolence of alcohol in law, in social research, and in the health-fitness movement—are ways of seeing drinking as a sign of weak and deficient character, which is itself a sign of illness. This is a view that the nineteenth century Temperance movement would have found congenial. It again unites the medical and the moral.

Science, the Temperance Ethic, and American Exceptionalism

For many Europeans the American Temperance ethic has seemed exceptional, a vestige of American Puritanism. The experience of Prohibition, the continuing and increasing legal constraints on drinking, the ambivalence of many drinkers about consumption, the cult of abstinence—all these stand in clear contrast with most other industrialized, modern societies, including Japan. Only in the United States, Scandinavia, and, to a much lesser extent, the United Kingdom have there been significant Temperance movements. How can this exceptional aspect of American culture be understood? How can its continuing presence in an age of scientific authority and discourse be explained? How has the moral meaning of drinking persisted in an age of the science of health?

The question is too broad for analysis in this chapter. In this final section I can offer only some aspects of an answer. It focuses on the relation between the moral meaning of self-control and the uses of leisure.

In a recent paper, Harry G. Levine (1993; see also 1978, 1979) has drawn on several of his studies to advance a theory to explain American exceptionalism. Using such comparative work as exists, he concludes that societies with Temperance societies are characterized by two conditions that differentiate them from other industrialized societies: the dominant mode of alcohol consumption is ardent spirits and the dominant religion is Protestantism, especially evangelical forms. In Levine's view, the clue to the impact of Protestantism on Temperance lies in the great importance that Protestantism gave to the necessity of self-control in a period of emergent industrial capitalism; internalized rules as distinct from the social controls of external authority.

In another recent paper, Craig Reinarman (1992), building on Levine's work, has suggested that the recent revivals of Temperance sentiment in the United States are sparked by conditions of postmodernity. The postmodern society manifests an intense preoccupation with mass consumption of goods. It appeals to and accentuates the desire for material goods and satisfaction of desires. Unhappiness is a cardinal vice. Under the temptations of a consumer-oriented culture and its institutions, the problems of maintaining control and discipline over desires are magnified.

> [T]here are increasing incentives for indulgence—more ways to lose self-control—and fewer and fewer countervailing capacities for retaining it. . . . People must continuously manage the contradiction between a Temperance culture that insists on self-control and a mass consumption culture which renders self-control continuously problematic. (Reinarman 1992, 21)

Playtime and Work Time:
A Theory of Culture Release

These analyses are stimulating and, in my judgment, go to the heart of the question. The difficulty with them is that they go only halfway there. Self-control is only part of the story because, for most drinkers, the loss of self-control under specified and patterned conditions is consistent with the reign of self-control in other specified and patterned conditions (LeMasters 1975; Gusfield 1993, 112–17; Williams 1951, chap. 10). This is the crux of the moral approval of the distinction between alcohol use and abuse. Many drinkers, if not most, can and do reconcile sobriety and insobriety; inhibition and disinhibition; restriction and release.

Understanding of leisure time and its diverse meanings is a necessary clue to the American Temperance ethic. By the time of the Civil War in the United States, the relationship between middle-class life and abstinence was in place. Drunkenness at work was no longer acceptable behavior. Alcohol was no longer an accompaniment to work. Drinking had become, if acceptable at all, an aspect of leisure time, of play, ceremony, and holiday. A "high culture" that prized sobriety and re-creation was in conflict with a "popular culture" that accepted, tolerated, and even prized an ethic of "tolerance for disorder." But the time for such disorder was standardized and encapsulated; it was part of playtime and not the "serious work" of familial and work responsibilities.

Many have noted a distinction in the use of alcohol in Scandinavian countries and in English-speaking countries compared to other European countries, especially the Mediterranean countries and Germany. Where alcohol is taken as beer and wine, it is understood as a food or an accompaniment to food. Its major usage and purpose is not that of mind alteration; it is not a contrast to the workday or to familial roles. Even where spirits are the customary drink, as in eastern European Jewish groups, there may be a similar meaning given to alcohol (Snyder 1958).

The concept of leisure is itself a product of modern, industrial life. Both as symbol and as actuality, modern life is displayed in the contrast between work time and playtime (Gusfield 1987; Marrus 1974). The periodization of modern life contrasts with the less definitive daily agendas of peasant societies. The various discussions of Saint Monday describe the bursts of work and nonwork often characteristic of preindustrial life (Gutman 1977, chap. 1; Kaplow 1980; Thompson 1967).

Leisure, however, can be directed by very diverse orientations. It can be conceived as "re-creation"; that is, as activity that strengthens and supports the work time and the "serious" in life. A sermon of a nineteenth-century American minister illustrates this in its title, "Christian Recreation and Unchristian Amusements." The minister warned against the stimulation and excitement of the stage and other enjoyments that "do not strengthen us for the work of the following day and lack spiritual value" (Gusfield 1963b, 30–31).

The ethical content of "re-creation" is in its continuity to the "serious" activity of daily work. I want to suggest an additional way of seeing leisure that is also a part of American society and often not noted. Another form of discontinuity is to see leisure as a time for even more "serious" activity: to re-creation I want to add spiritual pursuit. Here it is leisure that is reserved for the serious in life; whose discontinuity with "ordinary life" emphasizes the orderliness of action, its devotion to self-improvement, its dedication to the transcendental.

Still another point of view in regard to leisure lays stress on a different form of discontinuity; on the role of leisure as "playtime." In this formulation leisure that is play may be unserious and indifferent to the frame of mind and situation that is serious. In another form it may be precisely in opposition to the serious world but bounded by its own "territorial" rules (Bateson 1972; Callois 1961; Goffman 1974; Huizinga 1950).

Several students of drinking behavior have suggested one form of play as deeply inherent in many leisure actions. We can see in modes of cultural remission or cultural release what Sherri Cavan (1966) has labeled "time out." It is found in many places and at many times in modern as well as other periods in human history (Gusfield 1963a; Rieff 1966; Turner 1969).

Cohen and Taylor (1992) have described a wide variety of what they call "escape attempts." Holidays, social parties, vacations, picnics, and public drinking places are all instances marked by behavior that sets them apart from the daily round of serious work and human relations. They are ways in which people seek forms of culture release; a discontinuity between the "serious" and the "unserious"; between work time and fun time. In a phrase used as part of the title of their book, Cohen and Taylor have referred to such escapes as "resistance to everyday life."

It is important to recognize that such releases are not oppositions to everyday life, though they are antitheses to the demands of impulse restriction and the self-discipline of work and familial roles.

Many people are able to manage both—commitment to the serious and to play; to sobriety in particular times and places, and to drinking and drunkenness in other times and places. They can recognize and act upon the normative frameworks of both. When release breaks its accepted boundaries and intrudes on the serious, that is defined as pathological. It is not a matter of behavior but of behavior outside its normatively fixed borders.

Alcohol is, and has been, the classic "escape attempt." Cavan (1966) has described public drinking places for the contemporary American society, and MacAndrew and Edgerton (1969, chap. 6) for many primitive and peasant ones in these terms:

> The characteristic feature of these unserious times and places is that they grant the right to be indifferent about matters that would otherwise obligate concern by absolving them of the consequences they would otherwise be expected to have. They establish, as it were, a time-out period when the constraint and respect the social world ordinarily requires is no longer demanded and, hence, they permit even for the ordinarily prudent what would otherwise be considered social licentiousness. (Cavan 1966, 235)

Cavan's view, insightful as it is, lies in the assumption that such cultural release, though institutionalized, represents a consensus within the society about the proper form of impropriety. The history of drinking controls in United States as a source of political and social conflict indicates that the "toleration of disorder" is not uniformly shared; that "time out" is fun for some but abhorrent to others. For some, use is abuse, and "time out" is abuse of time. Health is a measure of character and consistency the mark of virtue. Illness that stems from the use of alcohol is illness produced by a flaw in character.

In the 1890s the Committee of Fifty, composed of members of the U.S. economic and political elite, attempted to bring a more detached attitude toward questions of alcohol use, one that was less bound by religious doctrine (Levine 1983). In the 1940s the Yale School of Alcohol Studies attempted to bring a scientific attitude toward alcohol use, one devoid of moral judgments. In the 1980s public health attempted to bring alcohol use more fully into the medical frame. These efforts to "sanitize," secularize, and objectify the drinking event have had little impact. If the evangelical churches no longer own the public problem of drinking in the United States, the ghost of that ownership still retains its hold in the assumption that the moral life is also the healthy life; that sobriety is virtue and drinking is villainous; that illness is a sign of sin and health the reward of virtue.

Notes

1. Here I am deeply indebted to Levine for his insights on the ideology of self-control, but I differ in the importance that he gives to a conception of addiction in the Temperance movement of the nineteenth century. While a concept of the drunkard as "out of control" and "enslaved" does appear, it is, in my judgment, subordinated to a general hatred of the state of drunkenness, whether in the habitual drunkard or in others (Levine 1978).
2. This section draws on part of chapter 3 in Gusfield (1996).

References

Arney, W. R. 1982. *Power and the profession of obstetrics*. Chicago: University of Chicago Press.

Bateson, Gregory. 1972. A theory of play and fantasy. In his *Steps to an ecology of mind*. New York: Ballantine Books.

Baumol, Jim. 1990. Inebriate institutions in North America, 1840–1920. *British Journal of Addiction* 85:1187–1204.

Berger, P., and T. Luckmann. 1967. *The social construction of reality*. Garden City, N.Y.: Anchor Books.

Bland, Sister Joan. 1951. *Hibernian crusade*. Washington, D.C.: Catholic University Press.

Blocker, Jack S. 1989. *American temperance movements: Cycles of reform*. Boston: Twayne.

Blumin, Stuart. 1989. *The emergence of the middle class: Social experience in the American city, 1760–1900*. Cambridge: Cambridge University Press.

Boyer, Paul. 1978. *Urban masses and moral order in America, 1820–1920*. Cambridge: Harvard University Press.

Brandt, Allan. 1985. *No magic bullet: A social history of venereal disease in the United States since 1880*. New York: Oxford University Press.

Brennan, Thomas. 1988. *Public drinking and popular culture in eighteenth century France*. Princeton: Princeton University Press.

Bruun, Kettil, et al. 1975. *Alcohol control policies in public health perspective*. Helsinki: Finnish Foundation for Alcohol Studies.

Burke, Peter. 1978. *Popular culture in early modern Europe*. New York: Harper.

Cahalan, D., I. Cisin, and H. Crossley. 1969. *American drinking practices: A national study of drinking behavior and attitudes*. Monographs of the Rutgers Center of Alcohol Studies, no. 6. Rutgers Center of Alcohol Studies, New Brunswick. New Haven, Conn.: College and University Press.

Cahn, Sidney. 1970. *The treatment of alcoholics: An evaluative study*. New York: Oxford University Press.

Caillois, Roger. 1961. *Man, play and games*. New York: Schocken Books.

Cavan, Sherri. 1966. *Liquor license*. Chicago: Aldine.

Cohen, Stanley, and Laurie Taylor. 1992. *Escape attempts: The theory and practice of resistance to everyday life*. London: Routledge.

Conrad, Peter. 1992. Medicalization and social control. *Annual Review of Sociology* 18:209–32.

Conrad, Peter, and Joseph Schneider. 1980. *Deviance and medicalization: From badness to sickness*. St. Louis: C. V. Mosby.

Crawford, Robert. 1979. Individual responsibility and health: Politics in the 1970s. In *Health care in America*, edited by S. Reverby and D. Rosner. Philadelphia: Temple University Press.

Duis, Perry. 1983. *The saloon: Public drinking in Chicago and Boston, 1880–1920*. Urbana: University of Illinois Press.

Fellman, Anita, and Michael Fellman. 1981. *Making sense of self: Medical advice literature in late nineteenth century America*. Philadelphia: University of Pennsylvania Press.

Fingarette, Herbert. 1988. *Heavy drinking*. Berkeley: University of California Press.

Foucault, Michel. 1965. *Madness and civilization: A history of insanity in the age of reason*. New York: New American Library.

Gillick, M. R. 1984. Jogging and the moral life. *Journal of Health Politics, Policy and Law* 9 (fall): 369–87.

Goffman, Erving. 1961. *Asylums*. Garden City, N.Y.: Anchor Books.

———. 1974. *Frame analysis: An essay on the organization of experience*. Cambridge: Harvard University Press.

Goldstein, Michael. 1991. *The health movement: Promoting fitness in America*. Boston: Twayne.

Greven, Philip. 1977. *The Protestant temperament: Patterns of child-rearing, religious experience, and the self in early America.* New York: Knopf.

Gusfield, Joseph. 1963a. *The 'double plot' in institutions.* Unpublished. *Patua University Journal* 18:1–9.

———. 1963b. *Symbolic crusade: Status politics and the American temperance movement.* 2d ed. 1986. Urbana: University of Illinois Press.

———. 1981. *The culture of public problems: Drinking-driving and the symbolic order.* Chicago: University of Chicago Press.

———. 1982. Prevention: Rise, decline and renaissance. In *Alcohol, science and society,* edited by E. Gomberg, H. White, and J. Carpenter. Ann Arbor: University of Michigan Press.

———. 1991. Benevolent repression: Popular culture, social structure and the control of drinking. In *Drinking: Behavior and belief in modern history,* edited by S. Barrows and R. Room. Berkeley: University of California Press.

———. 1992. Nature's body and the metaphors of food and health. In *Cultivating differences,* edited by M. Fourier and M. Lamont. Chicago: University of Chicago Press.

———. 1993. *The social symbolism of smoking and health.* In *Smoking: Law, policy and culture,* edited by S. Sugarman and R. Rabin. New York: Oxford University Press.

———. 1996. *Contested meanings: The construction of alcohol problems.* Madison: University of Wisconsin Press.

Gutman, Herbert. 1977. *Work, culture and society in industrializing America.* New York: Vintage Books.

Hamilton, Claire, and James Collins, Jr. 1981. The role of alcohol in wife beating and child abuse. In *Drinking and crime,* edited by James Collins, Jr. London: Tavistock.

Heath, Dwight. 1976. Anthropological perspectives on alcohol: An historical review. In *Cross-cultural approaches to the study of alcohol: An interdisciplinary perspective,* edited by M. Everett, J. Waddell, and D. Heath. The Hague: Mouton.

Huizinga, Johan. 1950. *Homo ludens: A study of the play element in culture.* Boston: Beacon Press.

Jellinek, E. K. 1960. *The disease concept of alcoholism.* New Haven, Conn.: Hillhouse Press.

Kaplow, Jeffrey. 1980. Saint Monday and the artisanal tradition in nineteenth century France. Lecture, University of California, San Diego, Department of History.

Keller, Mark. 1976. Problems with alcohol: An historical perspective. In *Alcohol and alcohol problems: New thinking and new directions,* edited by W. Filstead, J. J. Rossi, and M. Keller. Cambridge, Mass.: Ballinger.

LeMasters, E. E. 1975. *Blue-collar aristocrats: Life-styles at a working-class tavern.* Madison: University of Wisconsin Press.

Levine, Harry Gene. 1978. The discovery of addiction. *Journal of Studies on Alcohol* 39:143–74.

———. 1979. Demon of the middle class: Liquor, self-control and temperance ideology in 19th.-century America. Ph.D. diss., University of California, Berkeley.

———. 1983. The Committee of Fifty and the origins of alcohol control. *Journal of Drug Issues* (winter): 95–116.

MacAndrew, Craig, and Robert Edgerton. 1969. *Drunken comportment: A social explanation.* Chicago: Aldine.

Marrus, Michael. 1974. *The emergence of leisure.* New York: Harper & Row.

Moore, Robert. 1972. Comments on "The Alcohologist's Addiction." *Quarterly Journal of Studies on Alcohol* 33:1043–59.

Mulford, Harold, and Donald Miller. 1964. Measuring public acceptance of the alcoholic as a sick person. *Quarterly Journal of Studies on Alcohol*, 25:314–23.

Nissenbaum, Stephen. 1980. *Sex, diet and debility in Jacksonian America: Sylvester Graham and health reform.* Westport, Conn.: Greenwood Press.

Oldenburg, Ray. 1989. *The great good place: Cafes, coffee shops, community centers, beauty parlors, general stores, bars, hangouts, and how they get you through the day.* New York: Paragon House.

Pittman, David. 1991. Social policy and habitual drunkenness offenders. In *Alcohol: The development of sociological perspectives on use and abuse*, edited by P. Roman New Brunswick: Rutgers Center on Alcohol Studies.

Reinarman, Craig. 1988. The social construction of an alcohol problem. *Theory and Society* 17:91–120.

———. 1992. *The Protestant ethic, the spirit of capitalism, and the problem of pleasure in postmodernity.* Paper presented to the Society for the Study of Social Problems, August.

Rieff, Phillip. 1966. *The triumph of the therapeutic: Uses of faith after Freud.* New York: Harper & Row.

Rodin, Miriam. 1981. Alcoholism as a folk disease. *Journal of Studies on Alcohol* 42:822–35.

Roizen, Ron. 1991. *The American Discovery of Alcoholism.* Ph.D. diss., University of California, Berkeley.

Room, Robin. 1974. Governing images and the prevention of alcohol problems. *Preventive Medicine* 3:11–23.

———. 1983a. Sociology and the disease concept of alcoholism. In *Research advances in alcoholism and alcohol studies*, vol. 7; edited by R. Smart. New York & London: Plenum Press.

———. 1983b. Paternalism, rationality and the special status of alcohol in *Economics and alcohol: Consumption and control*, edited by Marcus Grant, Martin Plant, and Alan Williams. London: Crown, Helm; New York: Gardner Press.

Rorabaugh, Wiliam. 1979. *The alcoholic republic: An American tradition.* New York: Oxford University Press.

Rosen, George. 1968. *Madness in society: Chapters in the historical sociology of mental illness.* New York: Harper & Row.

Rosen, Ruth. 1982. *The lost sisterhood.* Baltimore: Johns Hopkins University Press.

Rosenberg, Charles. 1962. *The cholera years: The United States in 1832, 1849, and 1866.* Chicago: University of Chicago Press.

———. 1979. The therapeutic revolution: Medicine, meaning and social change in nineteenth-century America. In *The therapeutic revolution: Essays in the social history of American medicine*, edited by M. Vogel and C. Rosenberg. Philadelphia: University of Pennsylvania Press.

Rosenzweig, Roy. 1983. *Eight hours for what we will: Leisure in an industrial city, 1870–1920.* New York: Cambridge University Press.

Rothman, David. 1971. *The discovery of the asylum: Social order and disorder.* Boston: Little, Brown.

Ryan, Mary. 1981. *Cradle of the middle class: The family in Oneida, New York, 1790–1865.* Cambridge: Cambridge University Press.

Scull, Andrew. 1979. *Museums of madness: The social organization of insanity in 19th. century England.* London: Allen Lane.

Snyder, Charles R. 1958. *Alcohol and the Jews: A cultural study of drinking.* Glencoe, Ill.: Free Press.

Starr, Paul. 1982. *The social transformation of American medicine.* New York: Basic Books.

Stone, Deborah. 1986. The resistible rise of preventive medicine. *Journal of Health Politics, Policy and Law* 11:671–95.

Szaz, Thomas. 1961. *The myth of mental illness.* New York: Harper & Row.

Tesh, Sylvia. 1988. *Hidden arguments: Political ideology and disease prevention policy.* New Brunswick: Rutgers University Press.

Thompson, E. P. 1967. Time, work-discipline, and industrial capitalism. *Past and Present* 38:56–97.

Turner, Victor. 1969. *The ritual process*. Harmondsworth, Eng.: Penguin Books.

Tyrell, Ian. 1979. *Sobering up: From temperance to prohibition in antebellum America, 1800–1860*. Westport, Conn.: Greenwood Press.

U.S. Department of Health, Education, and Welfare. 1979. *Healthy people: The surgeon-general's report on health promotion and disease prevention*. Washington, D.C.: Government Printing Office.

Wertz, R., and D. Wertz. 1989. *Lying in: A history of childbirth in America*. New Haven: Yale University Press.

Whorton, James. 1982. *Crusaders for fitness: The history of American health reformers*. Princeton: Princeton University Press.

Williams, Robin. 1951. *American society: A sociological interpretation*. New York: Knopf.

Wrightson, Keith. 1981. Alehouses, order, and reformation in rural England. In *Popular culture and class conflict, 1590–1914*, edited by E. Yeo and S. Yeo. Sussex: Harvester Press.

Yale University Center of Alcohol Studies. 1945. *Alcohol, science, and society*. New Haven: Quarterly Journal of Studies on Alcohol.

Zola, Irving. 1972. Medicine as an institution of social control. In *The cultural crisis of modern medicine*, edited by J. Ehrenreich. New York: Monthly Review Press.

Morality, Religion, and Drug Use

David T. Courtwright

Moral and religious beliefs affect the ways in which people understand drug use and abuse, what they think should be done about it, and whether they themselves use illicit drugs. I say moral and religious beliefs because it is difficult, in the context of American history, to disentangle the two. Of all developed Western nations, the United States has been and still is the most overtly religious (Wills 1990, 15–17). The foundation of American morality is the Judeo-Christian tradition.

Religious Temperaments

Before discussing drug use, treatment, and policy, I would like to sketch a framework for understanding American moral and religious beliefs. It is based on the work of the historian Philip Greven (1977), who has described how early American religious experience was related to patterns of child rearing and attitudes toward the self. Greven argued that there were essentially three Protestant "temperaments": the Evangelical, the Moderate, and the Genteel.

The inner experience of the strictly disciplined Evangelicals was one of self-suppression, even self-obliteration. They believed that humanity was deeply flawed and that those who thought otherwise, who preoccupied themselves with earthly affairs and bodily pleasures, were headed for hell, to which God might dispatch them at any moment. Evangelicals hoped to escape this fate by virtue of their having been reborn. They had undergone a life-transforming religious experience rooted in the conviction of personal worthlessness and a resolve to subjugate their wills completely to that of God.

Not so the Moderates, who possessed a certain hard-won equanimity. Raised by parents who combined love and discipline, the Moderates acknowledged that the self needed to be watched and controlled but not annihilated. Moderates believed in sin but not that everything worldly was sinful. Grace and salvation might come to an individual gradually rather than suddenly; what mattered was the long, patient struggle to keep one's desires within reasonable bounds. Duty, restraint, order, balance—these were the guiding principles for both the Moderates' secular and religious lives.

Religion for the Genteel was more casual. They "took their state of grace for granted," Greven wrote, "when they cared about such matters at all, and were generally confident that the church and the sacraments, which they acknowledged, sufficed to ensure their personal salvation" (14). The Genteel led self-confident, self-assertive lives and displayed a fondness for high living that shocked the Evangelicals (Isaac 1974). The Genteel behaved this way because, in contrast to the Evangelicals, they had been raised by indulgent and, for the most part, wealthy parents who lavished affection upon them. The Genteel child thus grew up with a relaxed conscience, a benevolent conception of God, and a notion that church was a good place to catch up on gossip.

These three religious temperaments were not entirely distinct. Rather, they formed a continuum ranging from Genteel self-assertion on the left to Moderate self-control in the middle to Evangelical self-suppression on the right. This continuum still characterizes the divisions among twentieth-century American Protestants (Roof and McKinney 1987, 72–105) and, with appropriate changes in terminology, can be extended to Catholics and Jews as well:

self-dominant	self-assertive		self-controlled	self-suppressed
X————————	—X————————		—X————————	—X————————
Unchurched	Genteel	(P)	Moderate	Evangelical
Nonpracticing	Selective	(C)	Observant	Devout
Nonreligious	Reform	(J)	Conservative	Orthodox

Catholics and Jews, like Protestants, can be thought of as having temperaments. These I have labeled, imperfectly, as Devout, Observant, and Selective for the Catholics; as Orthodox, Conservative, and Reform for the Jews. Of course, there are also Jews who belong to no synagogue, just as there are Protestants and Catholics who attend no church. It is therefore necessary to extend the spectrum of belief—or, more precisely, nonbelief—to the left by adding a fourth category, the self-dominant. This would include people from all three religious backgrounds who do not attend any services, who doubt or deny the existence of God, and who expect that whatever meaning or pleasure life holds is to be realized in this world, not in the next. The number of such persons has grown in recent decades. Americans who told pollsters that they had no religion made up less than 3 percent of the population in 1957 but increased to 10 percent by 1988. (Religion in America 1982, 20, 41, 44, 45; Johnson 1985; McNamara 1985; Williamsburg Charter Foundation 1988, 34–35; Goldman 1991).

The further one is to the right of a given continuum—for brevity, let us call it the moral right—the more likely one is to believe in free will, sin, the appropriateness of punishment, and absolute moral standards as expressed in the Bible, in Canon Law, or in the Torah. (Or, for the Mormons, the Book of Mormon; for Muslims, the Koran; and so on.) Legislation against the violation of these standards is at once symbolic and instrumental. It reiterates conservative moral norms and discourages behavior that is thought to be reprehensible and destructive of family life. For moral rightists, the family is the fundamental, indispensable unit of society. Hierarchical rather than individualistic thinking predominates among them. Individuals should subordinate their desires to the wishes of familial, community, state, and other legitimate authorities, provided only that their orders do not countermand those of the Ultimate Authority.

Those who are on the moral left are inclined to question authority, to reject the concept of absolute (let alone divinely inspired) moral standards, and to oppose the prosecution of what they call victimless crimes. When confronted with a prohibition they typically ask, "Why not?" If no convincing secular answer, grounded in utilitarian or consequentialist ethics, is forthcoming, they assume that the prohibition is unjustified and should be repealed. This assumption is based upon another assumption, that human beings are fundamentally good and, if liberated from arbitrary and oppressive authority, they will flourish.

The further one is to the moral left, the more likely that one's moral thinking will be influenced by determinism and relativism. If

individual beliefs about truth and morality are conditioned by historical, social, and cultural circumstances, then there is reason to be
cautious about imposing any particular set of moral standards or
punishing persons who violate existing ones. This is not to say that
moral leftists deny the existence of evil. Far from it. They are inclined, however, to locate and condemn evil in systems or classes or
Weltanschauungen rather than in individuals, who, after all, are
products of their environments.

Those on the moral left are heirs of the Enlightenment (Hunter
1991, 131–32). They believe that harmful institutions, groups, and
attitudes, however deeply entrenched, can be analyzed, understood,
and ultimately eliminated. This is not a purely secular impulse. The
idea of targeting unjust social arrangements has become increasingly entrenched in liberal religion over the past 150 years, witness
the Protestant Social Gospel movement, the Jewish Social Justice
movement, and contemporary liberation theology. The corresponding deemphasis of individual sin, guilt, and repentance has drawn
the fire of religious traditionalists.

Disagreement over the nature and locus of sin is by no means a
peculiarity of the current American "culture wars," nor is the
United States the only country to have experienced moral polariza-
tion over the past three decades. Israel and India have been roiled
by religious controversies, as have Muslim countries like Egypt,
where there has been a widespread reaction against secularized
elites. Something is happening in widely separated cultures that is
expressive of a deep emotional reaction against liberalism, individualism, and other heterodox tendencies associated with enlightened
Western thought and behavior. Of late the war against the self, ancient in origin and perpetual in duration, has been escalating on several fronts.

Drug Wars

One of those fronts has been the drug war. The single most important fact about U.S. drug laws (and by "drugs" I narrowly mean
the opiates, cocaine, marijuana, and hallucinogens) is that they have
become much more police-oriented since the beginning of this century. Figure 1 illustrates the historical left-to-right movement of the
ideas that have governed U.S. drug policy (Gerstein and Harwood
1990, 43). Prior to 1909, even as more and more states were pro-

FIGURE 1

Ideas Governing American Drug Policy, 1850–1990

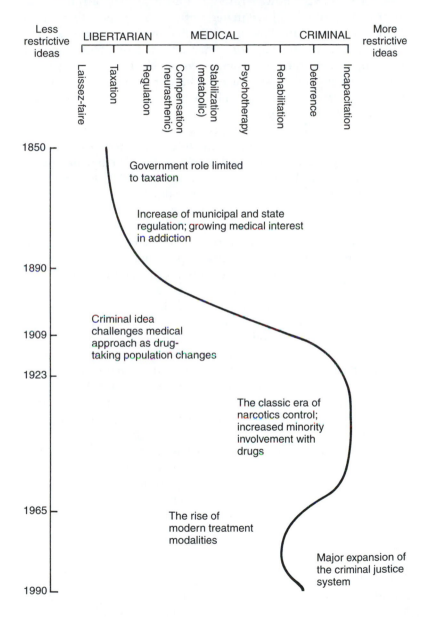

hibiting alcohol, drugs were simply taxed and regulated, generally by requiring a prescription for their possession. During the critical period 1909–1923, however, the various branches of the federal government, followed by state legislatures, began enacting, interpreting, and enforcing laws in a way that made it extremely difficult, in places impossible, for either addicted or casual users to obtain opium, morphine, heroin, or cocaine legally. The inevitable result of denying drugs to addicts was the creation of a large black market, which by the 1930s had become an important source of income to organized crime.

The list of forbidden substances was enlarged in 1937, when Congress passed, at the behest of the Bureau of Narcotics, the Marihuana Tax Act, actually a prohibition measure. The bureau and its director, Harry Anslinger, were active again in the 1950s, when they persuaded Congress to enact stricter penalties for narcotics-law violations, including the death penalty for those who sold drugs to adolescents.

There was a reaction against the punitive character of the drug policy in the 1960s and 1970s. Led by physicians, lawyers, and social scientists, reformers worked to reduce or eliminate the long, mandatory sentences prescribed by state and federal law and to develop treatment alternatives to the federal prison-hospitals at Lexington and Fort Worth, neither of which had been notably successful in rehabilitating addicts. The two most important treatment innovations were the second-generation therapeutic communities, modeled on Synanon, and long-term methadone maintenance, pioneered by Drs. Vincent Dole and Marie Nyswander. Methadone maintenance was the most radical departure, insofar as it directly challenged the fundamental principle of established policy, the denial of drugs to addicts.

In the late 1970s and the 1980s the pendulum swung back in the direction of the police approach. The turning point was the disgrace and resignation of Dr. Peter G. Bourne, President Carter's liberal drug adviser, who left the administration in July 1978 (Musto 1987, 265–73). Real funding for public treatment programs declined as additional billions were pumped into interdiction and enforcement efforts. Alarmed by the increased use of cocaine, and cheered on by moral conservatives, Ronald Reagan declared war on drugs and George Bush continued it. Congress responded with omnibus antidrug legislation in 1986 and 1988. These laws increased penalties for personal possession and use and reinstated the death penalty for some drug-related offenses. Although there have also been additional appropriations for prevention and treatment, the emphasis of the recent past has been on strict law enforcement and mandatory prison sentences—so much so that the drug war has spawned a countermovement, controlled legalization, which seeks a return to a more libertarian policy.

The key historical question is why U.S. drug policy veered so abruptly from left to right early in this century. Part of the answer is that the types of people who used drugs and the reasons that they used them changed dramatically. In the late nineteenth century the modal addict type was a native-born, white, middle-class woman who had become addicted to opium or morphine for medical reasons. In some instances her addiction originated in self-medication, but more usually she had been introduced to narcotics by a physician who was unable to treat the underlying cause of her disease and who resorted to the symptomatic relief of pain with injections of morphine. Patients with chronic diseases like arthritis or neuralgia were the most susceptible because their symptoms would return after an injection wore off and they would be tempted to resume the medication (Courtwright 1982, chap. 2).

Evangelicals conceive of the state as an extension of their own superegos and favor the energetic suppression of vice. So do the Moderates, although they are more concerned with imposing limits on the exercise of the police power. This tendency was as marked in the late nineteenth century as it is now. The difference, however, was that most cases of narcotic dependency were not then considered to be vicious. The sole exception was opium smoking, a practice popular among Chinese laborers and, after 1870, among some white gamblers and prostitutes. While opium smoking was universally regarded as a vice, the smokers were a minority among all opiate users. As long as medical users predominated, few Americans were interested in a broad-gauge war against narcotics. When legislators passed prohibitory narcotic laws, they did so only and specifically against opium smoking. Beginning in the 1870s, municipalities and some states passed laws aimed at closing opium dens (Courtwright 1982, chap. 3).

In pharmacological terms this policy was absurd. The morphine sold over the counter was ten times more powerful than the banned opium. Yet the legal distinction made moral and emotional sense, both because the Chinese laborers and white criminals who smoked opium were *personae non gratae* and because they had acquired the habit through self-indulgence rather than through the treatment of disease or painful symptoms.

This distinction was as evident in medicine as it was in law. When nineteenth-century doctors wrote about addiction, they generally regarded medical addicts sympathetically (as well they should have, given the high percentage of iatrogenic cases), while dismissing the opium smokers as sensuous idlers and reprobates. No scientific basis existed for this differentiation: an addicted opium smoker's withdrawal was symptomatically identical to that of a morphine addict. But for nineteenth-century doctors, as well as for laypersons, the moral antecedents of the disease and the personal characteristics of the patients mattered a great deal. They possessed a moral nosology that transcended the analysis and classification of physical symptoms.

The importance of the whos and whys of drug use is illustrated by the paradoxical case of the American South. As a result of widespread disease, poor sanitation, and the devastation of the Civil War, the South had an addiction rate among whites that far exceeded that of any other region. It also had a large and rapidly growing Evangelical movement. Church membership, overwhelmingly Baptist and Methodist, was up 51 percent in the period 1890–1906, compared to a 39 percent increase in population (Woodward 1971, 448–49). One would have thought widespread addiction shocking to these conservative churchgoers, and that they would have used their growing strength to lead a campaign against the southern narcotic problem, far and away the worst in the nation.

Nothing of the sort happened. Instead, Evangelical ministers and their congregants conducted a vigorous campaign against alcohol and saloons. By 1907 more than 85 percent of the counties in the former Confederate states were legally dry, a feat that was followed by statewide prohibition victories in Georgia, Oklahoma, Alabama, Mississippi, North Carolina, and Tennessee in 1907–1909 (Alcohol and Alcoholism 1989). Yet, in every one of these states it was possible to acquire legally medicinal opiates ranging in potency from paregoric to pure heroin.

The reason that alcohol rather than opium attracted the prohibitionists' attention was that southern opiate addicts were predominantly female, heavily sedated, disinclined to crime, and unlikely to spread the habit to anyone else. Their neighbors were often unaware that they used narcotics at all. The drunkards, by contrast, were predominantly male, irritatingly visible, and considered dangerous to themselves, their families, and society. Southern addicts also had the excuse that they had been introduced to drugs through the treatment or self-treatment of disease. Their relapses following detoxification could be partly attributed to the underlying physical disorder, such as neuroma or cancer or chronic diarrhea, over which the person had no control. Where there is no blame, there is no sin, and hence no basis for a moral or religious crusade.

All of this changed during the twentieth century. In both public perception and epidemiological fact opiate addiction moved from the upper world to the underworld, from the sickroom to the street. Physicians, who were becoming progressively better educated and more capable of managing illness, resorted less frequently to narcotics for symptomatic relief. The general public, alerted by muckrakers and the labeling of patent medicines mandated by the 1906 Pure Food and Drug Act, cut back on consumption of opiate-laced nostrums. Safer analgesics, such as aspirin, took the place of opiates in treating daily aches and pains. Fewer new narcotic addicts were being created, even as the ailing medical addicts were aging and dying.

This process is summarized in Figure 2, which shows the approximate ratios of medical to nonmedical opiate addicts at twenty-year intervals from 1895 to 1975. The outer circle, representing medical addicts, progressively shrank relative to the inner circle (morally, the "hard core") of nonmedical addicts. The nonmedical addicts, whose numbers remained roughly constant between 1895 and 1935, became heroin mainliners, opium having become expensive and difficult to obtain. Smugglers dropped opium for heroin, which was more compact, valuable, and easier to adulterate. But even heroin was largely unavailable during the early 1940s. World War II disrupted or diverted supplies, causing the number of active American addicts to drop to a twentieth-century low. Smuggling resumed after the war, however, and nonmedical addiction increased in the late 1940s and early 1950s, particularly in ghettos and barrios where the heroin traffic was concentrated.

Another, much larger increase in nonmedical opiate addiction began in the late 1960s. The number of heroin addicts went from roughly 100,000 in 1967 to perhaps half a million in 1975 (Ball, Englander, and Chambers 1970; Lingeman 1974, 111; Kaplan 1983, 2). This surge in narcotic use, which was part of the baby boom's polypharmaceutical experimentation and which was emotionally and ideologically tied to the rebellion against conservative institutions, was more broadly based than the surge in the 1950s. Although most addicts continued to come from the inner city, there were also middle-class white adolescents who had taken to using

FIGURE 2

Transformation of the American Opiate Addict Population, 1895–1975

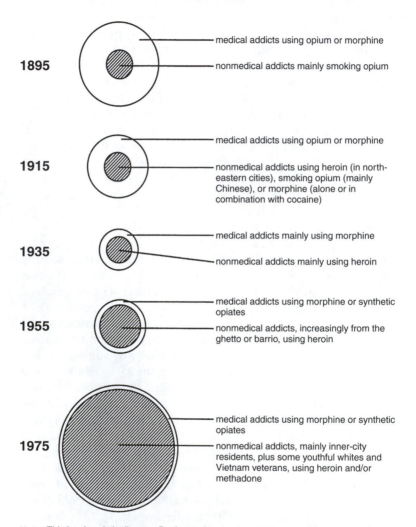

Note: *This is a heuristic diagram. Designated areas represent reasonable approximations, not exact numbers, which are unknown. Note also that medical addicts dependent on nonopiate drugs (e.g., Valium) are not included.*

heroin, and Vietnam veterans who had become addicted while stationed in Southeast Asia (Brecher 1974, 183–92). It was this rapid growth of heroin addiction, particularly among veterans, that alarmed Richard Nixon and led to his declaration of war on drugs in 1971. The Nixon administration's drug war was not blatantly punitive, as its predecessor had been and its successor would be, but stressed rehabilitation and treatment, including methadone maintenance.

What happened with cocaine use and addiction was similar to opiate use and addiction, although the process of stigmatization was telescoped into a shorter period of time. Cocaine, the principal active alkaloid of the coca plant, was one of the most enthusiastically touted new drugs of the 1880s. It was valued for its stimulating as well as its locally anesthetizing properties, and recommended for a wide variety of conditions. But physicians soon recognized the potential for abuse and dependence, and non-habit-forming substitutes like tropacocaine (1891) or stovaine (1903) or novocaine (1904) were developed as alternative local anesthetics. However, just as the comparatively minor problem of medical cocaine addiction was being brought under control, there was widespread and highly unfavorable publicity about the growing use of the drug as a stimulant by black laborers, prostitutes and pimps of both races, and assorted criminals, some of whom were said to go on violent sprees if they indulged in too much of the drug.

By 1915 cocaine had been restricted to the point of prohibition by local, state, and federal laws. Cocaine use persisted, though mainly as an expensive and exotic vice of show-business figures and big-city hustlers, something that might be found in Hollywood or Harlem but at few points in between. This was true until the 1970s, when improved supplies and favorable word of mouth led growing numbers of Americans to experiment with the drug. Cocaine's reincarnation as a middle-class drug was short-lived, however; the explosive epidemic of crack addiction in the mid-1980s reestablished its reputation as a hard inner-city drug and provided the catalyst for the Reagan-Bush drug war (Courtwright 1995).

Crack's emergence as a ghetto drug was a replay, racially if not pharmacologically, of the marijuana scare of the 1930s. In the nineteenth century, when cannabis was employed medically and included in the *U.S. Pharmacopeia*, it was not controversial. But when Mexican immigrants introduced recreational marijuana smoking in the early twentieth century; when the practice spread among black hipsters and musicians in New Orleans, Chicago, New

York, and other large cities; and when government officials like Harry Anslinger stressed that marijuana smokers committed horrible crimes, the stage was set for national prohibition, accomplished in 1937 through the Marijuana Tax Act (Bonnie and Whitebread 1974; Courtwright, Joseph, and Des Jarlais 1989, 23, 132–33 and passim; Jonnes 1996, 119–30).

Had these transformations in the opiate-, cocaine-, and marijuana-using populations not occurred, U.S. drug policy in this century would not—indeed, could not—have become so draconian. Jailing sick-old-lady addicts or patients whose prescriptions happened to contain certain drugs would have made no moral sense, even to those of Evangelical temperament. However, punishing junkies and crackheads and potheads (all pejorative terms of twentieth-century coinage) seemed morally dramatic and satisfying, a fitting end for the idle 'prentices of modern times.

Medical and Therapeutic Approaches to Narcotic Addiction

The historical transformation of the addict population also helps to explain changes in medical, as well as popular, conceptions of narcotic use and addiction. From the 1870s on, a growing number of physicians championed the idea that addiction, or at least morphine addiction, was a disease rather than a mere habit or a vice. They did not, however, agree on what sort of disease it was or who was most likely to contract it. One school held that some individuals were more susceptible to morphine because they had weakened nervous systems. The weakness stemmed from stress, or defective heredity, or both. Thus a brain worker who put in too many hours at the office or a highly strung society woman might resort to opiates to sooth frazzled nerves, develop a morbid craving, and then pass the predisposition on to offspring. Lamarckian ideas about the inheritability of acquired traits were then current.

Other physicians denied that either nervous weakness or predisposition played a role. Addiction specialists like Jansen Mattison and Charles Terry insisted that the majority of medical addicts were simply normal people who had become dependent on powerful drugs that had changed the chemistry of their bodies, as evidenced by tolerance and withdrawal symptoms. But they and their allies never demonstrated precisely how drugs altered somatic processes or showed that the change was permanent. Their failure to do so made possible the emergence of another, more sinister view of the problem: that addicts were really psychopaths.

The term *psychopath* described antisocial, pleasure-seeking individuals who acted without the least concern for conventional morality or the rights of others. In them the self was pathologically dominant—so dominant, in fact, that the original English term for psychopathy, coined in 1835, was *moral insanity*. Lawrence Kolb, a U.S. Public Health Service physician and administrator who popularized the psychopathy theory of addiction, argued that addicts, unlike normal people, experienced heightened pleasure from narcotics, continued to seek that pleasure regardless of the consequences, and ultimately came to depend on opiates as a kind of psychic crutch. The emergence of the street addict as the dominant type reinforced and gave credibility to Kolb's view that psychopathology was the fountainhead of narcotic addiction. By the 1940s the diagnosis of psychopathy in institutions like the Lexington Narcotic Hospital was almost a ritual.

By temperament Kolb was a moderate and a rationalist; by training he was a doctor and psychiatrist. He insisted, like some of his nineteenth-century physician predecessors, that compulsive drug-taking behavior was a manifestation of a genuine mental disease and that addicts were patients who ought to be supervised and rehabilitated in appropriate medical institutions rather than thrown willy-nilly into prisons. But Kolb ran into the cultural reality that there are good and bad diseases. Psychopathically rooted drug abuse was a bad disease, insofar as it was dangerous, morally tainted, and justified mandatory institutional treatment, if not necessarily in prison. Throughout his career Kolb argued for more humane treatment of narcotic addicts but did not get very far. Psychopaths did not seem much more deserving of sympathy than the merely vicious (Courtwright 1982, chap. 5).

Psychopathic addicts were certainly not sympathetic to Harry J. Anslinger, the head of the Federal Bureau of Narcotics from its inception in 1930 until his retirement in 1962. Anslinger was an outspoken hard-liner who thought that drug use and dealing were crimes and should be treated as such. Asked in 1957 why there was a resurgence of adolescent heroin addiction, he replied that the increase was almost entirely "among Negro people in police precincts with the lowest economic and social standards. . . . There is no drug addiction if the child comes from a good family, with the church, the home, and the school all integrated" (Anslinger and Chapman

1957, 189–90). Here, neatly summarized, is the basic worldview of the moral and religious right. Social problems like drug abuse are manifestations of bad character, and bad character develops when parents, teachers, and clergy are absent or inadequate to their disciplinary, instructional, and spiritual tasks.

Harry Anslinger's moral opposite was Dr. Marie Nyswander, the cofounder of methadone maintenance. Nyswander was an archetypal moral leftist. Raised in an academic household by a divorced, freethinking mother, Nyswander flirted with communism in her youth, graduated from Sarah Lawrence, enrolled in medical school, married and divorced, became a physician and psychiatrist, and specialized in the treatment of frigidity and drug addiction. In the early 1960s she began a collaboration with Dr. Vincent Dole, a medical researcher. They came to the conclusion that narcotic addiction was a metabolic disorder and that the most effective treatment was long-term maintenance with methadone, a synthetic opiate that, at a sufficiently high dose, blocked both the euphoric effects of heroin and the onset of withdrawal symptoms. Because methadone could be taken orally, because it was pure, and because it was legal, it permitted addicts to escape the deadly routine of hustling, scoring, and injecting adulterated black-market heroin.

But methadone was also a narcotic drug, and therein lay the rub. It was, detractors charged, just substituting one addiction for another, much like switching a scotch alcoholic to cheap wine. Criticism of methadone was voiced not only by conservative law-enforcement officials like Anslinger but by the pioneers of the therapeutic communities that mushroomed in the 1960s and 1970s. Men and women like Monsignor William O'Brien, cofounder of Daytop Village, and Judianne Densen-Gerber, founder of Odyssey House, held that the problem was the individual, not the drug. They understood drug abusers to be emotionally immature persons lacking in discipline, self-restraint, and other middle-class virtues. Instead of being rehabilitated, they had to be habilitated, that is, to develop "a socially productive, conventional lifestyle for the first time in their lives" (De Leon 1990–1991, 1540). The way for them to do so was to spend six to eighteen months in a structured, authoritarian family in which they played the role of children learning to emulate the responsible behavior of their parents and older siblings, often former-addict counselors.

The therapeutic community was, and remains, a moral hybrid. It is a psychotherapeutic and medical enterprise (enough so, at any rate, that many insurers will defray treatment costs), but it also combines elements of a Protestant camp meeting and the Catholic sacrament of reconciliation, as publicly practiced in the early church (Courtwright, Joseph, and Des Jarlais 1989, 317–18). A therapeutic community's goal is temperamental conversion, or, as George De Leon more neutrally puts it, "a global change in lifestyle," including abstinence from narcotic drugs (De Leon 1990–1991, 1538; De Leon 1995, 1608, 1638). Methadone treatment, which involves maintenance rather than abstinence, and which presumes that the problem is the drug and not the individual, contradicts both the philosophy and the goal of the therapeutic community movement. Although the methadone clinics and the therapeutic communities have reached a *modus vivendi,* there is a long history of mutual hostility and criticism. There is also a pattern: liberal rationalists have tended to champion, or at least to defend, methadone maintenance and needle-exchange programs, whereas moral conservatives have been actively involved with the therapeutic community approach.

The same is true of drug-abuse "boot camps," which are militarized versions of the therapeutic community, total institutions instead of merely authoritarian ones. Boot camps appeal to moral conservatives because they accentuate discipline and punishment. There is both a practical and an emotional logic here. If the drug abuser's real problem is lack of self-control, then a boot-camp milieu is one plausible way to instill it. But it is also deeply satisfying for people who have sacrificed themselves at the altar of God and family, who have lived the biblical message of death to self, to see those who have devoted themselves to illicit pleasures doing push-ups in the summer sun. This feeling is very close to what Nietzsche termed *ressentiment,* the festering resentment of others that can give rise to attempts to harm or degrade them.

The same point can be made with reference to the spectrum of ideas about drug policy in Figure 1. Beliefs about how strict drug laws should be are parallel to the continuum of religious temperaments. Moral rightists have strongly supported the coercive tactics associated with the drug war, whose stated ethical premise was that "the drug problem reflects bad decisions by individuals with free wills" (White House 1992, 2). Moral leftists, inclined to view addicts as victims of adverse social circumstances, have often favored less coercive medical approaches. "The great, largely unspoken argument for treatment instead of enforcement as the primary tool of drug policy," observes Mark Kleiman (1992, 187), "is that treatment expresses compassion for users while enforcement expresses only anger. To the moderate left . . . this is a powerful appeal."

Personal Drug Use

If the ways in which we argue and the conclusions we reach about drugs are influenced by our temperaments, the same should be true of the likelihood of personal drug use. Numerous empirical studies (summarized in Gersick, Grady, Sexton, and Lyons 1981, 44; Hawkins, Lishner, and Catalano 1985, 86) have shown that low religiosity is positively correlated with both drug experimentation and dependency. These studies also report that drug users are more likely to be self-centered than are nonusers. Marijuana smokers, for example, tend to have intra- rather than interpersonal values. "Intrapersonal values," explain Robert Carlson and William Edwards (1990),

> focus on the individual and on end-states of existence which take into consideration only personal benefit. These values are concerned with self-satisfaction and do not seem especially concerned with morality. Interpersonal values are other-centered and place greater importance on the good of all rather than on self-serving ends. (1399)

When Carlson and Edwards administered a questionnaire called the Wellness Activity Profile to more than 1,100 college students, they found that the marijuana smokers were more interested in pleasure, leading an exciting life, happiness, equality, self-capability, and imaginativeness. The nonmarijuana smokers were keener on salvation, family security, self-control, responsibility, and various other social and family values (see also Goode 1970, chap. 2, esp. 42–43; Brook, Lukoff, and Whiteman 1977, 388–99).

Although these and other empirical findings (Rokeach 1983, 178–89) dovetail with the notion of moral and religious temperaments, it is necessary to introduce some qualifications to the argument, which is overly tidy. The first caveat concerns the direction of causality. Temperaments may influence drug use, but the opposite is also true. A heroin or cocaine addict caught in the dog-eat-dog world of street hustling will test high on any scale of intrapersonal values, regardless of whether he was actually self-centered or psychopathic before the drug use commenced.

The second caveat is that moral and religious beliefs are by no means the only or even necessarily the most important reasons that people use or refrain from using illicit drugs. There are several other variables, the most critical of which is exposure. People cannot use psychoactive substances if they do not know about them or cannot acquire a supply. The experience of North American Indians with distilled alcohol before and after European contact is a well-known historical example.

Exposure plays an important role in marijuana use as well. Denise B. Kandel and Israel Adler (1982) report that although religious observance is negatively correlated with marijuana use in both the United States and France, having friends who use marijuana is the most important predictive variable. Of course, one's choice of friends might well be influenced by one's own or one's parents' moral and religious outlook. For example, the Amish have a minuscule drug problem both because they are intensely religious and because their religion leads them to isolate themselves in agrarian communities away from the drug-filled cities.

Technological change also has a bearing on the pattern of drug use. Opiates were widely available in the United States throughout the nineteenth century, but the big surge in consumption came during and after the 1870s, the period when hypodermic medication came into general use. Injections of morphine produced much more powerful sensations of pleasure and pain relief than did swallowing opium pills or laudanum, and hence were more liable to be repeated. Any innovation that makes the use of a psychoactive drug more intensely pleasurable, like injection, or more palatable, like flue-cured tobacco, will increase the frequency of its use, other things being equal.

All of this can be tied together by the concept of susceptibility. In any human group there are some people who are more likely to abuse drugs than others. They are more likely to do so because of their age, gender, marital and family status, health, education, income, and other, often correlative traits, such as personal values and moral and religious views. There may also be a genetic susceptibility, although this has not yet been established with any precision and probably varies from drug to drug. But susceptibility, whether environmental or genetic, does not matter in the absence of exposure. The most addiction-prone person in the world cannot abuse a substance that is unavailable. When historical and technological circumstances change, when drugs become more accessible, or affordable, or potent, or easily consumed, then the incidence of use and addiction will increase. If the new drug has important or numerous therapeutic applications, most of the initial cases of addiction will be iatrogenic, as was the case with morphine and cocaine. Eventually, however, abuse will become concentrated among those who are susceptible by reason of social circumstance or personality, including pleasure-seeking persons who ignore or reject conventional religious strictures. When that happens, their moral opposites, men and women of strict religious temperament, will be sure to object.

References

Alcohol and alcoholism. 1989. In *Encyclopedia of southern culture*, edited by C. R. Wilson and W. Ferris. Chapel Hill: University of North Carolina Press.

Anslinger, H., and K. W. Chapman. 1957. Narcotic addiction [interview]. *Modern Medicine* 25:170–93.

Ball, J. C., D. M. Englander, and C. D. Chambers. 1970. The incidence and prevalence of opiate addiction in the United States. In *The epidemiology of opiate addiction in the United States*, edited by J. C. Ball and C. D. Chambers. Springfield, Ill.: Charles C. Thomas.

Bonnie, R. J., and C. H. Whitebread, II. 1974. *The marijuana conviction: A history of marijuana prohibition in the United States.* Charlottesville: University Press of Virginia.

Brecher, E. M. 1974. *Licit & illicit drugs.* Boston: Little, Brown.

Brook, J. S., I. F. Lukoff, and M. Whiteman. 1977. Correlates of adolescent marijuana use as related to age, sex, and ethnicity. *Yale Journal of Biology and Medicine* 50:383–90.

Carlson, B. R., and W. H. Edwards. 1990. Human values and marijuana use. *International Journal of the Addictions* 25:1393–1401.

Courtwright, D. T. 1982. *Dark paradise: Opiate addiction in America before 1940.* Cambridge: Harvard University Press.

———. 1995. The rise and fall and rise of cocaine in the United States. In *Consuming habits: Drugs in history and anthropology*, edited by Jordan Goodman, Paul E. Lovejoy, and Andrew Sherratt. London: Routledge.

Courtwright, D. T., H. Joseph, and D. Des Jarlais. 1989. *Addicts who survived: An oral history of narcotic use in America, 1923–1965.* Knoxville: University of Tennessee Press.

De Leon, G. 1990–1991. The therapeutic community and behavioral science. *International Journal of the Addictions* 25 (special issue): 1537–57.

———. 1995. Therapeutic communities for addictions: A theoretical framework. *International Journal of the Addictions* 30:1603–45.

Gersick, K. E., K. Grady, E. Sexton, and M. Lyons. 1981. Personality and sociodemographic factors in adolescent drug use. In *Drug abuse and the American adolescent*, edited by D. J. Lettieri and J. P. Ludford. NIDA research monograph 38. Rockville, Md.: National Institute on Drug Abuse.

Gerstein, D. R., and H. J. Harwood, eds. 1990. *Treating drug problems: A study of the evolution, effectiveness, and financing of public and private drug treatment systems*, vol. 1. Washington, D.C.: National Academy Press.

Goldman, A. L. 1991. Portrait of religion in U.S. holds dozens of surprises. *New York Times*, April 10, nat. ed., A1, A11.

Goode, E. 1970. *The marijuana smokers*. New York: Basic Books.

Greven, P. 1977. *The Protestant temperament: Patterns of child-rearing, religious experience, and the self in early America*. New York: Knopf.

Hawkins, J. D., D. M. Lishner, and R. F. Catalano. 1985. Childhood predictors and the prevention of adolescent substance abuse. In *Etiology of drug abuse: Implications for prevention*, edited by C. L. Jones and R. J. Battjes. NIDA research monograph 56. Rockville, Md.: National Institute on Drug Abuse.

Hunter, J. D. 1991. *Culture wars: The struggle to define America*. New York: Basic Books.

Isaac, R. 1974. Evangelical revolt: The nature of the Baptists' challenge to the traditional order in Virginia, 1765 to 1775. *William and Mary Quarterly*, 3d ser., 31:345–68.

Johnson, B. 1985. Liberal Protestantism: End of the road? *Annals of the American Academy of Political and Social Science* 480:39–52.

Jonnes, J. 1996. *Hep-cats, narcs, and pipe dreams: A history of America's romance with illegal drugs*. New York: Scribner.

Kandel, D., and I. Adler. 1982. Socialization into marijuana use among French adolescents: A cross-cultural comparison with the United States. *Journal of Health and Social Behavior* 23:295–309.

Kaplan, J. 1983. *The hardest drug: Heroin and public policy*. Chicago: University of Chicago Press.

Kleiman, M. R. 1992. *Against excess: Drug policy for results*. New York: Basic Books.

Lingeman, R. R. 1974. *Drugs from a to z: A dictionary*. Rev. ed. New York: McGraw-Hill.

McNamara, P. 1985. American Catholicism in the mid-eighties: Pluralism and conflict in a changing Church. *Annals of the American Academy of Political and Social Science* 480:63–74.

Musto, D. F. 1987. *The American disease: Origins of narcotic control*. Rev. ed. New York: Oxford University Press.

Religion in America. 1982. *The Gallup Report*, nos. 201–2.

Rokeach, M. 1983. A value approach to the prevention and reduction of drug abuse. In *Preventing adolescent drug abuse: Intervention strategies*, edited by T. J. Glynn, C. G. Leukefeld, and J. P. Ludford. NIDA research monograph 47. Rockville, Md.: National Institute on Drug Abuse.

Roof, W. C., and W. McKinney. 1987. *American mainline religion: Its changing shape and future*. New Brunswick: Rutgers University Press.

White House. 1992. *National drug control strategy: A nation responds to drug use*. Washington, D.C.: Government Printing Office.

Williamsburg Charter Foundation. 1988. *The Williamsburg Charter survey on religion and public life*. Washington, D.C.: Williamsburg Charter Foundation.

Wills, G. 1990. *Under God: Religion and American politics*. New York: Simon & Schuster.

Woodward, C. V. 1971. *Origins of the new South, 1877–1913*. Baton Rouge: Louisiana State University Press.

Teenage Pregnancy and Out-of-Wedlock Birth

Morals, Moralism, Experts

Linda Gordon

Traditionally, teenage pregnancy and out-of-wedlock birth were two quite different matters, the former normal and even normative, the latter a matter of substantial social and moral concern. In the past century, out-of-wedlock birth, or "illegitimacy," has become, in addition, a subject of specialized expertise. In the past three decades, the two phenomena have been joined, often constructed as a single social problem. Either phrase—teenage pregnancy or out-of-wedlock birth—now stands for both in the popular and often also in the expert discourse.[1] In what follows I separate the two again, look at the historical path of the moral and expert discourses, examine how each was produced as a social problem, and conclude with some reflections on the contemporary discourse.

But first some historical context. The whole discourse, for at least a century and a half, has been shaped, first, by the development of the "helping" professions. Professionals asserted social responsibility for controlling reproductive practices as part of their search for collective status and financial security. Social workers were the first to claim this jurisdiction. More recently, social-science researchers, public health professionals, nurses, and even physicians have joined those whose expertise is based in part on this social problem. Second, the discourse has been state-centered. Teenage and out-of-wedlock sexual activity and reproduction became defined as social problems as a part of the expansion of the welfare state in the United States, a process in which several occupational groups used state-building as part of their profession-building agendas. Demands for state control of sexual immorality have been intermittently intense throughout this century, visible in controversies about prostitution, the age of consent, birth control, female juvenile delinquency, and censorship, as well as unwed motherhood. Third, although the teenage pregnancy problem had always been highly gendered, it became a major social problem within the early-twentieth-century context of political contestation about the proper behavior of women. Teenage pregnancy as a social problem signifies, of course, improper sexual behavior among girls, and sexual norms have shifted significantly, amidst great conflict, during the past century. But the definitions of teenage and out-of-wedlock pregnancy as social problems have been equally influenced by women's movements and particularly by women's struggles for a foothold in several helping professions. Fourth, most recently, teenage and out-of-wedlock pregnancy and reproduction have become a highly racialized issue, affected by a declining civil rights era and accelerating impoverishment and inequality. The current moralizing about teenage and out-of-wedlock pregnancy, for example, can fruitfully be interpreted as, in part, a backlash motivated by all four of these contexts: recoil against the authority of professionals; opposition to a welfare state; antagonism to feminism and sexual permissiveness; and conviction that moral failures, more than discrimination, lay behind deepened racial inequality.

Both issues have been somewhat medicalized, if not to the same degree as, say, alcoholism. Both are "epidemics," and although no one suggests that either is a disease, literally, nevertheless the discourse is characterized by metaphors of infection and plague, hereditary or ecological transmission, and individuals "at risk." The medical connection results partly from the medicalization of birth control in this century, partly from the public health aspects of the issue, and partly, no doubt, from the pervasive influence of a medical model on all professional discourses.

The politicization of this topic produced, ironically, a putatively apolitical reaction: the attempt to redefine teenage pregnancy in amoral, objectivist terminology. Denying the moral dimension of discourse has increasingly, in the twentieth century, been definitional to the professions, and in the past two decades that response has accelerated as traditionally liberal professionals faced strongly conservative political movements. This amoral style of discourse often remains covertly moralistic, however. I will argue here that public discussion of teenage and out-of-wedlock pregnancy cannot be removed from the realm of the moral. The regulation of sexual behavior and women's sexual and reproductive rights are essentially moral matters, inconceivable in the absence of ethical claims.

We can, however, usefully distinguish between *moral* and *moralistic* discourse. Although not often clearly distinguished, there are two different root adjectives in play here. The latter is often pejorative, the former rarely. Pregnancy and birth have never been amoral, outside a community moral system; few human practices have been as consistently subject to moral norms as these. Indeed, by the early seventeenth century, "moral" often referred specifically to sexual conduct. "Moralistic" literally came from the practice of a moralist, one who teaches or philosophizes about morality; and in a culture increasingly individualist, tolerant, or relativist, it came to refer to unwanted and objectionable moral judgments. Moralistic has a variety of meanings: preaching about the practices of others; being improperly rigid, lacking in the flexibility that acknowledges human variation and imperfection; being uncontextualized, offering judgments not based on a full examination of the actual universe of choice available to the one who is criticized. The attempt to disguise moral judgments, in fact, often produces moralism—the presentation of conclusions as scientific, universal, and objective because the moral assumptions on which they rest are dissimulated. I am arguing here that the attempt to produce "value-free" analyses often produces moralistic ones. "Moralistic" often refers, of course, to moral views to which the speaker is opposed. But difficulty in delineating intersubjective and universally specifiable definitions of the two terms does not at all vitiate the existence of two autonomous meanings in general usage. Although there have no doubt always been moralists, and moralizing prigs, it appears that in the past century and a half we have entered an era of heightened moralism because of the politicization of moral issues. Nowhere is this more evident than regarding questions of sexual, family, and reproductive behavior.

Out of Wedlock

Historically, the regulation of "illegitimate" *birth* has been rather separate from that of out-of-wedlock *pregnancy*. Traditional societies were usually far more concerned with births than with conceptions. Demographic historical research has demonstrated that in many premodern and modern communities, premarital conception was common, even the dominant pattern; no legal or ethical problem arose so long as the relation was legitimated by a marriage before or shortly after a childbirth. These systems of regulation were, evidently, primarily directed at protecting inheritance and providing for children, sometimes at protecting taxpayers.

The worry for "illegitimate" children was well founded, for even in very ancient and "simple" societies, children born without social fathers were often in trouble. (They would have been in worse trouble by far had they not had social mothers, but this was extremely rare.) In many cultures and legal structures, such offspring were without inheritance rights. Often considered outcasts altogether, bastards were much maligned. The meanings of the English word "bastard" express vividly what such a child was up against: mongrel, misbegotten or baseborn; blackguard or knave; threatening, carrying the "bar sinister"; ungenuine or inauthentic, spurious; *filius nullius*—a child with no family. There is evidence, however, of mixed feelings about illegitimacy in traditional societies, in the existence of a softer, sometimes even affectionate language: by-blow, catch colt, chance child, come-by-chance, *filius populi*, love child, woods colt, natural child. These phrases express the commonness and tolerance of illicit sex and the care for its offspring, a tolerance often based on a double standard, of course. They remind us of the flexibility of patriarchy as well as its rigidities. Reproductive wrongdoing was at the same time deviant and normal; not recommended, it was nevertheless expected (at least occasionally) and thus accepted as inevitable within the community if not of any given individual, handled not by ostracism but by inclusion. Illegitimacy was always a moral issue but less often an occasion for moralizing.

"Illegitimacy" does not seem to have taken on its modern, reproductive, meaning until the sixteenth century; before that it referred generically to illegal or unaccepted practice. The word's transformation indicates an increase in concern with out-of-wedlock births. This in turn was most likely related not to radical changes in sexual or reproduction-control behavior but to increases in indigence. Women alone with children were always likely to be among the poorest of a society. It was in this Elizabethan period that there arose also the modern "poor laws" regulating, and stigmatizing, social provision. In this context of escalating hostility to the poor, the hostility to illegitimacy was, so to speak, overdetermined—by misogyny, patriarchy, and resentment of the dependent poor. The modern meaning of illegitimacy, then, arose in the context of decline of community responsibility and the intervention of the state—a context in which immoral behavior created an occasion for a newly politicized moralizing.

The modern period also broke with traditional treatment of illegitimacy in another way: there was a gradual trend to the abolition of the disabilities and stigma attached to the illegitimate child. This included extending to illegitimate children the rights of the legitimate, and to fathers the same economic responsibilities. This reform pattern created individual paternal responsibility in an effort to protect the prosperous against claims by the poor. (Neither women's rights nor child welfare were at first evident among the motives for these changes in law.) In practice, however, male responsibility was not much enforced.

But the gains of once-illegitimate children did not mark an amoralization of the issue. The effect of creating greater equality among children was not to erase stigma but to transfer it from children to their mothers. In premodern society it was the bastard who was evil; in modern society it was his mother. Of course, condemnation of unwed mothers had never been entirely absent, given the ambiguity that long prevailed in attitudes about women's sexual activity. But this concern with women's morality greatly increased in the modern era, creating a widespread and distinctly moralistic alarm about unwed mothers and premarital sex. By the late eighteenth century a commitment to police women's morals seemed urgent among the newly urban middle classes.

This change in the meanings of illegitimacy produced a trend toward hypocrisy. Particularly in the prudish United States, hegemonic respectability required hiding unwed pregnancies and births in asylums to which the young women were sent for their "confinement." This was followed by a "charitable" version of concealment, providing some "rescue homes" for poor women, such as the Florence Crittenton Society. Despite the stubborn continuation of illegitimacy in the twentieth century, neither analysis of nor solutions to the problem were directed at men. This was in part due to the fact that the women's-rights movement in the United States, whose strength put it in a position to influence the discourse, did not much challenge conventional sexual moralism about the importance of women's purity and the inevitability of men's sexual predation.

In the 1890s in the United States, charity and social workers began a discussion about what to do with mothers without husbands, and there has been a continuous discourse about single mothers ever since. Its meaning has shifted from time to time, as the power to define the social problem shifted from liberals to conservatives, feminists to antifeminists, and back, in several waves, but the driving motives were always political. That is, the debate was always state-centered; its controversies were about what social policy regarding single mothers should be adopted. Until about 1910 the focus was on deserted wives, and the problem was usually defined in moral terms: feminists tended to blame irresponsible men, antifeminists the archetypical nagging wife, but to all a sin had been committed. In the period 1910–1920 widows came to dominate the discourse about single mothers, largely for strategic political reasons: social feminists were actively campaigning for mothers' aid laws, and they needed single mothers who were not morally culpable as their symbol. Never-married mothers began to figure importantly in this discourse only after about 1920. They were first spotlighted by social workers with several motivations: as progressive reformers, notably connected to the U.S. Children's Bureau, they sought to emphasize the child welfare aspects of the issue; as social workers fighting for the recognition and economic viability of their profession, they had an affinity for problems to which their work could provide solutions; often as feminists, they wanted to help impoverished and stigmatized mothers. The Children's Bureau's first investigations, after its establishment in 1912, centered on infant mortality and found that illegitimate babies died much more frequently. Soon psychiatric social workers directed their attention to illegitimate mothers, and specifically teenage mothers, finding psychological problems underlying their sexual misbehavior (Brush 1994; Gordon 1988).[2]

Throughout this early-twentieth-century discussion, and continuing today, runs an apparent tension between child welfare and sexual regulation goals. In the early twentieth century there was a running battle between antifeminist moralists and a social-feminist prowelfare network. On the issue of illegitimacy, the latter was represented particularly by the Children's Bureau, a pioneer in the early use of professional expertise—particularly statistical social surveys—to attempt to depoliticize and amoralize the issue. For example, the bureau promoted systematic birth registration for the first time, a minimal condition for studying the incidence of illegitimacy. Yet the Children's Bureau's vision of professionalism and social science was not at odds with partisanship. Its social scientific studies were designed to support convictions that predated the "data," such as expansion of the welfare state, decreasing inequality, and promoting women's political power. And it never lost its commitment to sexual chastity for women, so it is no surprise that it never succeeded in separating child welfare goals from the moralism surrounding illegitimacy (Gordon 1992). For example, many of the poor of the early twentieth century practiced a kind of secondary out-of-wedlock reproduction: children were born not to single women but to unmarried *couples*, often living together "in sin" only because one or both had been previously married and divorce was not accessible. In these cases the "illegitimate" children often lived with both their parents and were not necessarily worse off than those with married parents. The fact that such relationships were often common-law marriages, and recognized in law by many of the states, did not stop social workers from attempting to enforce either legal marriage or separation upon them (Gordon 1988).

Yet these reformers were challenging hegemonic moralisms. Periodizing the discussion about out-of-wedlock mothers allows us to see the continuities and discontinuities in the repeated reconstructions of the issue. By the 1920s an older, fundamentally Victorian line of thought, whose categories were sin and rescue, was strongly contested. Social workers questioned whether free moral choice was involved in illegitimacy, by looking both to environmental influences and biologistic deformations. In the 1920s unmarried mothers were frequently found to be led into sin by bad companions, unable to resist because they were feebleminded (Kammerer 1918). In the 1930s environmental analyses crowded out those based on mental deficiencies and the environment was interpreted more broadly. Social workers began to speak of the ecology of neighborhoods, thus blaming illegitimacy not only on "broken homes" but also on "disorganized neighborhoods" (Vincent 1961, 19). Throughout these reconstructions of unwed motherhood, it is clear that the experts were trying to position unwed mothers as victims in order to help them escape stigma and to justify welfare spending.

Underlying this tense combination of morals, moralism, medicalization, and social science was a simplistic class analysis. Aware of the widespread occurrence of illegitimacy in poor and immigrant neighborhoods, Progressive-era reformers perceived out-of-wedlock childbirth as a phenomenon primarily of poverty. This then stuck them with the task of explaining why some poor girls strayed and others didn't, without reverting to Victorian moralism. Their most common answer pointed to the combination of deprivation and bad neighborhoods and companions, which made girls seek "unwholesome" fun. (Their explanations continued a double standard by problematizing only girls', not boys', misbehavior.) Their analyses required rendering the girls as passive; any admission of agency on the girls' part led back to the traditional woman-blaming moralism they wanted to escape.

A class analysis of out-of-wedlock childbirth was, in the United States, hard to separate from racial analyses. In the Progressive era the racial "others" were not blacks but immigrants, mainly from southern and eastern Europe but including also the Irish. In reformers' analyses, up to the 1940s, out-of-wedlock births were commonly represented as peculiar to immigrants (Brush 1994, chap. 1).

Blacks were not widely identified in the out-of-wedlock birth discourse until the 1950s. Then the social work discourse began to name black reproductive behavior as a problem. In the late 1930s and 1940s social workers had begun to be influenced by the anthropological concept of "culture" as now applied to community studies in the United States, especially of southern blacks, and introduced an explanation of out-of-wedlock births as an "accepted way of life" in an alternative culture.[3] This analysis aimed to counteract stigma among poor blacks, although it also reflected ignorance about the complexity and variability of black patterns and racist assumptions about black "simplicity." Children's Bureau experts knew that southern African Americans had higher rates of out-of-wedlock births from at least the 1920s, but this phenomenon was then seen as a contained, rural, regional pattern, and thus unthreatening, so it remained a very marginal discourse until the "great migration" brought millions of blacks to the North.

For prosperous whites, there arose a different explanatory strategy. In the 1940s and 1950s psychiatric influences increased diagnoses of unmarried pregnancy and childbirth as resulting from emotional disturbance (for example, Young 1954). Black girls, by contrast, were not suspected of having individual motives for their sexual behavior—nor indeed were any signs of individual personality attributed to them; they were merely expressing the standard "low" culture and upbringing of their people (Gordon 1988, 89–92; Solinger 1992; Weatherley 1987; Young 1954). Thus as white unwed mothers became increasingly individualized, medicalized, and interesting, black ones remained a mass, objects not of medical but of sociological and anthropological investigation. In the late 1950s and 1960s, illegitimacy was for the first time associated with *young*, or teenage, childbearing, the latter problematized as it had never been before because, of course, there were by then expectations that girls from prosperous families would remain in school throughout their teenage years (National Council on Illegitimacy 1969; Vincent 1968).

Racial and class assumptions were also fundamental to how unwed births should be "managed." Nineteenth-century religious "rescue" workers had generally urged that young mothers, especially poor ones, keep their babies, believing that the responsibility would simultaneously punish and reform the mothers. More sympathetic to unmarried pregnant women, especially young ones, twentieth-century social workers in the field began to press for separating mother and child and putting the babies up for adoption. By the 1960s, about 90 percent of white illegitimate babies were adopted (Vinovskis 1981). But this was an entirely racial policy; at exactly the same time those who worked with black unwed mothers assumed that they would keep their babies and encouraged, even pressured, them to do so. Social workers assumed, of course, that there was no "market" for black adoptive babies but also that this aberrant reproductive behavior was "normal" among blacks and a sign of their cultural inferiority.[4] This complexly structured racial discourse included both white recognition of the existence of an autonomous African-American pattern of regulation of reproduction, *and* a racist reading of that pattern. It was not a benign but a discriminatory tolerance because it deprived black girls of opportunities (such as casework, counseling, and adoption services) whites got.

In the twentieth century, then, the meaning of "out of wedlock" was shifting rapidly. Children were decreasingly stigmatized, although because they were so often poor they continued to be seriously disadvantaged. Women, especially upper- or middle-class girls, were beginning to be "forgiven" through a professional, technocratic language, their sexual "fall" treated as a pathology to be cured. Meanwhile black out-of-wedlock motherhood was understood by experts as a mass, cultural rather than an individual psychological phenomenon, an understanding that contributed to excluding blacks from the family-policy side of the growing welfare state. The meanings have changed again, dramatically, since the 1960s, as a result of the intersection of several discourses about social problems: increasing welfare costs and higher AFDC rolls; a civil rights struggle that drew attention to racism and made blacks more noticeable to whites; a women's liberation movement that influenced attitudes about sex and family. In this late-twentieth-century period it is difficult to disentangle discussion of out-of-wedlock pregnancy from these other issues.

Today out-of-wedlock childbirth is usually associated with female-headed households. In the past "illegitimate" mother-child *families* were often integrated into *households* headed by others—by parents or siblings, for example (Gordon and McLanahan 1991). For many, unmarried mothers living alone with their children stimulate two different anxieties: one about women's immoral sexual and reproductive activity, and another about women's independence as householders, unconnected to men. For this reason, the construction of out-of-wedlock births as a social problem expresses political conflicts about welfare, feminism, sexual "freedom" for women, and ways to strengthen "the family." Most professionals respond ambivalently, trying not to blame the single mothers for their condition while documenting the disadvantages their condition produces for their children. The strategy, as that of Progressives, could be described as social scientific amoralization, but today's experts are much less willing to admit that their approaches rest on ethical opinions and policy preferences. They are more insistent that the nature of the problem is self-evident and that it can be solved by reliance on value-free research.

Before we examine this current discourse, however, we need to look at one of the newest meanings of out-of-wedlock birth: its virtual fusion with "teenage pregnancy." The two are run together in much of the discussion. Even many scholarly writers equivocate between the one and the other as if unaware that they are conceptually different.[5]

Teenage Pregnancy

Unlike illegitimacy, "teenage pregnancy" is a new idea. Although girls have been having babies since time immemorial, too-early pregnancy or motherhood did not arise as a *social* problem until the past few decades. The expression "teenage," in fact, was first used only in this century. It reflected the new concept of adolescence that originated late in the nineteenth century. In preindustrial societies the children of all except a tiny elite were incorporated into family labor as early as they could be useful. They were integrated into multigenerational groups and, because their transitions to adult responsibilities were relatively gradual and predictable, were not perceived by adults as normally passing through a time of difficulty.

Marriages often, depending on the wealth and inheritance patterns of the family and society and on the vagaries of good and bad economic times, occurred relatively early, in some societies commonly in the "teenage" years among girls.

With industrialism came several new patterns: prolonged education and age stratification that caused young people to form strong identifications with their exact age peers; for boys, the likelihood of entering work different from that of one's father; for girls and boys, a marriage "market" less formed by the adults of the community and more dependent on one's own resources and skills. Moreover, industrialism produced rapid cultural change, and young people often absorbed tastes and values different from those of their parents, thus creating generational conflict. In this context "teenager" took on a specific meaning: a person mature in body, often sexually active, but not economically prepared for formation of a new family and viewed by the adult community as not emotionally prepared, either.

With such an understanding of teenagers, teenage pregnancy and motherhood might be expected to appear problematic: teenage pregnancy signifies girls' early sexual activity, and teenage motherhood creates the danger of immature, single, and impoverished mothers. But in fact there was no widespread concern about these problems put together in this way until the past few decades, long after the spread of the notion of teenage itself as a problem. In fact, it is hard to think of any other social problem that is so at odds with the facts. Consider the following list of corrections to widely believed falsities about teenage pregnancy:

- Teenage pregnancy is not the same as teenage motherhood. Pregnant middle-class teenagers tend to have abortions; poor ones have babies (Weatherley 1987).

- Teenage childbearing is not increasing. Throughout the twentieth century the birth rate to those aged 15 to 19 was stable, until 1946; then it rose to a peak about 1957, and declined until the mid-1980s. Teenage pregnancy appears more noticeable because births to adults have declined even more, so that teenagers' *proportion* of all births has risen (Weatherley 1987; Zelnik and Kantner 1980; Children's Defense Fund 1986; Children's Defense Fund 1988, 27–29).[6]

- The decline in the rate of teenage births has been even steeper among blacks than among whites (Ladner 1986, 70).

- Teenage pregnancy does not contribute to an increase in abortion. On the contrary, teenagers constitute a declining proportion of those who get abortions—down from one-third to one-fourth since 1973 (Luker 1991).

- Teenage pregnancy is not the main cause of growing single motherhood. Only one-fourth of single mothers had their first births when they were teenagers (Ellwood 1988, 71).

- Teenage childbearing is not contributing to an increase in "unwanted babies." Although pregnancies that teenagers consider "mistimed" have increased, there has been an overall decline in the births of children reported as unwanted (Pratt and Horn 1985; Gordon 1990; Zelnik and Kantner 1980).

- Teenage childbearing is not, on the whole, a serious health risk to mother or child (Children's Defense Fund 1985, 3). Babies of teenage mothers are more likely to have health problems, but these disadvantages result mainly from the fact that teenage mothers are likely to be poor and therefore to have had inadequate prenatal care, poor diet, and so on (Schorr 1988, chap. 4; Luker 1991, 77).

- Teenage childbearing is not ruining teenagers' or children's lives. When teenagers of similarly poor and otherwise disadvantaged backgrounds are compared, the girls who don't have babies don't do much better. And children of poor teenage mothers do not fare any worse than children of poor adult mothers (Butler 1992; Furstenberg, Brooks-Gunn and Morgan 1987; Geronimus 1991; Geronimus and Korenman 1992, 1993). The myth derives from mistaking correlations for causes: that most teenage births occur among the poor does not mean that they *cause* poverty.

- Most teenage childbearing is only *partly* teenage: when teenage girls become pregnant, the fathers are usually not teenagers. For example, 14 percent of teenage white girls become parents, but only 5 percent of white boys; or 31 percent of black girls and 13 percent of black boys (Sandefur and McLanahan 1990).

Why, then, is there such a widespread impression that we have an "epidemic" of teenage pregnancy? Probably the most important intellectual reason is failure to distinguish between teenage and out-of-wedlock birth. Most teenage mothers in the first half of this century and earlier were married or got married. In 1970 babies born out of wedlock accounted for one-third of teen births; in 1986 they were almost two-thirds (Luker 1991, 75). Although the very concept of teenage implied someone immature, when girls got married, they somehow magically ceased being teenagers.

And out-of-wedlock pregnancy *has* increased. But here too there are many myths.

- Out-of-wedlock childbirth has increased only *relatively*, not absolutely. That is, it has increased mainly because married fertility has decreased.

- Among blacks, the apparent increase in out-of-wedlock childbirth is even more radically an artifact of a decline in marriage. The proportion of blacks ever married dropped from 72 percent in 1960 to 49 percent in 1988; among whites it went from 76 percent to 67 percent (Ellwood and Crane 1990).

- While the black teenage out-of-wedlock birth rate increased 25 percent, the rate quadrupled among white teens (Bumpass and McLanahan 1989; Luker 1991, 75).

- Although out-of-wedlock childbirth has increased generally, teenage motherhood has not increased as a proportion of out-of-wedlock fertility; adult out-of-wedlock births are increasing proportionately.

One useful way to characterize what is going on is as change in the situation and outcome of teenage pregnancies. We can categorize these changes thus: First, pregnant teenage girls are not getting married as much as they used to, neither before nor after their pregnancies. In 1984 only 6 percent of teenagers were married, compared to 12 percent in 1970. Thus, the proportion of teen pregnancy that becomes out-of-wedlock birth is growing. Second, unmarried teenage girls are now more likely to keep their babies than to give them up for adoption. Third, many more teenage pregnancies do not result in births because the girls have abortions—probably about half the teenage pregnancies end this way (Children's Defense Fund 1985, 4).

It is odd to find so many "experts" confusing teenage with out-of-wedlock childbirth. I would hypothesize that one reason is the search for an amoralized way of discussing the problem. The combined influence of feminism and a sexual revolution makes it no longer possible to assume that the error of nonmarital sex and reproduction is self-evident. The steady extension of childhood makes teenagers immature, while increasing immiseration and inequality make ghetto teenagers sometimes self-destructive and dangerous. To aid and control teenagers and their children seems, by contrast, a self-evident social need.

In both expert and popular discourse, the teenage pregnancy alarm fits so badly with "the facts" because it is actually about so many facts. The factual context includes a vast transformation in consciousness of and about women; a new religious secular/fundamentalist dichotomy; the developing of sexual liberalization to the extent that nonmarital sex is a norm; the enormous development of a market selling goods to teenagers—this list could be much longer. The teenage pregnancy moral panic *does* fit many such facts. It is a cluster of meaning, densely packed with a variety of extreme anxieties.

Because it is so packed, it is difficult to exhaust the meanings of teenage pregnancy, which could be analyzed along a variety of axes: attitudes toward welfare, toward marriage, toward sex, toward abortion, toward minorities, and so on. Teenage pregnancy may be effective as a symbol precisely because it can express so many different laments about society.

The discourse about teenage pregnancy offers not only a lament but also a variety of analyses and proposals in diverse discursive modes. Consider the phenomenon in class terms, for example. Much of the expert and political debate apparently focuses on the relation of teenage pregnancy to poverty. This is argued in terms of incentives and deterrents, causes and effects. Whether teenage pregnancy is more causal or more symptomatic is, of course, a version of an old dispute about characterological or environmental influences on behavior. Numerous commentators suggest that teenage pregnancy makes people poor and is responsible in part for the development of an "underclass"; the problem is caused, they charge, by immorality and irresponsibility on the part of parents if not girls. Those responsible should be punished. Experts respond by measuring incentive effects in an amoralized language. Punishment and responsibility are not in their vocabulary. Their universe of discourse is about intergenerational and intrafamilial transmission of out-of-wedlock pregnancy, opportunity costs, market insertion, labor-market attachment, long-term dependency, and the like. They are concerned to see what social policies correlate with what variations in teenage pregnancy rates. The fact that the research is almost entirely quantitative contributes to its positivist and unreflective foundations. David Ellwood (1988) pointed out a typical problem with this expert research and discourse: numerous expensive studies have demonstrated that "welfare" offers little if any incentive for unwed women to have babies, but the research has made no dent in public opinion, which remains sure that welfare encourages this kind of reproductive immorality and irresponsibility. Why do some formulations resonate with popular understandings while others do not?

In fact, most of the social scientific discussion of teenage pregnancy, popular or scholarly, rests on a variety of implicit value assumptions. For example, research about single motherhood usually accepts the premise that a large welfare state with many welfare recipients is a bad thing; the goal is to reduce it by getting single mothers "off welfare." It assumes that married teenage motherhood is not a problem. The research about whether welfare provides an incentive for women not to marry or to separate from their husbands assumes that these choices should be discouraged. My purpose here is not to conduct an argument about such premises but to show that they exist. Because the social scientific research about teenage pregnancy avoids articulating such hidden moral assumptions, it naturally has little impact on a political debate that is intensely moral and moralistic.

We would benefit from a moral discourse rather than a moralistic or an amoralized one. Experts as much as citizens have a responsibility to address explicitly what is wrong with teenage pregnancy and teenage and out-of-wedlock childbearing, ethically as well as medically and economically, in the context of the actual class and racial situations of the teenagers. For a middle-class white girl a pregnancy might be an emotionally painful and scary episode, but it would probably be an episode because it would probably not result in motherhood; if it did it would change her life enormously. For a poor black teenager the pregnancy might well create more positive emotions, would more likely yield a baby, and would not necessarily produce only negative consequences. Would this analysis then suggest that it was more justified for a middle-class than for a working-class girl to have an abortion? Obviously absurd. Certainly I am not defending teenage pregnancy; it would be preferable for all girls to have so many aspirations, so much to do, that they feel they must postpone childbearing. But research and policy experts need to analyze the context in which their own moral norms developed, and how applicable they are outside that context.

Moralistic as opposed to moral discourse, I have suggested, is created in part by failure to consider the entire context of decisions. One needed inquiry must ask, what are the real choices, and the self-interest, of poor teenage girls regarding sexual activity and reproduction? This question is blocked in part by the continued identification of teenage pregnancy with out-of-wedlock childbearing. Equally important are extremely limited understandings, found in popular and expert discussion alike, of how gender, race, and class position construct the options of actual individuals. For example, one rarely finds social science research about sexual and reproductive behavior that considers the actual degree of freedom that girls have in making sexual decisions, or the actual consequences of motherhood on an individual's range of choices. We lack nuanced comprehension of the blend of autonomy and coercion in girls' lives. For another example, the dominant discussion rarely integrates the two historical roots of high black out-of-wedlock birth rates. First, there is an African-American family system that does not stigmatize out-of-wedlock birth to the same degree that whites do. This sensibility does not honor or encourage out-of-wedlock pregnancy, but it is morally horrified by the Euro-American tradition of persecuting "illegitimate" mothers and children. Second, higher black rates of single motherhood and teen pregnancy also derive from racism, particularly in the form of economic discrimination in jobs and business. Not only do they represent the cutting off of education, career, and economic opportunities for many women, but they do so within a tradition that uniquely honors women's achievement. African-American notions of family and gender never adopted notions of women's domesticity to the extent that whites did; at the turn of this century, for example, a higher proportion of black than white women were professionals. Yet this tradition too has another cause: the greater likelihood of employment for black women was also an adaptation to race prejudice.

The social problem today called teenage pregnancy/out-of-wedlock childbearing/single motherhood has been historically constructed and drastically reshaped in the past few decades. This malleability suggests that the problem takes form from an entire context, including economic, social, cultural, and political matters. In contemporary society it is inevitably a moral and political problem, concerning fundamental values and relations of power between classes, races, generations, and the sexes. There is no way to avoid these moral and political questions and attempting to do so may result mainly in moralizing, which obscures the moral issues as well as the relevant facts, lowers the level of professional, political, and popular discussion, and makes it much harder to help the teenagers.

Notes

1. In fact, there are four categories here: teenage pregnancy, teenage childbirth, out-of-wedlock pregnancy, out-of-wedlock childbirth. In my discussion I will try to be specific, but sometimes I will use the phrases loosely, as they are used in the popular discussion, precisely in order to evoke the undifferentiated anxieties in play.
2. Divorced women became a part of this social problem only much later because until very recently, divorce was largely confined to the prosperous (Gordon 1988, 89–92; Gordon 1994, chap. 1).
3. The discovery of this separate "culture" among blacks was a contribution of an anthropological notion of culture, evident in a new spate of studies of southern negroes by, for example, Frazier (1939), Johnson (1934, 1941), Powdermaker (1939), and Myrdal (1944). See also Davis (1939).
4. This was evident as early as 1961: "The white unwed mothers, whose illicit pregnancies provide the means by which childless couples can have families, are not considered so great a social problem as the Negro" (Vincent 1961, 13).
5. The panic was strongly affected, if not started, by the Alan Guttmacher Institute (1976) pamphlet *Eleven Million Teenagers*. Among authors who fail to make this basic distinction: Furstenberg (1976), Kelly (1987), Weatherley (1987), and Vinovskis (1988).
6. Births to those fourteen years of age and under are small enough that statistically significant trends cannot be identified. Such births constitute 0.1 percent of all white births and 0.8 percent of non-white births. Not all publicists respect this limitation. For example, the pamphlet "Teen Pregnancy in Milwaukee" of the Wisconsin Association of Family and Children's Agencies (1988) reports a 200 percent increase in the birth rate among girls ten to fourteen years of age between 1980 and 1985, without reporting actual numbers. On rates of teenage sexual activity, see Hofferth, Kahn, and Baldwin (1987).

References

Brush, Lisa. 1994. Worthy widows, welfare cheats: Construing single mothers, constructing the US welfare state, 1900–1988. Ph.D. diss., University of Wisconsin.

Bumpass, L., and S. McLanahan. 1989. Unmarried motherhood: Recent trends, composition, and black-white differences. *Demography* 26(2): 279–86.

Butler, Amy C. 1992. The changing economic consequences of teenage childbearing. *Social Service Review* 66(1): 1–31.

Children's Defense Fund. 1985. *Preventing children having children.* Brochure. Washington, D.C.: Children's Defense Fund.

———. 1986. *Trends in teen births.* Data sheet. September. Washington, D.C.: Children's Defense Fund.

———. 1988. Adolescent pregnancy prevention: Prenatal care campaign. In *The health of America's children. Maternal and child health data book.* Washington, D.C.: Author.

Davis, Kingsley. 1939. Illegitimacy and the social structure. *American Journal of Sociology* 45:215–33.

Ellwood, D. T., and J. Crane. 1990. Family change among black Americans: What do we know? *Journal of Economic Perspectives* 4(1): 65–84.

Ellwood, David T. 1988. *Poor support: Poverty in the American family.* New York: Basic Books.

Frazier, Franklin. 1939. *The Negro family in the United States.* Chicago: University of Chicago Press.

Furstenberg, Frank F., Jr. 1976. *Unplanned parenthood: The social consequences of teenage childbearing.* New York: Free Press.

Furstenberg, Frank F. Jr., J. Brooks-Gunn, and S. Philip Morgan. 1987. Adolescent mothers and their children in later life. *Family Planning Perspectives* 19 (4):142–50.

Geronimus, A. T. 1991. Teenage childbearing and social and reproductive disadvantage. *Family Relations* 40:463–71.

Geronimus, A. T., and S. Korenman 1992. The socioeconomic consequences of teen childbearing reconsidered. *Quarterly Journal of Economics* 107:1187–1214.

———. 1993. The socioeconomic costs of teenage childbearing. *Demography* 30:281–90.

Gordon, L., and S. McLanahan. 1991. Single parenthood in 1900. *Journal of Family History* 16(2): 97–116.

Gordon, Linda. 1988. *Heroes of their own lives: The politics and history of family violence.* New York: Viking/Penguin.

————. 1992. Social insurance and public assistance. *American Historical Review* 97(1): 19–54.

————. 1994. *Pitied but not entitled: AFDC and the history of welfare.* New York: Free Press, 1994; Boston: Harvard University Press, 1995 (paperback).

————, ed. 1990. *Women, the state, and welfare.* Madison: University of Wisconsin Press.

Alan Guttmacher Institute. 1976. *11 million teenagers.* Pamphlet.

Hofferth, S. L., J. R. Kahn, and W. Baldwin. 1987. Premarital sexual activity among U.S. teenage women over the past three decades. *Family Planning Perspectives* 19(2): 46–53.

Johnson, Charles S. 1934. *Shadow of the plantation.* Chicago: University of Chicago Press.

————. (1941). *Growing up in the black belt: Negro youth in the rural South.* New York: Schocken.

Kammerer, Percy G. 1918. *The unmarried mother: A study of five hundred cases.* Boston: Little, Brown.

Kelly, James R. 1987. Numbers versus principles: Moral realism and teenage pregnancies. *America,* February 14. 130–36.

Kunzel, Regina. 1993. *Fallen women, problem girls: Unmarried mothers and the professionalization of social work.* New Haven: Yale University Press.

Ladner, Joyce. 1986. Teenage pregnancy: The implication for black Americans. In *The State of Black America, 1986.* New York: National Urban League.

Luker, Kristin. 1991. Dubious conceptions: The controversy over teen pregnancy. *American Prospect* 5(spring): 73–83.

Myrdal, Gunnar. 1944. *An American dilemma: The negro problem and modern democracy.* New York: Harper & Brothers.

National Council on Illegitimacy. 1969. *The double jeopardy, the triple crisis: Illegitimacy today.* New York: National Council on Illegitimacy.

Powdermaker, Hortense. 1939. *After freedom: A cultural study in the deep South.* New York: Atheneum.

Pratt, W. C., and M. C. Horn. 1985. "Wanted and unwanted childbearing: US, 1973–1982." *Advance Data from Vital and Health Statistics,* No. 108. Summarized in *Family Planning Perspectives* 17(6): 274–75.

Sandefur, G., and S. McLanahan. 1990. *Family background, race and ethnicity, and early family formation.* Discussion Papers No. 911–90. Madison: University of Wisconsin, Institute for Research on Poverty.

Schorr, Lisbeth B. 1988. *Within our reach: Breaking the cycle of disadvantage.* New York: Anchor Doubleday.

Solinger, Rickie. 1992. *Wake up little Susie: Single pregnancy and race before Roe v. Wade*. New York: Routledge.

Vincent, Clark E. 1961. *Unmarried mothers*. Glencoe, Ill.: Free Press.

———. 1968. Illegitimacy. In *International encyclopedia of the social sciences*, edited by D. L. Sills. Vol. 7. New York: Macmillan and the Free Press.

Vinovskis, Maris. 1981. *Fertility in Massachusetts from the Revolution to the Civil War*. New York: Academic Press.

———. 1988. Teenage pregnancy and the underclass. *Public Interest* 93(fall): 87–96.

Weatherley, Richard A. 1987. Teenage pregnancy, professional agendas, and problem definitions. *Journal of Sociology and Social Welfare* 14(2): 5–35.

Wisconsin Association of Family and Children's Agencies. 1988. *Teen pregnancy in Milwaukee*. Pamphlet.

Young, Leontine. 1954. *Out of wedlock*. New York: McGraw-Hill.

Zelnik, M., and J. F. Kantner. 1980. Sexual activity, contraceptive use and pregnancy among metropolitan-area teenagers: 1971–70. *Family Planning Perspectives* 12(5): 230–37.

Moralizing the Microbe

The Germ Theory and the Moral Construction of Behavior in the Late-Nineteenth-Century Antituberculosis Movement

Nancy Tomes

In September of 1893 a Philadelphia doctor named Lawrence Flick (1893) received a doleful letter from the husband of a consumptive patient. Husband and physician had agreed to tell the woman she had "a malignant tumor," a diagnosis they felt would be easier for her to bear than the knowledge she had an advanced case of tuberculosis—a grim reflection on the terrors associated with consumption. But the man had finally been forced to tell his wife the truth because other family members feared that she would unwittingly infect her little granddaughter by such loving intimacies as feeding the baby from her spoon. "Of course it became my duty to say so to Mrs. P and I have the usual credit of the bearer of bad news," her husband complained to Flick. To make her aware of the danger she represented to the child, the man gave his wife a brief lesson in the germ theory of tuberculosis: "that the mycrobes [*sic*] or bacilli might carry the disease to a young child and that for the sake of all of us she must not kiss the child or give it a chance of inhaling her breath or feeding from her plate of food."

This sad vignette attests to the relevance that new scientific conceptions of infectious disease came to have for a broad range of personal habits at the turn of the century. The germ theory of disease, which gained widespread acceptance after 1880, inspired mass health education crusades that intensified popular concerns about the contagious properties of the body and its by-products. Hygienic infractions once regarded as merely disgusting or ill-bred, such as indiscriminate spitting or coughing, now became defined as serious threats to the public health.

Nowhere was this intensification of concern about personal hygiene more evident than in the campaigns to prevent the spread of tuberculosis, the single most deadly disease of the period. The scientific revelation in 1882 that consumption, long thought to be a hereditary illness, was in fact caused by the tubercle bacillus prompted a great public health crusade to reshape the individual habits and social conditions thought accountable for its ravages. Until the discovery of effective drug treatments for the disease in the 1940s, prevention remained the central strategy of TB control.

In 1892 Lawrence Flick, who himself suffered from consumption, organized the first antituberculosis society in the United States: the Pennsylvania Society for the Prevention of Tuberculosis (Bates 1992). By 1916 more than thirteen hundred local and state groups were conducting aggressive propaganda campaigns under the direction of the National Tuberculosis Association (1916), founded in 1904. Municipal and state public health departments also made TB prevention a top priority of educational work. Together the private and public sectors of the antituberculosis movement mounted what constituted the first mass health education campaign in U.S. history. Through countless lectures, exhibits, posters, films, and pamphlets, millions of Americans from all walks of life were exposed to the same hygienic message: TB was a deadly communicable disease that had to be contained by hygienic measures such as spitting and coughing in a careful fashion, using individual drinking cups and dishes, and breathing fresh, clean air (Teller 1988).

Because of its unprecedented scope and intensity, the turn-of-the-century crusade against TB had a profound impact on what might be termed public health morality, that is, the responsibilities that ordinary people assumed to guard themselves and others against infection. Extremes of dirt and disorder had long been associated with the risk of contagious disease, but the hygienic transgressions identified by this new crusade were far more commonplace and subtle: acts as seemingly inconsequential as coughing without covering the mouth, sharing a drinking cup, or dusting the house incorrectly could endanger otherwise clean-living individuals. Invoking laboratory evidence about how TB spread, public health authorities used categorical statements about "good" and "bad," responsible and irresponsible behavior to promote the observance of exacting hygienic rituals.

The antituberculosis movement offers a revealing case study of the impact that a changing scientific theory, in this instance the reconceptualization of consumption as a germ disease, can have on the moral significance of health-related conduct. TB is particularly instructive in this regard because unlike other highly visible diseases of the period, such as typhoid and cholera, its identity as an infectious disease was not well established prior to Robert Koch's discovery of the tubercle bacillus in 1882. Moreover, the bacteriological investigation of TB focused attention on commonplace behaviors, from spitting and sneezing to sharing drinking cups and tolerating flies, that had not previously been linked to the spread of deadly disease (Rogers 1989). In other words, the newly moralized behaviors associated with TB prevention reflected a significant dependence on experimentally derived hygienic truths.

The history of the antituberculosis crusade also allows us to examine the frequently asserted but little investigated proposition that the germ theory of disease narrowed the social and moral vision of the public health movement. To be sure, older public health reformers resisted the germ theory because they felt that it made the course of disease too random, too divorced from personal and societal accountability (Stevenson 1955; Rosenberg 1992). But their apprehensions proved unfounded; far from narrowing the range of moral discourse about illness, the reconceptualization of TB as a germ disease opened up rich new veins of meaning regarding both individual and collective responsibilities for disease prevention.

These historical reflections on the antituberculosis campaign and its conceptions of public health morality are particularly timely, given the new concerns raised by what the media have christened "superbugs." Not only has the AIDS epidemic shattered the complacency about infectious diseases that developed after the antibiotic revolution of the mid-twentieth century, but also after years of decline, tuberculosis rates have begun to rise again in recent years (Grmek 1990; Ryan 1992). Health officials and the public generally are concerned once again about the potential risks of infection posed by certain personal behaviors. As I hope to demonstrate, the history of the early-twentieth-century antituberculosis campaigns provides insight into both the contagion beliefs and the moral expectations Americans bring to the contemporary resurgence of anxiety about infectious disease.

Public Health Morality and the Recognition
of Tuberculosis as a Germ Disease

The moralization of tuberculosis-related behaviors at the turn of the century built upon a long-term process of extending and intensifying popular responsibility for disease prevention. In times of epidemic, the public had traditionally been expected to observe certain precautions regarding personal and household cleanliness. Over the course of the nineteenth century, as both the rates of infectious disease and the scientific knowledge about their transmission increased dramatically, the range of those preventive duties expanded significantly. A hygienic vigilance once deemed necessary only when epidemic disease threatened became a daily requirement for urban living. This mid-nineteenth-century tradition of disease prevention, known as "sanitary science," provided the intellectual and moral foundation for the antituberculosis movement (Duffy 1990; Tomes 1990).

Early explications of the germ theory of disease built upon and reinforced the tendency, already apparent in sanitarian thinking, to highlight the role of the human body as a polluter. Whether conceived of as an organic poison or as living germs, invisible particles of contagion had awesome power to multiply in the human body and its immediate environment, according to late-nineteenth-century disease theory. Sanitarians and germ theory advocates alike stressed that under the right conditions, a single sick individual could start an epidemic. Thus, it was all the more essential that the public be educated about its responsibilities for disease prevention.

To this end, public health reformers promoted a new code of personal and domestic hygiene designed to control the disposal of dangerous human wastes, particularly fecal matter. In the 1870s and 1880s they conducted a vigorous campaign to get middle-class urbanites to open their homes to sunlight and fresh air, which were considered natural disinfectants; to install special plumbing to prevent dangerous "sewer gases" from polluting the household air; to isolate the sick and disinfect their bodily wastes, particularly fecal discharges; and to keep their homes and yards free of decaying organic matter (Tomes 1990).

Beginning in the late 1860s and 1870s, a small group of scientists, chief among them the French chemist Louis Pasteur, began to argue for a different explanation for why such hygienic measures worked to ward off contagion. Employing a new type of evidence, based on microscopic examination and laboratory experimentation, advocates of the so-called germ theory of disease posited that the real agents of infection were different species of living microorganisms, which entered the body through the nose, mouth, and skin. These living microorganisms spread from the sick to the well by means of the former's germ-laden discharges, either by direct personal contact or by diffusion into the air and water (King 1991).

Throughout the 1870s and 1880s the medical profession in Europe and the United States debated the validity of this new explanation for contagion. Accustomed to thinking of disease as the product of complex environmental and individual factors, many physicians found the new emphasis on bacteria to be too simplistic. But gradually, improved laboratory methods, including pure cultures, staining methods, and rigorous animal experiments, overcame objections to the germ theory. Moreover, its advocates were quick to emphasize that it supported the preventive measures adopted by the previous generation of sanitarians. For all their differences over etiological explanations, both sides in the controversy agreed that individual and civic cleanliness were the best means to contain the threat of contagion (Tomes 1990).

Initially, these widening expectations of vigilance against infection were not aimed at the prevention of tuberculosis. As did their western European contemporaries, American physicians firmly believed that consumption resulted from a constitutional tendency or "diathesis," which parents passed on to their children. Although traditional folk beliefs in the contagiousness of consumption persisted in the nineteenth century, doctors and educated laypeople alike never doubted that it was a hereditary disorder. Until the 1880s consumptives lived and died without the consciousness that they could infect others with their illness (Dubos and Dubos 1987; Rothman 1994).

In his autobiography, Edward Trudeau (1915), the founder of the famous Saranac sanitarium, vividly recalled the lack of concern about infection common in his youth. In the late 1860s, when he was in his early twenties, Trudeau nursed his consumptive brother through his final illness, even sleeping in the same bed with him, without the least thought of his own danger. "Not only did the doctor never advise any precautions to protect me against infection, but he told me repeatedly never to open the windows, as it would aggravate the cough," he remembered. Trudeau developed the disease himself soon after his brother's death, most likely as a result of his filial act of devotion.

The hereditary character of TB was so firmly established that

laboratory evidence to the contrary found little immediate acceptance. Even after Koch isolated the tubercle bacillus in 1882, many
physicians remained skeptical about the disease's contagiousness
(Dubos and Dubos 1987). Its pattern of spread simply did not con-
form to physicians' experience with epidemic diseases such as smallpox or cholera, which radiated quickly and more or less predictably
from a single infected individual or geographical location. Any doctor could think of households where relatives had lived closely with
consumptives for years yet never apparently developed the disease
themselves. In the words of one physician, TB simply did not con-
form to the "time-honored definition of a contagious disease"
(Morse 1919).

But slowly over the course of the 1880s and 1890s, painstaking
laboratory work and clinical observation began to unravel the complex identity of tuberculosis as a *chronic* infectious disease. First, researchers demonstrated that a wide range of seemingly disparate
diseases were caused by the same bacillus. Depending on how it
gained access to the body and where it lodged, the tubercle bacillus
(and more rarely, the bovine strain of the disease) attacked different
structures, producing phthisis, or tuberculosis of the lung (the most
common form of the disease); scrofula, or tuberculosis of the lymph
nodes; Pott's disease, or tuberculosis of the bone; and "galloping"
or miliary consumption, a massive, generalized infection spread
through the bloodstream. Furthermore, autopsies of individuals
who died from other diseases frequently revealed healed TB lesions,
suggesting that many people had mild cases of the disease without
ever being aware of it (Dubos and Dubos 1987).

Second, investigators found that the tubercle bacillus could be
found abundantly in the household environment, in house dust and
fly droppings, on drinking vessels and skirt hems. Subsequent research showed that the microorganisms so cultured had little infective power, but *at the time*, these fledgling bacteriological
investigations seemed to confirm that infective particles were everywhere present in the air, dust, and foods such as milk and meat. As
the distinguished physician William Osler (1905) observed, "The
germ of tuberculosis is ubiquitous; few reach maturity without infection; none reach old age without a focus somewhere." He concluded, "That we do not all die of the disease is owing to the
resistance of the tissues; in other words, to [the] unfavorable, i.e.,
the rocky soil on which the seeds have fallen."

The key to understanding why not everyone developed tuberculosis was "resistance," that is, the body's capacity to resist the germ

invasion. In these early discussions of what we now call the immune system, turn-of-the-century researchers posited various factors that contributed to the individual's "resisting power." Some people inherited a stronger physique, which allowed them to throw off the germs of disease, a position that nicely harmonized with older traditions of constitutional medicine. In addition, Edward Trudeau's animal experiments (1887) suggested that overcrowding and malnutrition dramatically lowered the body's ability to resist invasion by the tubercle bacillus. Thus, scientific research seemed to confirm that personal regimen could either protect or predispose one to tuberculosis.

The strategy for containing the dangers of tuberculosis that researchers deduced from this experimental evidence was twofold, as Dr. James Tyson (1894) of Philadelphia declared: "[F]irst, the contagion must be destroyed as far as possible with the means at our disposal, and second, we must seek to change the soil on which it is known that the bacillus flourishes, by improving the general health of the individual, and thus increase his ability to repel the invader." The antituberculosis crusade promoted both lines of action, that is, reducing the number of tubercle bacillus in the environment by teaching everyone preventive hygienic measures; and improving general resistance by providing adequate housing, nutritious food, fresh air, and ample sunlight for every citizen.

Despite the growing quantity and sophistication of bacteriological evidence attesting to its infectious nature, many American physicians remained unconvinced that TB was more than mildly communicable. The idea of classing consumption with smallpox or typhoid, and applying the same rigorous measures of isolation to those who suffered from it, generated considerable resistance. The disease's course seemed so clearly dependent on factors other than exposure to the tubercle bacillus that emphasizing its contagious nature might be counterproductive. When during a debate at the College of Physicians of Philadelphia in 1894, Lawrence Flick argued for registering TB as a contagious disease, Solomon Solis-Cohen (1894) summed up the general sense of opposition to the proposal: "If we direct our attention too strongly toward germicidal measures we shall lose sight of the more important measures that relate to the general sanitation of cities, of houses, and of individuals."

But the fear that representing TB as a germ disease would result in a narrower range of preventive measures against it proved to be unfounded. The very fact that the bacilli's impact on the body depended on so many other factors, from personal hygiene to housing conditions, made it a splendid vehicle for late-nineteenth-century public health activism. Unlike venereal diseases, whose rising rates also concerned reformers in this period (Brandt 1985), the TB menace could be discussed openly and aggressively. As cholera and typhoid had supplied the previous generation of public health leaders with a generous mandate for attacking urban filth, recognition of TB as a germ disease allowed Progressive Era reformers to promote an expansive new spirit of individual and collective responsibility for disease.

Tuberculosis "Religion"

Addressing the Warren, Pennsylvania, Academy of Sciences in 1909 on the subject of "Preventive Measures Against Tuberculosis," Dr. M. V. Ball (1909) said of the "doctrine" of tuberculosis contagion, "When . . . one has this conviction strong in his heart he becomes as zealous in the promulgation of what he calls 'the light' as the most devout convert of some new religious truth. The antituberculosis campaign has in it much of the fervor of a new religion." This fervor was explicitly grounded in the popular veneration of science so common among Progressive Era reformers (Burnham 1987). They believed that the scientific method, as they variously construed it, would produce an ever more accurate understanding of why diseases occurred; through popular education, the public would be shown the "light" and thereby be freed from disease and death. Pasteur, Koch, and Trudeau were often invoked as modern-day saints whose courage and scientific skill had finally exposed the infective nature of the deadly white plague. Playing up the heroic dimension, a postcard designed to advertise the 1909 International Tuberculosis Exhibition in Philadelphia bore the legend "The two emancipators: Lincoln wiped out slavery. Science can wipe out consumption" (Yeager 1909).

Although science was certainly their touchstone, TB workers invoked religious language and symbols in their hygienic exhortations as well. The recurrent use of terms such as *salvation*, *gospel*, and *crusade* along with the symbol of the double-barred cross imbued their work with a sense of spiritual mission. TB pamphlets were often referred to as "tracts" or "catechisms," and the rules of health they contained were called "commandments." One circular for consumptives distributed by the Illinois State Board of Health (1908–

1910) began with the admonition "FOLLOW THE GOLDEN RULE: 'Do unto others as you would that they should do unto you,' " followed by a list of more prosaic injunctions such as "DON'T EVER SPIT ON ANY FLOOR, BE HOPEFUL AND CHEERFUL, KEEP THE WINDOW OPEN." The National Tuberculosis Association's (NTA) Modern Health Crusade, an innovative child health education program begun in the 1910s, enlisted the young in a quasi-holy war against TB, reminiscent of the role nineteenth-century evangelicals accorded the "redemptive child" (Welter 1976). Observing the parallel with the medieval Christians' crusades against the infidels, one young crusader observed in her prize-winning essay, now "the germs are the Turks" (Modern Health Crusade Department 1918).

If not as overtly as their sanitarian predecessors, TB workers still equated their hygienic code with God's natural law. The same Illinois State Board of Health (1908–1910) circular that began with the "Golden Rule" explained,

> God gives man an abundance of fresh air and sunlight for his daily use. Man, with the perversity which characterizes the human race, immures himself behind wooden or stone walls, and excludes or grudgingly admits even that air and light which is necessary for his well-being. The sickness or death resulting from this violation of the laws of nature is invariably attributed to "the will of God."

Reformers asserted that TB resulted not from divine providence but from human ignorance and stubbornness, or a kind of hygienic original sin.

Tuberculosis "religion" required rigorous adherence to a set of stringent rules designed to contain the dangers of contagion. This hygienic code envisioned the infective human body at the center of a series of concentric circles, moving outward from the individual body to the house to the public spaces of streets and buildings. Each circle of contagion posed its own special dangers and required its own special hygienic precautions. The TB workers' conception of these circles incorporated older sanitarian mappings of the body's dangerous attributes. Prior to the 1890s, the main focus of hygienic precautions against infection had been the breath, feces, vomit, and skin particles of the sick, bodily by-products that had been implicated by long clinical and epidemiological experience with eruptive fevers such as smallpox and "filth diseases" such as cholera and typhoid. TB prevention reformulated older fears of the infectious breath into more specific concerns with the saliva, sputum, and droplets expelled by coughing and sneezing, which had not been so closely linked with lethal disease. In other words, the bacteriological investigation of tuberculosis intensified the dangers associated with discharges from the mouth and nose (Tomes in press).

Spit was by far the most lethal new element added to late-nineteenth-century conceptions of bodily contagion. Etiquette and health authorities had long condemned spitting, especially of tobacco juice, as a breach of manners and general cleanliness (Elias 1978; Kasson 1990). But prior to the 1880s, they had portrayed the negative moral and health consequences of spitting as limited to the transgressor himself; spitting was not condemned as a mode of spreading diseases to others. Only after microscopic investigation located the tubercle bacillus in the consumptive's sputum did the spitting habit become defined as a serious menace to the public health.

The antituberculosis literature waxed eloquent on the perils posed by the consumptives' mouth discharges. An NTA (1916) circular warned, "The germ, which is a microscopic rod, is found in millions in their spit from very early in the disease, and it is through this spit almost alone that it reaches others." The antispitting slogans taught schoolchildren constantly affirmed the habit's deadly consequences. A pamphlet distributed in the public schools by the New York City Department of Health (1908) affirmed the precepts "Spitting is dangerous, indecent and against the law" and "No spit, no consumption."

These beliefs about the infective properties of the consumptives' bodily discharges, particularly their spit, led logically to an emphasis on the home as a source of disease. In frequently styling TB as a "house disease," Progressive reformers adopted and adapted older sanitarian preoccupations with home hygiene. The same zones of danger outlined in domestic manuals of the 1870s and 1880s, such as damp cellars, unaired bedrooms, and upholstered furniture (Tomes 1990), persisted in TB pamphlets for decades later (Tomes 1997).

The infective matter of TB was endowed with extraordinary abilities to fly through the air for great distances, to attach itself to common objects, to mingle with dust and dirt, and to taint liquids such as water and milk. A 1910 TB "catechism" prepared for eighth graders in New York City schools described its persistence and mobility: "The germs will live in the darkness and dampness for a long time, and are stirred up in dusting and sweeping these rooms, and float in the air and may be breathed into the lungs, or may fall upon articles of food and be taken into the body in that way" (New York City Department of Health and the Committee on Prevention of Tuberculosis of the Charity Organization Society 1910). At times the infective power of germs seemed almost supernatural, "an ever present demon" and an "insatiable, microscopic destroyer," in the words of one tract (Salmon 1889).

Although antituberculosis reformers saw the home as the primary site of infection, they also emphasized how contagion lurked in the outside world as well. Any public space or social interaction where human bodies and their by-products mingled represented a potential site for spreading the disease. Anxiety about preventing TB led to changes in the conduct of diverse institutions, including hotels, funeral parlors, commercial laundries, and public schools. For example, occupying a steamship cabin, a Pullman berth, or a hotel room involved the risk of inhabiting a space previously contaminated by a consumptive. Thus, the owners of such establishments had to take pains to assure clients that the room and its contents had been thoroughly cleaned and disinfected (Tomes in press). To avoid the dangers of contaminated blankets, the *Pennsylvania Health Bulletin* advised in 1910, "The careful traveller will . . . insist that the blanket be covered by a fresh clean sheet the turn down of which shall cover it for a distance of two feet from the top" (Pennsylvania Department of Health 1910), a custom that persists in many hotels to this day.

The fact that TB sufferers were often able to maintain a normal routine until their disease was far advanced made such vigilance especially important. Unlike cholera or smallpox victims, consumptives could move freely in society and spread the seeds of disease for many years. In an 1888 talk entitled "The Hygiene of Phthisis," Lawrence Flick conjured up a chilling vision of "consumptive tailors and dressmakers, consumptive cooks and waiters, consumptive candy-makers, consumptive bakers, consumptives indeed in every calling of life. These people do not suspect for a moment that they are spreading the disease, and take no precaution against doing so."

The dangers of contagion were all the more insidious because of the invisible, insensible nature of germs. Unlike the older, more straightforward concept of "filth," which usually announced itself by foul odor and squalid appearance, the menace of bacterial enemies was far harder to detect. Antituberculosis writings constantly repeated the warning that things were not as they seemed, conjuring up images of the quaint wooden dipper laden with deadly germs or the seemingly healthy-looking dairy cows infected with bovine tuberculosis.

"Worries and Torments": Hygiene as Moral Regeneration

To counter this all-pervading danger, popular health education aimed at a "sort of moral regeneration," in the words of one anti-tuberculosis worker. As he put it, "What the tuberculosis propaganda seeks to do is not to stamp facts and figures on the public mind but to infuse life into them and make them into so many thousand worries and torments to prick the public conscience into action" (Hamman 1910). Antituberculosis work required that the everyday world of objects and habits be made problematic: familiar ways of disposing of one's spit, cleaning one's rugs, and serving one's food had to be infused with new significance and urgency. In translating the cosmology of germ dangers into a concrete code of hygienic behavior at both the personal and collective level, the conceptions of what constituted faulty behavior were cast exceedingly wide.

Here again, the TB crusade built upon sanitarian conventions of public health morality. In and of themselves, the intensity and scope of their hygienic exhortations were no greater than the previous generations' efforts to avoid foul air and sewer gas. Where the TB movement clearly outdid its sanitarian predecessors was in the superiority of its mass educational methods: using the best of Progressive Era advertising techniques, TB workers exposed a much broader range of Americans to their "worries and torments" (Tomes in press).

The pedagogical techniques used by TB workers were morally heavy-handed, to say the least. They devised endless lists of "dos and don'ts," covering a multitude of behaviors: there were "right" and "wrong" ways to mop the floor, blow one's nose, prepare a baby's bottle, and set a table. Health exhibits specialized in "good" and "bad" rooms that laid out the proper floor coverings, drapes, and furniture styles to combat the scourge of the tubercle bacillus. The tone of admonitions was fierce, brooking no deviation: "It should be an absolute rule," intoned one author, "never to put a baby or a young child on the floor to play, as is so generally the custom" (Vietor 1905). The extraordinary range of behaviors identified as potentially dangerous, from licking stamps to handling paper money, reinforced the message that even the tiniest infraction could lead to death. "We are each one of us in hourly danger," warned the Pennsylvania Department of Health (1910) in an article entitled "Little Dangers to Be Avoided in the Daily Fight Against Tuberculosis."

At the same time they stressed elaborate rituals of germ avoidance, antituberculosis writers took pains to emphasize the other side of the preventive equation, namely, maintaining the body's "resisting power." Each individual had a responsibility not to provide the omnipresent TB germs with a susceptible host. The "seed-and-soil" metaphor, drawn from the New Testament parable about the soil needed to nourish the seeds of sin, was a favorite metaphor for making this point. The individuals who led a healthy life and kept their homes clean provided the tubercle bacillus only a "rocky soil" for propagation (Osler 1905). The metaphor had the added merit of reconciling the germ theory with older hygienic traditions that stressed the importance of maintaining a strong body and a clean environment (Nutton 1983). In this fashion, TB workers easily incorporated the time-honored emphasis on the "nonnaturals"—good food, fresh air, sufficient rest, and mental balance—in their preventive regimen, and linked TB control with the temperance and mental hygiene movements.

The Socialism of the Microbe

The moral framework for explaining why some people caught tuberculosis and others did not clearly emphasized individual responsibility: each person had an impelling duty to attend to public health directives and to practice protective rituals against consumption. But this emphasis on individual responsibility did not preclude more collective conceptualizations of health morality in the war against the white plague. The tuberculosis movement constantly acknowledged the interconnectedness of health behavior: imprudent behavior endangered not only the individual but those around him as well. Given the mobility and vitality of tuberculosis germs, there could be no simple dividing line between the potentially contagious self and the rest of society.

As in its conceptions of individual responsibility, the tuberculosis movement built upon older hygienic conventions of public health morality. Both in the older sanitarian tradition and the early formulations of the germ theory, nineteenth-century hygiene writers constantly emphasized how a better scientific understanding of contagion transformed and broadened one's civic responsibilities to prevent disease. As Harriette Plunkett (1885) wrote in her quaintly titled treatise *Women, Doctors, and Plumbers*, a neighbor was no longer just the man who lived next door, "but he also is the man whose premises the breeze may sweep, and bear its particles to our lungs and blood, at whatever distance, or at whichever point of the compas [*sic*] he abides." Germs were no respecters of persons, she concluded, and would fasten on a man "whether he be a millionaire or a shillingaire, with a perfectly leveling and democratic impartiality."

Progressive Era public health reformers repeated and elaborated on this interdependency theme endlessly. A particularly fine explication of the argument appeared in an article provocatively entitled "The Microbe as a Social Leveller," written by New York City Health Commissioner Cyrus Edson (1895). "The microbe of disease is no respecter of persons," he wrote; "it cannot be guarded against by any bank account, however large." Wealth might protect the individual by allowing him to be "well nourished, warmly clad, and properly housed." But in this day and age, Edson warned, the "Socialistic side" of the microbe required that the wealthy be concerned for the poor.

> The former cannot afford to sit at his well-covered table and forget the absence of food in the latter's poor room, because that absence of food means, sooner or later, that disease will break out in the room, and the microbes or their spores will in time pass the heavy curtains on the windows of the mansion to find their prey inside. This is the Socialism of the microbe, this is the chain of disease, which binds all the people of a community together.

The "chain-of-disease" concept naturally led to the recognition that many poor Americans lacked the material resources to avoid the known risk factors of tuberculosis. When TB workers tried to explain why some people seemed more liable than others to contract the disease, many acknowledged that conditions such as low wages and poor housing were often outside the individual's control. New York City's (1910) TB catechism explained the problem in simple terms: "The kind of people most likely to get tuberculosis are those who are run down or ill from poor or insufficient food, from living in dark, overcrowded or ill-ventilated rooms, or from overwork, or during convalescence from other exhausting diseases."

As did many Progressive Era reformers, TB workers equated the insufficiency of adequate food, rest, or housing for working-class Americans with the moral failings of their affluent neighbors. Discussions of the TB problem often included spirited condemnations of builders who put up shoddy, unsafe tenements, landlords who failed to provide adequate water supplies or toilet facilities, factory owners who paid their workers poorly, and shopkeepers who sold unclean food. Poverty and TB were obviously related; the same greedy "special interests" who depressed the living conditions of the working classes made them fertile soil for the tuberculosis bacillus.

The rhetoric of the antituberculosis crusade had many elements in common with the larger Progressive movement, especially the emphasis on the social costs of poverty and the state's overarching responsibility for the public's health. Much as reformers in general were attacking laissez-faire notions of economy and welfare, TB workers criticized the tendency toward rugged individualism in health-related matters. In their view, scientific revelations about the invisible world of germs required a new sensitivity to the interdependence of all members of society.

The recognition of collective responsibility for tuberculosis impelled many activists to endorse a broader agenda of social reform. As M. V. Ball (1909) explained to the Warren, Pennsylvania Academy of Sciences, "The fight against consumption is a fight against bad environment, in the home, in the city, in the workshop, and in the school." The elimination of TB became a powerful justification for strengthening municipal boards of public health, regulating tenement housing, inspecting sanitary conditions in factories, and providing school health services.

While encouraging concern about "how the other half lived," the TB crusade also expressed the infinite variety of ethnic and racial prejudices that abounded at the turn of the century. From the 1880s on, statistics collected by public health boards made increasingly evident that poor, immigrant, and nonwhite Americans were more likely to contract the disease than their affluent, native-born, white peers. As did Progressive reformers in general, TB workers disagreed over whether individual behavior, hereditary defect, or environmental conditions were most to blame for these group differences in the incidence of TB (Teller 1988). Their conception of collective moral responsibility for infectious disease reflected a fundamental tension between portraying the diseased "other" simultaneously as victim and menace.

Predictably, some reformers saw high rates of TB as a poor reflection on the cleanliness and temperance of specific ethnic and racial groups. In his talk "The Home in Its Relation to the Tuberculosis Problem," the influential Johns Hopkins physician William Osler (1905) provided a chart comparing the "personal and household cleanliness" of tuberculous patients treated at a Baltimore clinic, purportedly showing that 70 percent of the Russian Jewish homes, 56 percent of the "colored" homes, and 30 percent of the "white" homes were not clean. In his talk, Osler stressed the importance of personal cleanliness even though his chart demonstrated the importance of other factors, such as "bad sanitary location," "insufficient light and ventilation," and "overcrowding," that the immigrants clearly had little or no control over.

Discussions of the "Negro problem" in the South exemplify the varied causal hypotheses and moral judgments that TB workers could derive from the often repeated observation that "germs knew no color line" (Galishoff 1985; Gamble 1989). In explaining why African Americans suffered higher rates of tuberculosis, conservative whites emphasized their intellectual and moral inferiority, and pushed for special measures to segregate the "colored consumptive." In contrast, African-American reformers and their liberal white allies pointed to the same disease statistics as evidence of the race's heavy economic and social disadvantages. In cities such as Atlanta, black antituberculosis societies used white fears about the disease to press their case for improved educational and municipal services for minority neighborhoods (Tomes in press).

Gender issues figured less prominently in the rhetoric of the antituberculosis movement. Although sex differences in mortality rates were noticed as early as the 1850s (Rosenkrantz 1987), contagion and resistance were represented as bodily processes that affected women and men alike. In practice, the burden of the preventive cleanliness promoted in the name of disease control clearly fell more heavily on women than men; yet the rhetoric of the antituberculosis movement emphasized the crusade as one in which both sexes had an important role to play (Tomes 1997, Tomes in press).

Although the TB crusade certainly appealed to common stereotypes of the "other" as dirty and dangerous, and the woman citizen as social housekeeper, its public rhetoric tended to emphasize the integrative, as opposed to factionalizing, mission of health education.

Certainly, compared to contemporary efforts to prevent disease by immigration restriction and eugenics legislation, the antituberculosis movement chose a more inclusive strategy. Its stated goal was not to ostracize groups at high risk for the disease but, rather, to bring them within a protective circle of hygienic knowledge. In a society split by ethnic, class, and racial differences, the crusade portrayed the common fight against an invisible enemy—the tubercle bacillus—as a positive means of redefining what it meant to be an American.

No aspect of the movement better symbolized the reintegrative role assigned the new codes of public health morality than the many antituberculosis parades and pageants staged in the early twentieth century. These community rituals recast nineteenth-century parade forms, which had displayed the serried ranks of society by class and occupation (Davis 1986; Ryan 1989), into an army of citizens marching against disease. Conducted with circus-style promotional flourishes, antituberculosis parades were often led by children, befitting their special role as "evangelists" of health reform, and included delegations and floats from local businesses, labor unions, women's clubs, and the YM and YWCAs, in other words, the whole panoply of Progressive Era reform groups. In these symbolic public health demonstrations, disease prevention furnished a seemingly uncontested good whose pursuit cut across painful lines of difference (see, for example, Memphis Pageant 1919).

In the ideology of the TB movement, the "socialism of the microbe" undergirded a new democratic society in which good health, particularly freedom from TB, could be identified as the birthright of every citizen, regardless of gender, ethnicity, class, or race. In the context of the Progressive Era, the TB menace had a unifying as well as a fragmenting effect on a diverse society: the yardstick of health morality could be used to compare different groups and chart the path of their reclamation, both in personal and social terms.

At the same time, the recognition that TB was a germ disease undoubtedly contributed to a harsher condemnation of those who contracted the disease. Social problems such as poor housing or low wages proved far harder to correct than individual deficiencies in hygienic knowledge and control. As the Committee on Tuberculosis of the U.S. Public Health Service (1904) concluded,

> The simplest, most efficacious, and the most readily executed [method] is to prevent the opportunity of infection. . . . The tu-

berculous must be taught that they are not only capable, but are at the present time the most prolific source of the spreading of consumption. They must also be taught that they are in duty bound to protect the rest of humanity from their disease.

The TB crusade reserved its harshest moral language for the so-called careless consumptives, that is, individuals who knew they had the disease and refused to abide by the necessary precautions concerning their germ-laden discharges. For all TB workers' criticism of irresponsible landlords and factory owners, when it came time to personify the causes of tuberculosis, they almost always chose the homes and the habits of the consumptives themselves. In the NTA's stock lantern-slide lecture for the public, the only human faces shown to whom blame could be readily attached were "ignorant" consumptive parents exposing their innocent children to the disease (A Stock Lecture on Tuberculosis 1915).

In effect, the reformers communicated a double message about the tuberculous. On the one hand, they repeatedly insisted, as the brochure jointly issued by the New York City Department of Health and the Charity Organization Society (1910) explained, "It is not dangerous to live or work with a person who has tuberculosis if he is cleanly and is very careful to destroy all the sputum which he coughs up." On the other hand, the endless warnings about the ubiquitous bacteria to be found in the consumptives' vicinity invariably created a revulsion toward their company. "If we know that a friend has tuberculosis, we shall be wise if we avoid shaking hands with him, and we shall be extremely careful whom we kiss or whom we ALLOW OUR CHILDREN TO KISS," warned the Pennsylvania Health Department (1910) in "Little Dangers to Be Avoided in the Daily Fight Against Tuberculosis."

Not surprisingly, the "careless" or "unteachable" consumptive was usually poor, uneducated, and foreign-born or nonwhite. As the public health nurse Ellen La Motte (1909) wrote, "The day laborer, the shop girl, the drunken negro belong to a class which, *by reason of the very conditions which constitute it a class*, is unable to make use of what it learns" (emphasis in original). No matter how often TB workers acknowledged the "socialism of the microbe," their emphasis on both education and careful observance of sanitary rituals as the key to prevention invariably bounded the sphere of effective action along class lines. Thus, consumption inevitably became associated with not only the moral failings of individuals but also the sanitary defects of the so-called lower orders.

Conclusion

As this account of the moral lessons spun out by turn-of-the-century TB workers makes clear, the reconceptualization of tuberculosis as a germ disease did not diminish personal or collective responsibility for its prevention, as some nineteenth-century observers had feared. On the contrary, scientific revelations about the invisible menace posed by the tubercle bacillus led to a vigorous effort to define a new public health morality for both the individual and the larger society. Because the bacteria's inroads depended on so many individual and social factors, TB provided ample opportunities for moralizing about the lessons of disease.

That the public health movement eventually adopted a more restricted vision of its social mission in the 1920s did not reflect a moral narrowness inherent in the germ theory of TB. Rather, declining rates of infectious diseases, changing conceptions of disease control, and a more conservative political climate combined to dim the reformist zeal of the antituberculosis movement (Tomes in press). Deaths from tuberculosis began to decrease in the late 1800s, for reasons that historians and demographers still hotly debate (Smith 1988). Improved nutrition and housing, as well as greater efforts to isolate the ill, probably all played a role in its decline. By the late 1920s, cancer and heart disease had displaced TB as the leading causes of death. The antituberculosis societies broadened their scope to include prevention and research concerning lung diseases in general, including lung cancer. The National Tuberculosis Association renamed itself the American Lung Association in 1954.

Regardless of how much public health education actually contributed to the decline of tuberculosis, the turn-of-the-century crusades clearly transformed personal and household habits of disease avoidance. By the 1920s the antituberculosis movement had done a remarkable job of making Americans of all backgrounds feel responsible for preventing the spread of infection by attending to the minutiae of personal behavior. These contagion rules continued to be passed on from parent to child, teacher to student, long after TB ceased to be the leading cause of death; with surprisingly little modification, they inform what adults teach children about avoiding germs and staying well to this day. Most people still think in terms of using their own cups, avoiding others' sneezes, and keeping up their resistance as the best means to avoid contagion (Tomes in press).

The history of the early-twentieth-century TB crusade underlines the importance of appreciating the generational nature of popular health beliefs. Many Americans over the age of fifty today learned the explicit rules for avoiding contagion in an era when diseases such as TB were still common causes of death, and no "magic bullets" had been discovered to cure them. Not surprisingly, these survivors of the preantibiotic era in American medicine often have a greater fear of germs and devotion to hygienic rituals than their offspring, who grew up in a era when cancer, not infectious diseases, was the more fearsome threat. Phobias about dirt and germs seem to be especially strong among second- and third-generation ethnic women, whose mothers and grandmothers were the particular target of Progressive Era public health crusades (Tomes in press).

This historical understanding of the connection between generational health beliefs and past disease experiences helps to illuminate the complexity of popular health beliefs. Contagion fears and rituals forged in one high-risk disease environment were passed on to children who came to adulthood in a very different disease environment. For example, turn-of-the-century public health educators linked flies to the spread of infectious diseases such as TB and typhoid when those diseases were serious threats to the public health. The aversion to flies lighting on one's food remains strong today, even when fly-borne cases of disease are comparatively rare. No doubt children growing up today in the midst of the AIDS epidemic will transmit a very intense and specific set of fears and rituals to their children and grandchildren who may be at little risk for HIV infection.

The persistence of older layers of knowledge and behavior helps to explain why a new infectious disease such as AIDS, which has a radically different pattern of transmission than tuberculosis, originally provoked such deep anxieties about casual infection. In the face of a new and unknown infectious disease, many people regressed to an earlier era of fears and rituals designed to ward off a pervasive microbial threat rather than a disease spread primarily by the exchange of blood or semen. For example, fears of AIDS patients' saliva and spit may well have reflected the old formulation of "spit and death" so often repeated in the antituberculosis campaigns. Because of the success of these earlier public health movements, the early public health efforts against AIDS had to counteract a deeply ingrained layer of contagion beliefs with a campaign of "negative" education, that is, explaining that the disease is *not* spread by drinking glasses or shaking hands (Tomes in press).

The legacy of previous popular health crusades against infectious diseases such as TB is only one element complicating modern-day understandings of AIDS and its avoidance (Martin 1994). Still, the history of the antituberculosis movement suggests that the conceptions of public health morality adopted in the wake of the germ theory have had a long-lasting influence on American habits of disease avoidance. Perhaps with a greater awareness of the historical persistence of popular health beliefs, we can better calculate the impact of contemporary crusades to moralize the microbe.

Note

The research for this chapter was supported in part by the Rockefeller Foundation, the National Endowment for the Humanities (Grant No. RH–21055–92), and the National Library of Medicine (Grant No. RO1 LM0579–01). Its contents are solely the responsibility of the author and do not necessarily represent the views of these granting agencies. I want to thank Joan Jacobs Brumberg, Christopher Sellers, and the members of the Health and Morality working group, particularly Allan Brandt, Paul Rozin, and Keith Thomas, for their helpful comments on earlier drafts of the paper.

References

Ball, M. V. 1909. Preventive measures against tuberculosis. *Tuberculosis Pamphlets*, vol. 106, no. 28. Lawrence Flick Papers, College of Physicians of Philadelphia.

Bates, B. 1992. *Bargaining for life*. Philadelphia: University of Pennsylvania Press.

Brandt, A. M. 1985. *No magic bullet: A social history of venereal disease in the United States since 1880*. New York: Oxford University Press.

Burnham, J. C. 1987. *How superstition won and science lost: Popularizing science and health in the United States* New Brunswick: Rutgers University Press.

Davis, S. G. 1986. *Parades and power*. Philadelphia: Temple University Press.

Dubos, R., and J. Dubos 1987. *The white plague*. New Brunswick: Rutgers University Press.

Duffy, J. 1990. *The sanitarians*. Urbana: University of Illinois Press.

Elias, N. 1978. *The civilizing process: The history of manners.* Oxford: Basil Blackwell.

Edson, C. 1895. The microbe as social leveller. *North American Review* 161:421–26.

Flick, L. 1888. The hygiene of phthisis. Philadelphia: William J. Dornan. Pamphlet Collection, College of Physicians of Philadelphia.

————. 1893. WMP to Lawrence Flick, 22 September 1893. Tuberculosis Letters, Lawrence Flick Papers, Historical Collections, College of Physicians of Philadelphia.

Galishoff, S. 1985. Germs know no color line: Black health and public policy in Atlanta, 1900–1918. *Journal of the History of Medicine and Allied Sciences* 40:22–41.

Gamble, V. N. 1989. *Germs have no color line: Blacks and American medicine, 1900–1940.* New York: Garland.

Grmek, M. D. 1990. *History of AIDS: Emergence and origin of a modern pandemic.* Princeton: Princeton University Press.

Hamman, L. 1910. The prevention of tuberculosis. *Journal of the Outdoor life* 7(2): 29.

Illinois State Board of Health. 1908–1910. Consumption: [Circular] Recommended by the central board of health for general distribution. In *Tuberculosis Pamphlets*, vol. 106, no. 24. Lawrence Flick Papers, College of Physicians of Philadelphia.

Kasson, J. 1990. *Rudeness and civility.* New York: Hill & Wang.

King, L. 1991. *Transformations in American medicine.* Baltimore: Johns Hopkins University Press.

LaMotte, E. N. 1909. The unteachable consumptive. *Journal of the Outdoor Life* 6(4): 105–7.

Martin, E. 1994. *Flexible bodies: Tracking immunity in American culture from the days of polio to the age of AIDS.* Boston: Beacon Press.

Memphis pageant. 1919. *Bulletin of the National Tuberculosis Association* 5(14): 7.

Modern Health Crusade Department. 1918. *Bulletin of the National Tuberculosis Association* 4(9): 3.

Morse, L. B. 1919. Tuberculophobia—Can it longer be excused as an adult entity? *Journal of the Outdoor Life* 16(2): 45–48.

National Tuberculosis Association. 1916. *What you should know about tuberculosis.* New York: National Tuberculosis Association.

New York City Department of Health. 1908. *Do not spit: A tuberculosis (consumption) catechism and primer for school children.* New York: Board of Health.

New York City Department of Health and the Committee on Prevention of Tuberculosis of the Charity Organization Society. 1910. *What you should know about tuberculosis.* New York: Board of Health.

Nutton, V. 1983. The seeds of disease: An explanation of contagion and infection from the Greeks to the Renaissance. *Medical History* 27:1–34.

Osler, W. 1905. The home in its relation to the tuberculosis problem. *First Annual Report of the Henry Phipps Institute.* Philadelphia: Phipps Institute.

Pennsylvania Department of Health. 1910. Little dangers to be avoided in the daily fight against tuberculosis. *Pennsylvania Health Bulletin* 7:1–5.

Plunkett, H. M. 1885. *Women, plumbers, and doctors.* New York: Appleton.

Rogers, N. 1989. Germs with legs: Flies, disease, and the new public health. *Bulletin of the History of Medicine* 63(4): 599–617.

Rosenberg, C. E. 1992. Florence Nightingale on contagion: The hospital as moral universe. In *Explaining epidemics and other studies in the history of medicine.* New York: Cambridge University Press.

Rosenkrantz, B. G. 1952/1987. Introductory essay. In *The white plague,* edited by R. Dubos and J. Dubos. New Brunswick: Rutgers University Press.

Rothman, S. 1994. *Living in the shadow of death: T.B. and the social experience of illness in American history.* New York: Basic Books.

Ryan, F. 1992. *The forgotten plague.* Boston: Little, Brown.

Ryan, M. 1989. The American parade: Representations of the nineteenth-century social order. In *The New Cultural History,* edited by L. Hunt. Los Angeles: University of California Press.

Salmon, D. E. 1889. The origin and prevention of tuberculosis. *Sanitary Volunteer* 1(4): 81–86.

Smith, F. B. 1988. *The retreat of Tuberculosis, 1850–1950.* New York: Croom Helm.

Solis-Cohen, S. 1894. Discussion on the advisability of the registration of Tuberculosis. *Transactions of the College of Physicians of Philadelphia* 3d ser., 16:21.

Stevenson, L. 1955. Science down the drain. *Bulletin of the History of Medicine* 29:1–26.

A stock lecture on tuberculosis. 1915. *Journal of the Outdoor Life* 12(8): 262–63.

Teller, M. 1988. *The tuberculosis movement.* Westwood, Conn.: Greenwood Press.

Tomes, N. 1990. The private side of public health: Sanitary science, domestic hygiene, and the germ theory. *Bulletin of the History of Medicine* 64(4): 509–39.

———. In press. *The gospel of germs: Men, women, and the microbe in American life, 1880–1930*. Cambridge: Harvard University Press.

———. 1997. Spreading the germ theory: Sanitary science and the home economics movement. In *Rethinking women and home economics in the 20th century*, edited by S. Stage and V. Vincenti. Ithaca: Cornell University Press.

Trudeau, E. L. 1887. Environment experiment in relation to bacterial invasion. *Transactions of the American Climatological and Clinical Association* 4:131.

———. 1915. *An autobiography*. Philadelphia: Lea & Febiger.

Tyson, J. 1894. Discussion on the advisability of the registration of Tuberculosis. *Transactions of the College of Physicians of Philadelphia*, 3d ser., 16:18.

U.S. Public Health Service. 1904. Report of the committee on Tuberculosis. *Transactions of the Second Annual Conference of State and Territorial Health Officers with the United States Public Health and Marine-Hospital Service*, Appendix B. Washington, D.C.: Government Printing Office.

Vietor, A. 1905. Tuberculosis in everyday life. *Journal of the Outdoor Life* 2(7): 163–67.

Welter, B. 1976. Coming of age in America. In *Dimity convictions*, edited by B. Welter. Athens: Ohio University Press.

Yeager, F. N. 1909. Post cards as educational agents. *Journal of the Outdoor Life* 6(6): 172.

Contemporary Perspectives on Morality and Health

Secular Morality

Solomon Katz

The complete ban on cigarette smoking on domestic flights in the United States went into effect in October 1989. As early as January 27, 1989, when the temporary ban was still in effect, David S. Davis wrote the following on the op-ed page of the *New York Times*, in a piece entitled "Selfish, Sanctimonious Anti-Smokers":

> Recently, I boarded a flight from Boston to New York. As I sat down, the attendant announced that the flight was scheduled to take less than two hours (it actually took four hours) and consequently "in accord with Federal Aviation Association regulations this is a nonsmoking flight." A large number of the passengers cheered and applauded.
>
> There was something so sanctimonious about this outburst that I spent the remainder of the flight trying to understand why. I concluded that I had witnessed a self-righteous exhibition of moral superiority. This is not something most people, in these days of subjective moral values, have much opportunity to do. However, smoking has now become a sin, so opposing it has taken on a sanctioned and religious quality.

This description of the moral fervor surrounding smoking does not represent an impression held by Davis alone. In an address in Philadelphia in 1989, Secretary Louis Sullivan of the U.S. Department of Health and Human Services labeled R. J. Reynolds Tobacco Company "immoral" for targeting inner-city blacks in its advertising campaign for a new cigarette called Uptown. Sullivan said: "Uptown's message is more diseases, more suffering, and more death for a group already bearing more that its share of smoking-related illness and mortality" (*Philadelphia Inquirer* 1989). Within days, the company withdrew its plans to test market the new product in Philadelphia. Since the initial ban in 1987, the movement to stop smoking in public places has acquired such strong overtones for both nonsmokers and recent quitters that it has become a *moral issue.*

The Emergence of Public Secular Morality

A new kind of morality is supplementing the traditional moral code. The traditional Judeo-Christian ethic deals with sin and redemption from sin, which are defined by basic moral codes such as the Ten Commandments, the Golden Rule, various biblical sources, and their derivatives. The secular moral code, expressed in the context of health, is built on many of the same principles, but the specifics of their application depend on the new moral prescriptive and proscriptive behaviors associated with the health and fitness movement. In other words, the new code is a complex syncretism of contemporary beliefs overlaying the old framework. Thus, the same social pressures inherent in sin and redemptive sacrifice within the structure of the *traditional* code become an important means for applying the new *secular* moral code. For example, any acts that tend to violate the prescribed code are seen in moral terms, which then become transferred into the already-established model of morality (which includes concepts of sin, punishment, and redemption as a means to label and deal with transgressions). In this system eating a fattening food becomes a sin to be redeemed by eating a fat-free food in the next meal. Smoking a cigarette in private is sinful, but in smokers' minds it can be redeemed by jogging each day. The same phenomenon is evident in our health-conscious society: exercising every day or in a prescribed manner is viewed as proper, but being slothful as immoral. Ironically, however, some individuals carry their exercise morality to extremes and suffer major disabilities due to the excessive practice of their new "moral code." Jogging, when carried to excess, can become a significant source of both orthopedic injuries and cardiovascular deaths. Thus, the various forms of behavior that directly influence the health of many individuals assume a language of sin and redemption that can ultimately become a self-fulfilling prophecy of guilt, in itself having serious negative health consequences (when carried to an extreme).

Although the exact statistical effects of this new morality on smoking behavior remain to be determined, there is no doubt that the social power of this movement is so great—in contrast to other planned measures designed to discourage initiation and encourage quitting and control of smoking—that the rise of this new social phenomenon warrants careful analysis and understanding. In matters of health and health-related behaviors, this new movement toward a *secular as opposed to a religious morality* represents a departure from the reluctance of the public to adopt a strong secular moral position in our society that has seldom been seen in modern times. It may have enormous implications for the cessation of smoking in the future, as well as for other similar lifestyle behaviors that impinge upon public health, such as drunk driving or gun control. In a society that is increasingly pluralistic and relativistic secular moralities serve as a lowest common denominator in the moral realm upon which most people will agree. Even if, as Davis implies, we do not like the politically correct tone of this new morality, the fact that it is arising in the secular context of health issues—and provides such a powerful motivation for behavioral change—is sufficient for us to evaluate its pros and cons carefully. The purpose of this chapter is to explore the origins, development, and implications of secular morality as it applies to smoking and, more generally, to develop a model that is applicable to a broad set of related health problems, planning, and policies.

To accomplish these goals, the chapter is divided into three parts. The first deals with principal factors that undergird the *potential* for this social movement. The second develops a more complete analysis of the major social institutions involved, assessing the roles of each in shaping the rapid use of this new morality. The third part presents an integrative model of the interactions among the various institutional players, agencies, and political structures; briefly tests its validity for the interpretation of closely related examples in the field of disease prevention and health promotion; and sketches an agenda for further research in this realm.

Part 1. The Emerging Role of Epidemiology in Shaping Public Health Policy and Public Awareness of Attributable Risk

The modern epidemiological analysis of the risk of cigarette smoking did not begin until the release of the Surgeon General's report of 1964. This report, more than any other single event, made an enormous difference in the public perception of *risk analysis.* The report demonstrates an important new dimension of epidemiology for the public: the ability of the developing epidemiological methods and data to inform us about a new way to look at cause and effect, even when the exact mechanism for that cause is not entirely understood (as was the case with the causes of cancer among smokers). This approach has been developed even further over the past two decades with the advent of sophisticated methods in biostatistics and their implementation using computer-assisted processing technology. Without the development of the knowledge of how to collect, accurately compute, and project these findings to the public, public health authorities would have had to rely on the individual assessments that would tend to downplay the risks at lower levels, so that we would be largely ignorant of one of the largest single causes of mortality in modern times.

It is increasingly possible to extend the meaning of cause-and-effect relationships from the proximal terms of individual experience over short periods to population profiles over life-cycle time periods. For example, we may have a series of very strong proximal responses, physiological or behavioral, for rejecting spoiled or highly toxic food. However, food that contains excessive amounts of cholesterol could be harmful over the lifetime of the individual, yet it fails to elicit a similarly immediate response. The rise of the ability to attribute risk to behavior associated with the development of chronic disease much later in the life cycle has enormous impact on the lifestyle of the individual: sophisticated new knowledge enables us to make rational decisions about the ways in which we want to lead our lives. The tangible development in our ability to integrate our knowledge of long-term health risks, environmental problems, and other demographic projections in meaningful ways demands that we integrate this knowledge into our society as a whole. Of course, moving from understanding the problem to implementing the changes suggested by this approach will require a substantial extension of knowledge about how communities operate when confronted with the new information being developed from such epidemiological studies of chronic disease and related problems.

To some extent, the shift from understanding to action at the social level is already occurring. Since the Surgeon General's 1964 report, the science of epidemiology as a "new" source of understanding about "risk" has come of age for the American public. It is now publicly accepted that epidemiologists can describe risk factors associated with health outcomes far in the future. This allows us to extend the cause-and-effect relationship between behavior or exposure to various environmental factors and the subsequent development of chronic disease at a later point in life. The fact that this relationship has been largely accepted by the sophisticated lay public suggests that the credibility of the epidemiologist has reached new highs in terms of informing the public about risk reduction in the prevention of chronic disease. However, this brief overview of the development of the epidemiological approach does not tell us how epidemiology became so involved in answering certain questions and not others. To address this issue, we have to examine the interactions between epidemiological science and the public's understanding of and interest in its own health as they influence those social and political institutions that mediate research priorities.

The Development of the Health and Fitness Movement

A second factor in the new smoking morality has been the enormous shift in the public attitude about health-promoting information. A wide segment of the population has come to believe that they can change their behavior and reap the benefits of a healthier lifestyle. Statistics support it, and results over the past several decades show dramatic declines in mortality from cardiovascular disease. This can be associated with improvements in diet, exercise, hypertension detection and pharmacological control, and decreases in smoking. The net effects in the face of these facts produce a deep belief in the message, and a multibillion dollar health and fitness industry to satisfy this social phenomenon. In fact, the health movement can be considered competitive with religion: the "good life" is extended life, not necessarily by religious morality but by a new belief in the new secular mythology (notion) about health and fitness.

Thus, a shift in the social fabric away from traditional religious sources of eternal value has complemented a drive toward a "here-and-now" secular value system. This secular code emphasizes a high-quality life that is extendable in years well beyond the lifespan of the previous generation—a relative immortality, won by a redoubled commitment to the health and fitness lifestyle. The combination of the new means of publicizing scientifically established facts about preventing diseases through shifts in behavior, and the medical evidence for the efficacy of changing these behaviors has reinforced an enormously powerful social movement in which the expectation of a long and healthy life is attainable. The movement becomes enmeshed in a variety of overlapping circumstances. These include eating "healthy" foods; prescribing and proscribing the dietary intake of specific nutrients; protecting the quality of the water supply; being sure that foods are not "contaminated" by insecticides or by additives that corrupt the foods' "natural" goodness; protecting the quality of the air we breathe and the overall balance of our ecosystem; keeping nondegradeable environmental contaminants to a minimum; daily exercise; avoiding smoking and smoke; decreasing our consumption of alcoholic beverages; maintaining lower weight; wearing seatbelts in cars; using safety equipment of all kinds in sporting activities; practicing safe sex by decreasing the number of partners; reducing the escalating costs of health treatment, which (as opposed to prevention) unnecessarily deplete everyone's financial resources; devouring all kinds of physical and mental self-help books; distrusting the anonymous "government" or "scientific" statistics that appear to be slanted politically to protect various industries that violate occupational safety or contaminate the environment; and trusting groups that share the "believers" perspective.

Although this social movement characterizes a substantial portion of white middle-class Americans, it also functions within a pluralistic society with various ethnic minorities who at least partially share this view of health and welfare. To be sure, there are other less *enfranchised* individuals—with more immediate priorities for survival—who do not share the future-oriented values of the urban and suburban elite who have the financial capacity to participate in this process and plan out their lives far into the future. However, the communication media, social networks, and sports icons ensure that the less fortunate aspire to the lifestyles of the more fortunate, and thus identify with the broader goals of this movement. Although the movement provides for a common value system within which more traditional values fit, for some it becomes the major source of values, which results in a tremendous identification with its overall goal of attaining a "touch of immortality."

Libertarian and Communitarian Traditions That Shape Social Policy in the United States

As powerful as this social/health movement is in demanding conformity of individual behavior by encouraging a healthy lifestyle, it runs the risk of directly confronting the long-established tradition in our society that reserves for individuals the basic freedom to lead their lives as they see fit. Thus, even though it is appropriate to believe in the value of a life of health and fitness, our tradition insists that is not appropriate to impose this belief upon the rights of others. It is all right to persuade others to join if they want to, but it is not acceptable to force them into joining by economic coercion or other means. There is a fine line between what constitutes ethically appropriate persuasion and incorrect persuasion that is publicly acceptable. This sense of rights that pervades much of our society can be traced back most clearly to John Stuart Mill's (1989) essay "On Liberty," in which he sets forth the principle that the inalienable rights of the individual always take precedence over those of society, except in cases where others might be clearly harmed as a direct result of the individual's abuse of personal freedom.

It is manifest that the philosophical and political history of the United States reflects a tremendous concern for the rights of the individual as opposed to society. Thus, it is not considered proper for "society" to intervene in the affairs of the individual even if there are long-term negative consequences of his or her behavior to himself or herself. In this framework, when one's health fails it is because of some flaw or behavior in the individual rather than the community or social framework for preventing, or even treating, health disorders. Of course, healthy individuals are looked upon with admiration because they are "in control." Therefore, if an individual smokes, and we believe that the social and economic costs of extended treatment of illnesses directly connected with the smoking are so high that we would like to require the smoker to quit, we cannot. Thus, the long-established and highly respected libertarian traditions of our society have been the major *impediment* to the legal codification of the newly emerging secular morality involving health and fitness.

The concept of secular morality differs morally from this paradigm of individual responsibility because it brings into focus another dimension of social control of behaviors that are unhealthful to others. It has the elements of ostracism for the potential transgressor, and guilt and shame for the actual transgressor. These are powerful motivating forces, which if modified to also include social inclusivity to the former transgressor, become a powerful social mechanism not unlike religious conversion groups. The other dimension of social morality is that it calls for the formation of advocacy groups, each usually formed around a single focus (for example, Mothers Against Drunk Driving (MADD), antismoking groups, specific disease-prevention groups, and so forth). These groups give rise to another social force in counterbalancing both the aspects of the health system that are market driven and the aspects of the more general economic system that may seek to make environmental issues profitable while causing individual health problems. In essence, the advocacy groups help to promote healthful behavior and forcefully identify health-endangering environmental issues that no individual could ever regulate alone. They compensate for the lower level of communal responsibility that our traditional system of values about the rights of the individual provides for us. Thus, because in our society most health-advocacy groups are nonprofit, they are not constrained by the same balance of political forces that regulate groups that seek financial profit.

Given the health risk of smoking and the tremendous social and individual emotional investment in the health and fitness movement, it is not surprising to see a new forcefulness emerge among nonsmokers, especially with the recent documentation that smoking is directly harmful to the nonsmoker in a smoke-polluted environment. In addition, the growth of this knowledge about risk factors and preventive health behaviors has had an enormous impact on cardiovascular disease. The general reduction in mortality rates from the chief cause of mortality in our society has directly reinforced the value of pursuing a healthy lifestyle. However, to attain the new level of fitness and health required a degree of sacrifice and discipline that reinforced a new kind of secular morality involving health issues. Smoking was clearly not part of this new lifestyle but was protected by our libertarian traditions. As soon as it became clear that smoking was harmful to others, however, this health-driven secular morality unleashed an enormous tide of public opinion against it. It is not surprising, given the magnitude of the health and fitness movement and the new morality accompanying it, that the findings on sidestream smoke should produce such a strong response: it appears as if the majority immediately seized upon the concept of harming the innocent and changed its attitude regarding the rights of the smoker. However, understanding how this process played out in our society requires further analysis of the various institutional domains and their interactions.

Part 2. The Institutional Framework Underlying the Expression of Secular Morality

The Surgeon General

This analysis begins with the two most important factors that appeared to account for the knowledge that set up the social conditions for this rapid and powerful change. The first is the original Surgeon General's report of 1964, which transformed public understanding about the deadly effects of smoking on the health of the smoker. The second was the Surgeon General's report of 1989, which produced new evidence that smoking was also life-threatening for the people who shared the smoker's environment. The scientific findings appear to have provided the initial impetus toward the development of this secular morality about smoking. But in the past, most moral issues have not developed in response to scientific findings. In this case it is reasonable to suggest that the 1964 report was so well received that the 1986 report assumed the same credibility in the eyes of the public. There have been many other reports issued by the Surgeon General over the past twenty-five years, but few (if any) have received the attention that these have received. Hence, although it is clear that the reports are the source of the major shift in public attitude, a number of other factors had to play crucial roles in this process. These include, inter alia, the basis for the public response; the reliability and trustworthiness of the epidemiological data and the scientific interpretation; the role of the Surgeon General in engendering that trust; the role of the mass media; the basic social conditions in our society that allow for the development of a new kind of secular rather than religious morality; the political system and how it worked in this process; the legal system and its dimensions; and the roles and responses to these diverse social developments by the cigarette manufacturers, smokers, nonsmokers, and previous smokers.

Beginning with the Surgeon General, it is evident that some individuals, such as Dr. C. Everett Koop, by the power of their vision, the integrity with which they pursue it, and their ability to communicate their message effectively, take on a charismatic quality that tends to add extra weight to the significance of the epidemiological findings. Once a leader has crossed the threshold of attention and maintained a position of authority, vision, and integrity, that leader gains public acceptance of his or her name and the believability of his or her message. In this regard, Koop became well known first as a famous surgeon but then as a conservative, fundamentalist physician who, as Surgeon General, acted to immediately release the report on sidestream smoke, and then appeared to put aside his own beliefs to tackle the problem of AIDS. In the eyes of many, his response showed a degree of courage and leadership, none more important than the mere title of Surgeon General. However, initially it earned him few friends and supporters.

Thus, when Koop, who had always been an opponent of smoking, issued the Surgeon General's report on sidestream smoke, he had not yet earned support for his established integrity for his record on AIDS. This strong position of leadership initially established on smoking, and subsequently on AIDS, provided him with an enormous public willingness to continue to attend to the findings. Although it is difficult to know the degree to which Koop's role contributed to gaining rapid and widespread acceptance, it is important to examine the data in some depth. This is especially so in light of the relatively small increase in the risk of passive smoking as opposed to the overwhelming risk of active smoking in producing fatalities.

In addition, the data supporting the risk of sidestream smoke were much less clear than the report issued almost a quarter of a century earlier. In the subsequent National Research Council report that corroborated the Surgeon General's conclusions, the relative risks for lung cancer from passive smoke exposure (for example, as a result of living with a smoking spouse) were much smaller than a regular smoker's risk rates, ranging from 1.32 in females (95 percent confidence interval of 1.16 to 1.51) to 1.62 in men (95 percent confidence interval of 0.99 to 2.64). However, unlike the previous reports based upon large studies, the NRC judged that only 13 studies provided sufficient data to be pooled. This data set showed 643 cases of lung cancer in women, 34 cases in men. Thus, the results could have been confounded by other factors and the NRC report called attention to factors associated both with lung cancer itself and with assumptions about living with a smoking spouse (Byrd, Shapiro, and Schiedermayer 1989). The net effect of this lowered the relative risk from 1.34 to 1.25 for both sexes. Although sidestream smoke does, in all probability, have some effects on both cardiovascular health and other pulmonary diseases that result in mortality, this was not considered the risk assessment because they are more difficult to prove as direct and causal effects. In one study about the relative risk of cardiovascular disease, published subsequent to the NRC report, Sandler and colleagues (1989) find that other risk factors that are known to alter significantly the risk of cardiovascular disease, such as alcohol consumption and certain dietary habits, are also highly correlated with cigarette-smoking households. However, even with these caveats about the cardiovascular disease data and the very small sample of males upon which the sidestream smoke attributable risk estimates were made, Byrd and colleagues (1989) point out that if the attributable risk were to be as low as 1 to 5 percent of the attributable risk of active smoking, there would still be 3,000 to 5,000 deaths per year attributable to sidestream smoke.

Given the relative weakness of the data, we are led to question why the response to the Surgeon General's report was so overwhelming. Brandt(1990) has concluded that the public is willing to "assume" large risks personally where there is a modicum of free will involved in the decision (as with the decision to smoke), but is willing to allow only very small risks to be imposed by others. The data also suggest that the pronouncement by a very highly respected spokesperson had a powerful influence on the public acceptability of the results. This points to the modern problem of credibility of government agencies, and the need to attract outstanding and trusted public figures to lead them.

Health Advocacy Groups

Although the Surgeon General has had a large role in influencing public opinion on the issue of smoking, he is not by any means the only advocate of health issues in the public arena. One of the most interesting social developments over the past two decades is the rise in the number and variety of patient-advocacy groups, originally established to help patients and their families cope with the effects of devastating diseases such as tuberculosis, polio, and cancer. More recently two new phenomena have transformed patient-advocacy groups. Their number has increased to include many rare and previously unrepresented groups, and they have become much more politically active than they were in the past. In the increasingly politicized and economically regulated health care industry, patient advocacy groups also attempt to influence the *quality* of care from the medical community; to sensitize the general community to their special needs; and to influence the flow of money for treatment, research, and education about the disease. In fact, they have increasingly become advocates to represent the needs of patients and their families who are too helpless or overburdened to assist themselves in obtaining necessary health care services.

The advocacy groups are also adopting the highly effective lobbying practices that large industries like the tobacco industry have successfully engaged in for several decades. In addition, these lobbying groups assume the mantle of social rectitude; they believe that they occupy the moral high ground on smoking and other behaviors. Thus, the various disease and health advocacy groups have been more and more effective in influencing congressional action on a variety of important legislation, especially in relation to health and safety in the workplace. Their modus operandi includes support networking, activist forums, public education programs, and even dramatic hyperbole. They have come to provide a stimulus to the activation of the government bureaucracy, first demanding attention to the problem and eventually becoming part of the support underlying the actions and decisions of the Surgeon General.

The Tobacco Interests

In the interest of self-preservation, the tobacco companies have been the major force behind attempts to slow the process of legal codification against smoking. Self-interest has also led them to take steps to fund smoking and health research, allowing them to contest the findings of studies that show the negative effects of smoking. Tobacco manufacturers continue to assert that the evidence on the hazards of smoking is not conclusive, and to propose (and fund) yet more research. They also take every opportunity to play up the viewpoints of dissenting scientists.

By questioning the status of smoking as a known health risk and protesting that no one is forced to initiate smoking or barred from ceasing to smoke, tobacco manufacturers have avoided being successfully sued to date. And while they insist that cigarettes are not a proven health risk, they cater to an increasingly disbelieving society, selling filtered and low-tar products, as well as smokeless tobacco. Insisting that the fully informed adult consumer has the right to make his or her own choice, has been their main defense when they have had the opportunity to testify before Congress. Of course, the reason they have been as successful in congressional hearings as they have is the tremendous political and economic clout that the tobacco lobby has wielded in the past, although this is waning significantly.

In addition, current cigarette advertising focuses on combating the negative health image of smoking and getting more people to smoke by depicting attractive, healthy-looking role models in their ads. These clever advertising campaigns are often targeted at particular groups within society who are at risk for initiating and becoming habituated to smoking.

The At-Risk Segments of Society: Changing Risk Patterns

Curiously, the statistics on trends of smoking prevalence show substantial shifts in almost every sector of males but none among females. Overall, male frequency is down, per capita consumption is down, and the rate of initiation is lower than ever in this century. However, trends are less promising among the less well-educated, and worse among females. Overall initiation among young females did not decline between 1974 and 1985, although there is some indication of a decline beginning in 1987 (Pierce et al. 1989). When the data for both sexes are disaggregated by educational level, the effects are more dramatic: Pierce and colleagues report a ninefold difference in the rates of smoking between the highest- and lowest-educated American women aged twenty years and over. In fact, there is no evidence of any decline among the males and females of the lowest-education group. Considered with the data on smoking initiation among twenty- to twenty-four-year-olds (showing a tenfold greater rate of decline among males versus females from 1974 to 1987), this strongly suggests that the principal growth in the number of new smokers consists of lower-educated women. Among the cigarette manufacturers, this market of young, relatively uneducated females is apparently already well known and exploited. Their marketing would target the young white woman who is content with her lack of education. She is part of a subculture that prefers high-action entertainment; that is tilted to male-dominated family, young marriage, early childbearing; has low aspirations for socioeconomic advancement, careers, and education; and identifies with the television character Roseanne.

In the case of the young white male, the classic Marlboro man, for example, epitomized a combination of outdoor freedom, a retreat from modern life, a chance to be like the rugged individualist cowboy working outdoors in the last American frontier; he was idealized in films, free from modern urban complications, a throwback to the earlier good old days. This engineered icon captured the imagination of millions of mostly young white males, and was enchanting enough to draw them into smoking. Proudly, they identified with the mythical dream this brand represented, and in this macho context, disregarded the label that warned them about the health hazards of smoking.

This description of young white males characterizes one marketing strategy. There was another approach to the women who did *not* identify with the macho male image associated with the Marlboro man, nor with those young males who did identify with the sexy cowboy. Simultaneous with mass communication's wide dissemination of the real and suspected health effects of smoking was a powerful new movement of liberation for women, occurring in all sectors of American society and in some extent throughout much of the developed countries of the world. The old patriarchal hegemony in every sector of life was being challenged, and the older myths of the feminine "mystique" that spurred the turn-of-the-century idea that "good" women did not smoke was turned on its side when Virginia Slims told the newly liberated women that smoking was a way of expressing what a long way they had come. Once again the manufacturers had tapped into a lucrative consumer dream; they had only to market cigarettes as a symbol of liberation. They even began seriously supporting women's sporting events, becoming a force in the move to free the sports world from its male focus. The health data fit the success of this changing image of women and smoking extraordinarily well. Lung cancer and cardiovascular disease associated with smoking in women are rising very rapidly. In fact, within the decade lung cancer is expected to exceed breast cancer as the leading cause of mortality in women (U.S. Department of Health and Human Services 1988).

The manufacturers assert that their advertising targets are smokers who are switching brands (Waterson 1982). Part of these efforts involved clever approaches to various ethnic minorities who might not otherwise identify with one particular approach. In marketing cigarettes to the U.S. black population, advertisers promoted Afrocentrism rather than the melting pot, prompting greater ethnic autonomy, pride, and self-identification. For example, Blacks were successfuly tapped in the movement away from Kool cigarettes, popular in the 1940s and 1950s, to other cool (mentholated) cigarettes in the 1960s and 1970s. Thus a study in Philadelphia found a young urban black population that smoked Newport (100 percent of surveyed Philadelphia adolescents aged fifteen to nineteen who reported smoking indicated that they smoked mentholated cigarettes) as a way to be "cool" and a member of a modern generation. So even as public health education authorities stressed the need to get confirmed smokers to quit, the actual consumption of cigarettes per American climbed steadily as a result of marketing strategies that extensively identified smoking as a means of satisfying unmet social or psychological needs.

In examining the two sides of the smoking issue, it becomes quite apparent that the cognitively oriented public-health type of educational approach emanating from the interactions of the Surgeon General's recommendations and various units of government dealing with health, and the various nonprofit health and disease advocacy groups was fairly effective in reaching a significant segment of the public. Faced with this onslaught of health information, the tobacco interests chose to target the segments of the population least likely to care about or be influenced by the approach that worked so well with the older and more-highly-educated segments of society. What is particularly interesting in the context of this rising secular morality is the degree to which the new rules about smoking are so fundamentally changing the social context in which the smoking was traditionally practiced; so strong is it now that it may undo much of the effectiveness of the traditional advertising of the cigarette companies. Today, one cannot find the Marlboro man smoking, or even holding a cigarette.

In the context of everyday life, there is no better evidence that the new secular morality about smoking is having a profound effect on smokers than the variety of evidence supporting the willingness of smokers to be ostracized. The social effect is so strong that Philip Morris has supported new "smoker's bills of rights" that are now being passed in the various state legislatures. As of June 1, 1991, twenty-five states have such bills either pending (twelve) or passed (thirteen). An organized backlash has formed against the new secular morality. The ACLU, labor unions, and tobacco interests are working side by side to turn attention away from the morality and health issue to a "rights" issue that allows for greater freedom in smoking.

Because smoking has become highly regulated and labeled as immoral and, increasingly, as illegal by society, smokers will undoubtedly seek the company of other smokers with whom to commiserate

as they continue to smoke. Two responses are likely among these individuals: some may respond negatively by continuing to be hardened
smokers; others will decide that the habit is not worth the effort and
will quit or attempt to quit. Under these circumstances it is not difficult to imagine that the more recent evidence in the Surgeon General's
1988 report that nicotine is highly addictive will cause smoking to be
labeled as an even more undesirable element in society.

The Role of the Mass Media

The media are integral in promoting knowledge about the problem to the public. Yet, often the media also accept advertising from
the very same cigarette manufacturers that they speak against. Although this paradox has been troubling to some, advertising of any
kind by the tobacco industry has come increasingly under the
scrutiny of the regulatory powers of Congress ever since the controversy over television commercials resulted in their withdrawal in
the late 1960s. The widespread public belief was that the absence of
cigarette advertising on television would lead to a rapid decline in
smoking, but the results did not confirm this. On the contrary, the
industry turned to print media, sponsored special sporting events
(for example, Virginia Slims tennis tournaments), and used extensive billboard campaigns that effectively targeted its chosen audi-
ences (Davis 1987).

Although the tobacco companies said their intentions in using this
sophisticated advertising were simply to get current smokers to
switch brands, the net effect was to encourage persons in the various
targeted groups to smoke and become habituated. In this case the
companies emphasized social identification to initiate new smokers.

The mass media have also been able to magnify the effects of secular morality in a highly effective way by helping to accelerate the
formation of a consensus on this topic. However, they did not create consensus so much as create the potential for a strong public response to Koop's announcement. It had the elements of a dramatic
confrontation: Koop, a powerful, well-respected, and trusted figure,
at the center of a story that involved the effects of smoking on the
"innocent" nonsmoker. The established smoker was guilty of polluting the environment, and the manufacturers were villains to be
attacked as Health and Human Services Secretary Sullivan attacked
them for marketing cigarettes to the naive public.

Advocacy groups cannot have an impact without being able to appeal broadly to various constituencies. The mass media have profoundly influenced the social psychology of the public response to smoking. Weis (1968) summarizes the general effects of the mass media on three levels of processing and action: cognition and comprehension; attitude and value change; and behavioral change. With respect to cigarette smoking, there was a highly effective media campaign mounted by the manufacturers to challenge indirectly the health information developed in the Surgeon General's report of 1964. However, following the successful bid by the health promotion agencies—both governmental and private—to challenge the smoking advertisements on the broadcast media with counteradvertisements, there was a rapid retreat of the manufacturers, which occurred after smoking declined by 19 percent between 1966 and 1970 (Warner 1981) and the manufacturers acquiesced to a legislative ban on television advertising.

In a cognitive sense it was obvious there was sufficient authoritative information being transmitted to effect value change and result in reduced smoking rates. The confrontation on the broadcast media between the two groups was, itself, news. However, the news tended to reflect the authoritative sources from the health sciences more than the manufacturers' claims, which were presented as advertising. This entire episode in the freedom of the broadcast media quickly resulted in the manufacturers switching to other markets and media: in this case youths, who were least likely to be influenced by the cognitively-oriented reports appearing in the print media about the hazards of cigarette smoking (and less likely to watch or comprehend the television news against them). Even though the label on the pack provides warning, the teenager and young adult targeted as potential smokers are well known to disregard risks due to a very strong belief in their invulnerability, particularly life-threatening effects that may not become actual for decades.

Another effect of the mass media is to encourage privately held attitudes and beliefs to become sufficiently public as to provide consensus for moral action (Lazarsfeld and Merton 1960). By exposing, for example, the problem of smoking on planes, and allowing a public condemnatory response, the incipient antismoking morality becomes more solidified. By giving approval to enforcement of the new antismoking rule as a result of the attention given to the problem, the mass media reinforce the strength of the existing values and attitudes to the point where they can become so widely shared that the people are fully confident in expressing them more forcefully in public.

Legislative Codification

The combined impact of a well-respected figure such as Dr. Koop and the increasingly effective lobbying by the health advocacy groups was substantial on the legislative process. Perhaps one of the best examples of the moral power of this issue is reflected in the change in congressional politics between the time of the initial "limited" ban on cigarette smoking in planes on flights of two hours or less in 1987 and the approval on October 16, 1989, of a permanent ban on all but a few domestic flights. In May of 1991 a bill was proposed to extend the ban to all international flights.

Alyson Pytte (1989) suggests that the limited ban was expected to produce a severe political backlash among voters (and even their political parties). However, she points out, none of the expectations materialized; instead, a large majority of the public, in poll after poll, supported extending the two-year ban. A combination of the flight attendants' union and other health advocacy groups worked against the tobacco industry in a lobby that has been described as one of the most powerful in modern times. In fact, recent polls show that this consensus is growing (see Pytte 1989, 29) and providing strong support for future legislation.

Senator Frank Lautenberg (D-N.J.), a former two-pack-a-day smoker, managed to steer the extension bill away from the subcommittee that should have handled it, but which was chaired by a senator from a tobacco state. Not only was Lautenberg's action controversial in the subcommittee to which it was sent, it also produced a remarkable defeat of a Senate filibuster by tobacco-state senators. One argument was that a congressionally mandated study of cabin air quality was due in April 1990 and the Senate ought to use it to make decisions about extending the ban. But this was countered by "supporters of the broader ban [who] said more than enough studies had been done to demonstrate the hazards of passive smoking" (Pytte 1989). What was unusual, given this defense and filibuster, was the degree to which the previously strong tobacco lobby was defeated: 77–21, considerably above the 60 needed for cloture. The majority included senators from the traditional tobacco states Georgia and Tennessee, as well as well-known heavy smokers who would be personally inconvenienced by the smokeless planes.

Two elements were particularly evident in the cloture vote. One was the large number of senators who quite correctly read that voting to extend the ban was a safe choice in regard to their constituencies. The other was the strong stand that Lautenberg took when the House-Senate conference committee could not choose between the more moderate House bill, which only permanently extended the two-hour-flight ban, and the Senate version, which called for the nearly total ban. However, Lautenberg held fast and won, saying, "I don't know how you can compromise on people's health." Thus, there is no doubt that the legislative process in this case closely resembled the will of people made deeply aware of the dangers of continuing to respect the rights of smokers when smokers' behavior impinges on their right to protect their health. Although smoking had always been looked upon skeptically by the nonsmoking flying public, the airlines catered to smokers. Now the need to do so was no longer there. This case shows, even more than the tobacco industry's surrendering of television advertising in 1969, that the antismoking lobby has been able to communicate to the lawmakers that the tide of public opinion has changed.

In a major review of the legal issues surrounding the medical effects of passive smoking, Byrd and associates (1989) concluded that the current direction of codification is a slow process of state and local legislative-level initiatives to bar smoking in various restricted environments such as the workplace and restaurants. Even though the major exposure has been in the home, unless parental smoking in a home with children is classified as a form of child abuse, it is unlikely to become the arena for further legal initiatives. However, Byrd and associates are quick to point out that if an individual "who [had] never smoked but developed a smoking-related illness and can prove his or her only exposure to tobacco smoke was in the workplace," "such a verdict against an employer would likely lead to dramatic legislative and private sector action" (213). In 1989, when they sketched the above scenario, Byrd and his associates believed this kind of dramatic legal precedent very probable, but the recent discovery of a gene associated with lung cancer that is responsive to the toxic effects of cigarette smoke changes the scenario. It holds the promise of satisfying the key condition for directly linking lung cancer and smoke in the environment. The potential of screening lung-cancer victims who are positive for the gene, have the specific tissue response to smoke, and have been exposed to smoke only in the workplace narrows the cause-and-effect relationship to the point where a precedent's being set is greatly enhanced. The direction of scientific progress and trends in public opinion both point to increasingly successful legal restrictions on smoking.

It is evident that no single factor has accounted for the immense increase of legislation in Congress and in the states. However, it is clear that the public supports increased curbs on smoking and that industry attempts to pass smokers' bills of rights will continue against the tide of morally righteous restrictions.

Part 3. Modeling the Development of Secular Morality

New Questions

The preceding pages have documented that no single factor is responsible for secular morality's substantial impact in response to the effects of sidestream smoke. A whole series of interacting institutional factors and scientific developments had to be in place for this response to grow and become so powerful. This social phenomenon raises a series of important questions: Are there similar phenomena involving other health issues that could also produce a secular moral response? What are the risks and benefits of using secular morality as a way of promoting healthy behaviors? We know secular morality is powerful, but does it produce too many opportunities for social stigma and maladaptive social adjustments in the current context?

More generally, can secular morality be controlled? Can its emergence be predicted based on our understanding and modeling of examples?

A Heuristic Model of Secular Morality

From the preceding analysis of the secular morality encompassing smoking, two basic sources of morality in modern societies are apparent: religious and secular.

The religious realm provides a source of moral codes or rules from long-standing traditions. Morality stemming from traditional

religious sources is powerful and highly motivational of specific behaviors. Deviance from the accepted moral behavior seldom occurs
without serious risk of social and even physical ostracism or individual guilt. Traditional religious morality works in part out of a
concern for consequences of transgressing the moral code.

The secular source of morality usually comes into play when new
social conditions arise that previously were not part of the moral
expectations stemming from a particular religious tradition. A more
recent form of secular morality in the United States is constructed
from the amalgamation of a wide range of moral systems. This kind
of secular morality comes from a national tradition of religious
and ethnic pluralism that comprises negotiated lowest-common-
denominator values such as "do no harm to others." (In some cases
a secular morality does not arise because of the inability of the different traditions to negotiate a moral position when there are fundamental disagreements with one another's definition of the moral
behavior—such as in the case of abortion.) A related source of secular morality is rapid technological change that produces a series of
novel problems not previously encountered or adapted to by the
traditional religious systems of the society.

In contemporary U.S. society, both religious and secular sources
of morality are involved in the responses to various problems associated with health care and disease prevention. In cases where the
morality works, that is, the behavior it promotes makes a substantial difference in the natural course of the disease, there is a powerful feedback effect to support further development of the morality.

The basic model of secular morality as it pertains to health
matters is constructed from an analysis of smoking since the 1986
Surgeon General's report on effects of smoking on the health of
nonsmokers. It is as follows:

1. There is the continuing development of a body of scientific
   facts that are well documented epidemiologically, that produce consensus among scientific experts, and that have a basis
   in common knowledge, in consequence of which it becomes
   appropriate to recommend an intervention of some kind.
   Such action appears to be especially justifiable if the facts
   contain data on the harmful effects of one person's behavior
   upon others. If the effects are upon the person only, the problem that develops is much more difficult to address because
   of the long tradition of individual libertarian values in our
   society.

2. Given the enormous amounts of data that can be developed (pro and con) about any issue, it is very difficult to arrive at a consensus upon which a moral stance can be built. Consequently, the emergence of a person of considerable status promotes effective presentation of data to the public. Using the data as the source and the charisma of the person as the means to communicate them in an unequivocal way provides sufficient authority to reach consensus on social mobilization and action.

3. There has to be a mechanism for transmitting the information to a wide public, using the media. Sullivan's critical stance vis-à-vis the cigarette industry gave him a new kind of folk moral authority status. Koop gained his status from his courageous and pragmatic stand on AIDS. It is only a matter of impressing the media; they translate the findings into a story, which becomes part of the public understanding of the health problem.

4. The nontransgressor(s) adopt a morally sound position. This gives rise to the opportunity for individual and social mobilization and group action. Advocacy groups already formed or in formation often have an enormous effect on the transgressing behaviors by providing a moral definition, which is communicated by the mass media and helps to define the basis of legal codification of the secular morality.

5. Transgressors can be analyzed at several different levels. These include the individual, the financial interest group or company who profits from the sale of the materials, and the society of the transgressors as a whole. At the individual level, the evidence of the behavior's inflicting harm on others creates a sense of guilt, which is enhanced by the reproachful responses of the nontransgressors. The company profiting from cigarettes uses the libertarian argument and a variety of public media to justify its position. At the cumulative level, the overall shift in behavior of other transgressors has a powerful effect on the continuance of the behavior of the more resistant individuals as they become more and more in the minority. There is a self-fulfilling-prophecy aspect of the social movement involving decreased rates of initiation as well as increased rates of quitting of smoking as a habit.

6. Processes of codification at the social level (laws and regulations) and internalization at the individual level begin to take

place. Secular moral commitments are amenable to legal codification only because the fundamental nature of the tobacco industry is to make "legal" profits rather than go out of the business of selling cigarettes. Another principal source of values equivalent to the "harm" principle is the concept of privacy. Thus, for the most part the laws govern behavior in public places and not in private spaces. Moreover the laws provide a basis for adjudication in times of public disagreement, that is, before a total smoking ban.

7. Maintenance and continuity of the secular morality occurs as a final stage of the process of codification. It may be useful to contrast religious with secular morality in terms of the expectations and consequences when the rules are disobeyed. The media play an important role in the continuity of the rules and expectations of secular morals, whereas traditional religious practices systemically play a role in religious morality.

The data supporting this model of secular morality indicate the power of this social movement. Many factors account for the powerful moral response to smoking. Within the broad context of the social traditions of the past several decades, there has been an increased sense of loss of control of the social environment. For many, this was evidenced by accelerated big-business takeovers, a spoiling of the environment, increased international political instability, broad economic decline, and loss of some of the pride of world leadership (especially in the post-Vietnam years). At the same time there was a profound look inward toward personal and individual betterment, epitomized physically by the tremendous interest in fitness, health, and life extension.

This social movement needs also to be seen in the context of the tremendous pluralism of religious and secular sources of values in the United States, which actively separates church from state and allows for a much wider source of moral values to be developed. In the case of life extension, however, religious values can easily embody the same desire as the nonreligious constituency. There is a great range of historic and modern evidence of the association of sin with inappropriate dietary, physical, and sexual behavior. It is not surprising to see wide consensus on the power of this movement regarding self-betterment. Whether the movement also gives rise to a preoccupation with self that appears to characterize the "me" generation is not clear. Perhaps in this context, the moral outrage that is manifest about smoking is directly related to the intrusion that the smoker makes on the nonsmoker, who in every avenue of life is trying and sacrificing by dieting, watching food intake, being careful not to pollute the environment, and otherwise leading a sanctimonious life (as defined by the modern gurus of technology who tell the public how to extend the good life). This is due to the combination of our ability to define the behavior as an abrogation of the rights of others as much as it is to any inherent power ascribed to the rights and themselves. In other words, the motivation for the "moral" issue may come more from a broader context of the prevailing dynamics of the particular times rather than in an inherent break in the rights issues. Thus, it appears to be a matter of how the issue is framed rather than the particular issue. It is because of this that social issues such as smoking can be pushed hard, and others, such as gun control, are more resistant.

In the midst of the huge gain in personal control offered by the health and fitness movement, there has been the increasing frustration of the healthy at having to pay higher health care costs because of the lifestyle behaviors of the "unhealthy." Since 1964, it has been well known that smoking is very risky and can be deadly. However, in a society that lives according to the libertarian tradition of not interfering with the freedom of people to pursue whatever they want (provided they are informed about the attendant risk), there was tremendous reluctance to restrict the rights of smokers, even though there was tremendous concern about what smokers were doing to themselves, and annoyance on the part of those who had to endure their habit.

Previous to the 1986 Surgeon General's report the obnoxious quality of smoking could be addressed by appropriate "separate but equal facilities," in planes, buses, restaurants, offices, and public places. Now, however, smoking had changed from a nuisance to menace. The threat to health prompted a powerful moral confrontational response from nonsmokers who were already sacrificing to attain an improved quality and quantity of life. Their response was predictable. Sabini and Silver (1982, 35–53) have proposed that in order for moral reproach to occur, there has to be clear consensus on what constitutes a transgression; that is, there must be an accepted norm for behavior. The consensus concerning sidestream smoke and the need to regulate smoking fits this concept well. In addition, Sabini and Silver point out that the transgression has to be objectively definable, to the point where observers would easily recognize the behavior as breaking the code (which is obvious in the case of smoking). Finally, there has to be an appropriate social relationship to the wrongdoer. It is interesting to note that ordinarily there would be a potent inhibiting force, but when it comes to smoking, the moralistic tone is so intense that most nonsmokers, and especially former smokers have little compunction about brazenly confronting a transgressing smoker.

While this broad social explanation may account for the phenomenon of secular morality, it is so strong, and has had such profound effects, that analysis of all of the parameters of the model appears to be warranted for several reasons. Smoking and other lifestyle variables have been some of the most difficult to change; perhaps a more formal understanding of this process will yield other insights. Because nicotine addiction is one of the most difficult addictions to overcome, it is important to know the extent to which secular moral pressure actually affects rates of cessation. Although it is too early to measure the pressure's effects on initiation, we can evaluate its codification into law as the best indicator of the substantive change in public attitudes about smoking. There is a need to comprehend the limitations of secular morality so that the emerging secular morality of the majority does not overzealously remove the rights of those who do not practice the same lifestyle, which is exactly one of the fears that motivated John Stuart Mill to write his influential essay.

We already know that the threatened mandatory testing in the case of AIDS would have driven it further underground early on, and that the current movement to test all health professionals for AIDS is equally controversial. Likewise, the social ostracism of committed smokers may also have negative consequences. Furthermore, given our social history of rugged individualism, freedom of choice, and emphasis on individual responsibility, it is important to determine the impact secular morality may have as a result of placing too much psychological guilt on individuals who are labeled as "immoral." Such labeling could have other adverse effects, such as being denied insurance coverage and other support because of their "legal" habit. The less scrupulous segments of the health industry that operate largely on a profit motive could eventually attempt to take advantage of the antismoking movement by also blaming the smoker, and thereby excuse themselves from providing adequate coverage of a health problem. Another possible result of this secular moral movement would be allowing business to deny employees benefits for health problems associated with chronic smoking. This is hardly idle speculation: in 1991 twenty-five states were considering and/or approving bills to prevent this eventuality (*Philadelphia Inquirer*, May 24, 1991).

The success of the secular morality movement in mobilizing the moral response against smokers may spread to other similar behaviors. For example, drinking and drunk driving appear to fit the same model, although in this case there are notable exceptions, such as the enlightened attitude of the alcohol industry in encouraging responsible drinking and designated drivers. Similarly, the enormous response to adverse publicity about ALAR in apples, which was fueled in part by scientific misinformation, fits the model, especially when the harmed are helpless babies being fed potentially tainted applesauce. And currently, the risk of the transfer of AIDS and hepatitis by health workers appears to fit the social dynamics of this model. Such incidents also have been substantially influenced by increasingly powerful health advocacy groups that have studied the way of the business lobbies and consciously use similar kinds of political persuasion to help a private interest group, usually organized around a single disease. The former resemble the latter in the belief that they work from the moral high ground; their righteous vigor is usually unmatched even by the best-paid business lobbyists.

Given the power of the secular moral response, it is important to reexamine the more traditional approaches to the modification of health-risk factors. It is becoming increasingly well known that education and knowledge alone are not sufficient to change behaviors. For example, sex education programs for teenagers have increased knowledge but have not had a significant impact on the incidence of sexually transmitted diseases. Addictions also appear to follow this phenomenon. Yet, when a much more inclusive and *morally persuasive* treatment program is instituted, as in the case of the twelve-step Alcoholics Anonymous program, there is a much greater success rate. However, secular morality as a social movement may have too heavy a social-psychological cost in terms of a loss of freedom and therefore may not be politically viable in any more organized form. Nevertheless, a thorough understanding of the significance of this model provides us with the best opportunity to avoid its potential misuse in the future. Furthermore, there may be a number of new insights about measures that could improve the contemporary health education approach for the dissemination of health-promoting behaviors. The model also has the potential for gaining new insights into other major health problems. For example, spitting in public was such a common practice prior to the turn of the century that restaurants put sawdust on their floors to keep them from becoming too wet, and spittoons were a regular feature in every bar. By the turn of the century, however, with the discovery of the infectious nature of tuberculosis, spitting became immoral and illegal. Today spitting in public is usually regarded with disgust. Similarly, the sale of semiautomatic firearms may also be another classic example of this same phenomenon operating in contemporary society.

Prospects for the Future

Another sphere in which there is a rapidly emerging secular morality relates to the rapid advances in new technologies that stretch the definitions of personhood and life. Thus, as each new technology impacts on the traditional, fundamental value systems stemming from the religious traditions, there is an enormous attempt to adjust the traditional values to the resulting problems. The outcome appears to be a type of postmodern cultural relativism that accepts the social imperatives of having moral systems to regulate human behavior, and simultaneously respects their traditional religious and ethnic origins and development. This emerging relativism may provide a more comprehensive means to integrate the values of the traditional religious-based moral pluralism with the issue-by-issue fragmented character of the contemporary sources of secular morality—which are at best negotiated lowest common denominators for the basic values upon which the society is built.

This state of affairs, with its fragmentary secular morality, exists in contrast to the coherent type of morality that emanates from revitalization movements. The latter involves an initial stage of increasing social anomie and loss of purpose, which becomes so severe that it leads to widespread deviant behavior, breakdown of social law and customs, a high rate of suicide, and a pervasive sense of a meaningless existence. This results in either a generalized disintegration of the society or in the pronouncements of a prophetic and charismatic leader with a vision of how a society can be reintegrated with a new theme and sense of purpose. As this visionary gains adherents, there develops a secondary group that also communicates the vision, which almost always includes a new religion with its own code of morals and value distinctions. Once this occurs, these new values assimilate into routine and a new equilibrium is established in the place of the recent disorder (see Wallace 1965). This kind of revitalization movement took place in Iran under the charismatic leadership of the Ayatollah Khomeini, but it is not likely to take place in our society, which values and upholds its widely based pluralism and deeply embedded libertarian tradition.

In fact, in health promotion there is a powerful self-fulfilling prophecy of becoming a "follower" because the positive feedback of adherence can be more objectively measured by using more sophisticated techniques than those used to evaluate the strictly religious revitalization. Thus, if exercise and dieting work to reduce cardiovascular disease, their effects can be measured physiologically and epidemiologically by emerging technologies. This procedure, in fact, is the sine qua non of the evolving health movement: the highly sensitive and specific ability to detect changes in health due to socially induced changes in behavioral practices. Accordingly, a central portion of the model that accounts for this phenomenon is the epidemiological ability to enumerate and account for these changes in health phenomena.

The emerging epidemiological synthesis that attributes risk within populations has provided a powerful new scientific methodology to confirm or deny the truth claims of these new health and fitness movements. In summary, if the appropriate lifestyle factors are identified and are validated by modern methodologies that have high visibility, then the overall credibility becomes so enhanced that the reward for the strict adherence built on trust and faith in the fitness movement is the potential for a longer, more fulfilled life.

Social Rights and Responsibilities

The moral element in the social response to smoking comes about both as a response to the evidence that smoking is harmful to the innocent and that the harm is life threatening. Under these circumstances, it is justifiable on moral grounds both to declare smoking in public as immoral and to support strongly the legal sanctions to regulate its use in areas where it may be harmful to others.

The moral side of the argument, however, goes further. It not only provides legal means of regulating the behavior, it also provides strong social sanctions that make the smoker feel that he or she is harming others by the habit. This removes one of the primary pleasures of smoking: enjoying the presence of others while smoking. The moral issue calls into question smoking in homes (where it is unlikely that the legal restraints, except in cases of children who cannot care for themselves, will be called into place) where non-smokers might reside. Smoking in the workplace is also the responsibility of the employer, who under current legal precedents must eliminate hazards (of which smoking is now one) from the workplace.

This analysis of *secular* morality also raises another series of questions about the syncretism of the religious practices associated with morality. Essentially, in the religious model violating a moral stipulation equates with sin, which can result in some kind of harm coming to the individual as a result of the transgression. In this religious model it is appropriate and even expected that the community will step in and address the sinner by admonishing him or her not to sin. However, in the secular model of this society, the community is not expected nor in many cases even allowed to step in and admonish the risk taker. The rights of the individual to make up his or her own mind stand sacrosanct, and the community has no right to interfere with the freedom of the individual. Moreover, the individual is supposed to know that his or her behavior is risky because it is up to the "government" to warn him or her, usually through various public health messages.

Conclusion

As our society approaches some form of nationalization of health care, preventing smoking, which is still the largest single source of preventable mortality in the country, becomes a key issue for the communitarian perspective. In trying to improve the cost-effectiveness of health care, erecting barriers to smoking initiation, particularly among the young, and creating the social circumstances to encourage and support quitting become two of the most prominent preventive steps to emphasize.

In this light the public and preventive health impact of the new secular morality on the reduction of smoking is enormous by any measure; it is eliminating barriers that were traditionally present and allowing new kinds of effective healthy behaviors to emerge. Countering this public health perspective is the libertarian argument that such restrictions come at too great a cost to society because they limit our traditional freedom of choice. Furthermore, the new antismoking regulations constitute a morally slippery slope. Specifically, rules to coerce smokers to change behaviors that afford them relaxation and comfort and that they do not perceive to be significantly harmful to themselves constitute a remarkable invasion of privacy, particularly in environments where the effects of smoking are not harmful to others. From the libertarian perspective, such regulation may represent a Draconian measure.

If we weigh and investigate the alternatives, one question is immediately apparent: Do the smokers who decide to quit want to change? The communitarians argue that if smokers desire to quit and cannot, principally because of the addictiveness of smoking, then it is morally appropriate to assist them to quit. Under these circumstances, the loss of freedom of choice is not as much an issue as helping someone to quit. Likewise, in the case of discouraging initiation among children and adolescents, it is only helping the innocent avoid a highly risky habit.

Couched in these terms, this sounds easy—too easy. It is all right for the smoker who desperately wants to quit and needs the extra support to do so. But what about the smoker who has not made up her or his mind? Or even more invasively, what about those who do not want to quit and get real pleasure out of smoking but now find themselves consigned to sometimes inhospitable spaces when they smoke? Is this equal treatment? Does this fit our libertarian tradition?

Yet, restricting smoking works; smokers do submissively stand outside smoking. Suppose for a moment that this movement could spread to other cases. Will our rights be further eroded? Or even worse, will secular morality turn to *secular moralism*? In other words, will we have to endure a new kind of political correctness in health issues where the Bill of Rights is benignly neglected in exchange for a "healthier" population and therefore less costly insurance for all?

Examining the data on drinking and driving reveals a fairly hefty trend. The rates of drunken driving have declined significantly in the past several years. With both the liquor industry and the public responding, particularly under the pressure developed by Mothers Against Drunk Driving (MADD), there has been a significant decrease in the rates of highway fatalities. On the face of it, the emergence of the secular morality encapsulated in "Don't drink and drive," or in the idea of designated drivers is working. No one is publicly defending drinking and driving anymore, and a new optimism about the problem is emerging.

Suppose for a moment we accept the status quo and agree that regulating both smoking and drinking and driving are worth the social price, are there other secular moralities emerging that are not worth the price? *And* if they are not worth the price, how do we control them so that new issues do not become fodder for new kinds of moralistic movements that undermine our basic freedoms?

Perhaps it is even naive to suppose that secular moralities are programmable. The underlying social equation or calculus is complicated and, further, any attempt to plan a strategy for eliminating a particular behavior may be seen as too paternalistic on the part of planners or business people or policy makers. Still, such movements can and do arise, if initiated in the arena of public activist leader and group concerns. This puts a special burden on both the activist leader and others, including the public health official, the policy maker, and individuals of the media in the chain that generates the secular morality.

If the decades of the 1960s, 70s, and 80s were associated with individual rights and the emergence of the "me" generation, then the 1990s will probably be looked upon as the decade in which individual and corporate responsibility resulted in the "us" generation. In these terms will the powerful kinds of secular morality that emerged in the beginning of the 1990s become more powerful as the populace recognizes the social costs of the excesses of the previous decades?

As we look back at the past several decades, there is an increasing awareness that our basic rights are not free, but are part of a social contract that requires individual social responsibility. Thus, activist leaders must frame issues in a socially responsive manner or risk losing their own credibility and that of their peers in the process. Public health authorities and scientists must also be responsible and continuously vigilant in providing as accurate and complete a picture as possible in order to eliminate the possibility of error that will undermine their current credibility and the future of their establishment in the process. Public policy makers must be willing to understand and use the data developed by epidemiologists and other scientists or risk falling prey to special interest groups. Media professionals must assume responsibility for understanding the significance of agreement and disagreement in the scientific community in reporting accurate and reliable information.

And what is our role in this movement? Is it to understand, watch, listen, and act more responsibly? Most of us are aware of the history of overreaction in these areas. The ALAR scare permanently wiped out many fruit growers; Chilean grape growers are still re-covering from their difficulties; and cyclamates are no longer sold, even though saccharin is still marketed. Where will the next battle-ground be? Who knows?

The U.S. Department of Agriculture recently revised its dietary guidelines; its "Nutritional Pyramid" lists the relative amounts of foods that should be eaten daily for balanced nutrition. Because the emerging evidence implicating the risk of a high-fat diet is sub-stantial, the USDA lowered the recommended saturated-fat intake to levels well below those now consumed. Yet, another branch of the USDA still pays subsidies to dairy farmers for milk that must contain at least 4 percent dairy fat. Moreover, the public no longer desires so much fat in milk and milk products. Enormous quanti-ties of fat are consequently removed from milk, which the USDA buys, stores, and eventually gives to school lunch programs—which feed it to our children and insidiously undermine the Nutri-tional Pyramid.

Needless to say, the butterfat issue is awaiting the secular moral process. The ingredients have a familiar look, including unsuspect-ing children, saturated fat epidemiology, outmoded commodity subsidization, and the USDA being caught up in the controversy about special interest groups influencing the new definitions of what is nutritionally sound. The story will unfold in the morning papers.

Note

This paper was written in 1994 before the enormous success of the legal battles against the tobacco companies and before the well spring of new scientific evidence concerning the hazards of sec-ondary smoke became well established.

The most important public health development during the past few years relates to our making cigarettes a legal forbidden fruit of the 1990s. In so doing we may be unwittingly creating a whole gen-eration of newly addicted smokers.

While the adult nonsmokers and ex-smokers of our society have had a secular moral field day with labelling, ostracism, and outright hostility toward smokers, the adolescent youth, typically sensitive to the "injustices" and social labelling this movement has created, have taken up smoking. This current trend may be in part similar to the period following the end of television advertising in the late 1960s. At that time most foes of cigarettes believed smoking would end with the absence of television advertising. However, far from the expected decreases, the smoking rates for women actually increased as a part of women's countercultural statement in the 1970s. Before history repeats itself with the nation's youth, we need to counter the subtle and not so subtle messages of "sinful" behavior directed toward smokers that are fueling this new adolescent expression of countercultural identity.

References

Brandt, Allan M. 1990. The cigarette, risk, and American culture. *Daedalus*, fall, 135–76.

Byrd, J. C., R. S. Shapiro, and D. L. Schiedermayer. 1989. Passive smoking: A review of medical and legal issues. *American Journal of Public Health* 79(2): (February): 209–15.

Davis, R. M. 1987. Current trends in cigarette advertising and marketing. *New England Journal of Medicine* 316(12): 725–32.

Mill, John Stuart. 1989. *On liberty*, edited by S. Collini. New York: Cambridge University Press.

Pierce, J. P., M. C. Fiore, T. E. Novotny, E. J. Hatziandru, and R. M. Davis. 1989. Trends in cigarette smoking in the United States. Projections to the year 2000. *Journal of the American Medical Association* 261(1): 61–65.

Pierce, John P. 1989. International comparisons of trends in cigarette smoking prevalence. *American Journal of Public Health* 79(2): 152.

Pytte, Alyson. 1989. Total smoking ban on airlines faces big fight in Senate. *Congressional Quarterly Weekly Report* 47:2310, September 9.

Sabini, J., and M. Silver. 1982. *Moralities of everyday life*. New York: Oxford University Press.

Sandler, D., G. Comstock, K. Helsing, and D. Shore. 1989. Deaths from all causes in non-smokers who live with smokers. *American Journal of Public Health* 79(2): 163.

U.S. Department of Health and Human Services. 1988. *Surgeon General's report, the health consequences of smoking: Nicotine addiction.* DHHS Publication No. (CDC) 88–8406. Washington, D.C.: Public Health Service.

U.S. Department of Health and Human Services. 1989. *Surgeon General's report, reducing the health consequences of smoking: Twenty-five years of progress.* DHHS Publication No. (CDC) 90–8411. Washington, D.C.: Public Health Service.

Warner, Kenneth E. 1981. Cigarette smoking in the 1970s: The impact of the antismoking campaign on consumption. *Science* 211 (February 13): 729–31.

Waterson, M. J. 1982. *Advertising and cigarette consumption* (December). London: Advertising Association.

The Legal Regulation of Smoking (and Smokers)

Public Health or Secular Morality?

Lawrence Gostin

It was said during the civil rights era that the state could not change individual or public attitudes about African Americans by enacting antidiscrimination legislation. The retort of civil rights leaders was that they were concerned not merely with how people think but how they behave. Law surely was an effective tool in altering behaviors. Whether the law ultimately affects personal beliefs and behaviors is probably unknowable. But the legislative, perhaps even the judicial, process is certainly sensitive to public beliefs. Thus, legislators and judges are influenced in their decisions by their perceptions of what the public believes. This influence can lead lawmakers to restrict or punish behaviors that are widely regarded as immoral, whether or not they truly threaten the health of others.

The interrelationships between law, public belief systems (here called secular morality), and behavior have seldom been studied. I will examine these interrelationships using the paradigm of the regulation of smoking and smokers. Seldom has a behavior whose health risks are primarily directed toward the individual him or herself been the subject of such intense public and private regulation. Regulation has taken the form of bans and restrictions on advertising, strict package-labeling requirements, tort litigation against manufacturers, restrictions on engaging in the activity in public places, and private restrictions on engaging in the activity at work or even at home or while pregnant.

The assumption made in this chapter is that these public and private regulations of lawful behavior are justified if they are supported by a well-developed body of scientific knowledge showing that the intervention will improve the public health. The intervention must also be no more restrictive than necessary to achieve the public health objective. If behaviors are regulated in the absence of a well-targeted public health strategy, the consequences are that other powerful personal and social values are needlessly undermined. These values include the right to autonomy and self-determination, the freedom of expression and action, and the right not to be discriminated against on the basis of health status. Whenever strict regulation is pursued with public zeal in the absence of scientific evidence of risk to others or efficacy of response, then the impetus is likely not the public health but the public morality.

The Regulation of Cigarette Advertising

Public beliefs that advertising of hazardous products such as cigarettes and alcoholic beverages is dangerous, even immoral, have nearly reached the proportions of a social movement. Congress has already banned tobacco advertising on radio and television. Many public health officials would go further by banning all cigarette advertising in magazines and billboards as well as sponsorship of sports events. The Surgeon General and the American Medical Association (AMA) called on the R.J. Reynolds tobacco company to withdraw all advertising in which the cartoon character Joe Camel appears. They also urged advertising agencies, the media, and retailers not to accept this advertising campaign (Elliot 1992).

The antitobacco lobby's most frequently voiced assertion is that cigarette advertising is misleading and is intended to encourage children, adolescents, and other vulnerable groups to purchase cigarettes. Although the industry denies that it advertises to minors, antitobacco advocates point out that advertisements in teenage and sports magazines reach a predominately youthful audience (R.J. Reynolds 1984). Advertisements directed toward young people make use of images conveying adventure and risk taking (Altman 1987). Sponsorship of sporting events also associates smoking with vigorous athletic pursuits. Young viewers see brand name cigarettes prominently displayed on television (such as on racing cars), without any health warning and despite the statutory ban on broadcast advertising (Ledwith 1984). Marketing toward young people is exemplified in the "Old Joe" campaign of R.J. Reynolds with an animated camel (Dagnoli 1988). "Old Joe knows how to have a good time; that is the kind of message that turns a lot of younger people on" (Old Joe 1990). Despite the health concern about smoking by children, shareholders of one major tobacco company overwhelmingly rejected a proposal to study the impact of advertising on young people (Proposals fail 1991).

Courts are beginning to recognize the dangers inherent in cigarette advertisements that are directed toward young people. In *Mangini v. R. J. Reynolds Tobacco Co.* (1993, 1994) the California Court of Appeals held that the "Old Joe" campaign is an unfair trade practice. The court found that targeting children is oppressive and unscrupulous, causing children substantial bodily injury. Around the same time, the attorneys general of twenty-seven states asked the Federal Trade Commission (FTC) to ban the campaign, and the staff of the FTC recommended the prohibition (Elliot 1993; Auerbach 1993).

Concerns about the marketing of cigarettes to minors has resulted in regulations by the Federal Food and Drug Administration (FDA) to restrict advertising and promotions that disproportionately affect minors (60 Fed. Reg. 41314 1995j). Specifically, the regulations require a text-only format for advertising to which minors are exposed; ban the sale of nontobacco products such as hats and T-shirts; and allow the use of only the manufacturer's corporate name when sponsoring events. The objective of the regulations is to reduce by half the use of tobacco products among minors.[1]

Antitobacco advocates point to cigarette brands that are marketed specifically for a particular population, such as Virginia Slims for women, Kool for African Americans, and Dorado for Latinos. R.J. Reynolds succumbed to pressure by the secretary of the Department of Health and Human Services not to market that Uptown brand, which was specifically geared toward African Americans (Editorial 1990; Dagnoli 1990).[2]

Women's magazines receive significant revenue from tobacco advertising (Kessler 1989). The use of "slim" and "thin" in cigarette advertising suggests the weight-losing effect in women (Davis 1987). Models in the ads are said to have a powerful influence on young women's evaluation of the attractiveness and persuasiveness of cigarette ads (Loken and Howard-Pitney 1988).

Antitobacco campaigners complain about the economic power of the tobacco industry. Magazines may find it difficult to turn away extensive advertising revenue and may even self-censor health coverage and antismoking editorials (Kessler 1989; Villarosa 1991).

Manufacturers of cigarettes, in an uneasy alliance with civil libertarians, have fought back, wrapping themselves in the banner of the Constitution and the ideal of personal freedom. They argue that the regulation of advertising violates the commercial free speech doctrine. They assert a First Amendment right to run whatever advertising campaign they think will best promote their product. Manufacturers and civil libertarians even argue that informal calls by government officials to cease particular advertising campaigns pose a chilling effect on free expression. Regulatory agencies themselves have hidden behind the commercial free speech doctrine as an excuse not to exercise their powers over advertising (Killroy 1990, 88).

Commercial Free Speech

The U.S. Supreme Court has yet to hear a major First Amendment case involving restrictions on tobacco advertising. The Court, however, is likely to uphold regulation of tobacco advertising, provided it is carefully considered.

The Court has defined commercial speech as "expression related solely to the economic interests of the speaker and its audience" (*Virginia State Board of Pharmacy v. Virginia Citizens Consumer Council* 1978). Advertisements by manufacturers of cigarettes or alcoholic beverages inviting consumers to buy their product are examples of commercial speech. The Court initially found that commercial speech deserved no protection under the First Amendment (*Valentine v. Chreatensen* 1942). The failure to protect commercial speech made it possible in 1972 for the Court to uphold a congressional ban on tobacco advertising on radio and television (*Capitol Broadcasting Co. v. Acting Attorney General* 1972; *Capitol Broadcasting Co. v. Mitchell* 1971).

In 1975, however, the Court held for the first time that commercial advertising was entitled to First Amendment protection (*Bigelow v. Virginia* 1975). It has since defended commercial speech in cases involving advertisement of abortion referral services and of the price of pharmaceuticals (*Bigelow v. Virginia* 1975; *Virginia State Board of Pharmacy v. Virginia Citizens Consumer Council* 1976). Its jurisprudence has emphasized, however, that "commercial speech [enjoys] a limited measure of protection, commensurate with its subordinate position on the scale of First Amendment values," and is subject to modes of regulation that might be impermissible in the realm of noncommercial expression (*Ohralik v. Ohio State Bar Ass'n.* 1978; 425 U.S. at 771–72).

In recognizing this limited protection the Court in *Posadas de Puerto Rico v. Tourism Company of Puerto Rico* (1986) upheld a prohibition on advertising of legal gambling casinos to the residents of the commonwealth. It said that because the legislature could have prohibited gambling altogether, it could take the lesser step of banning advertising: "It would surely be a strange constitutional doctrine which would concede to the legislature the authority to totally ban a product or activity, but deny to the legislature the authority to forbid the stimulation of demand through advertising" (478 U.S. at 346).

This language was highly apposite to advertising cigarette and alcoholic beverages. Because government unquestionably has the right to ban outright the sale of hazardous products, the Court appeared to be granting the government considerable discretion to reduce demand for cigarette or alcoholic beverages through restrictions on advertising, and said so quite explicitly in *Posadas*:

> Legislative regulation of products or activities deemed harmful, such as cigarettes, alcoholic beverages, and prostitution, have varied from outright prohibition on the one hand . . . to legalization of the product or activity with restrictions on stimulation of its demand on the other hand. To rule out the latter, intermediate kind of response would require more than we find in the First Amendment" (478 U.S. at 346–47).

Notably, the Court cited cases upholding restrictions on the advertisement of alcoholic beverages and cigarettes as precedents for its decision in *Posadas* (*Dunagin v. City of Oxford, Miss.* 1983, 1984; *Capitol Broadcasting Co. v. Mitchell* 1971, 1972).

Many have seen *Posadas* as the evisceration of First Amendment protection of commercial speech. Two antithetical visions emerge from the commercial free speech doctrine: the "free market of ideas" vision and the "consumer protection" vision. The latter underlies much social welfare legislation and points to a need for state regulations that protect individuals from the hazards of a free market ("Leading Cases" 1986; "Comment" 1987). With *Posadas*, the Court appeared to be moving toward upholding social welfare regulation designed to protect the health of the public.

However, more recently, the Supreme Court struck down a provision of the Federal Alcohol Administration Act (FAAA) that prohibited beer labels from displaying alcohol content (*Rubin v. Coors Brewing Co.* 1995). The government had argued that the labeling ban was needed to prevent "strength wars" among brewers, who would seek to compete based on the potency of their beer. The Court found that the government did have a significant interest in protecting the public's health and welfare, but the government failed to show that the prohibition advanced the government's interest "in a direct and material way" (115 S.Ct at 1592). This burden could not be satisfied by "mere speculation and conjecture"; rather, the government must show that "the harms it recites are real and that its restriction will in fact alleviate them to a material degree." Applying this standard, the Court found that the FAAA's regulatory scheme was irrational: countervailing provisions undermined the government's purported purpose and several less intrusive alternatives were available.[3]

In a further move away from its decision in *Posadas*, the Court invalidated Rhode Island statutes prohibiting the advertising of liquor prices. The state argued that the prohibition promoted temperance (*44 Liquormart, Inc. v. Rhode Island* 1996). The Court, however, in looking at the informational worth of the speech found that the statutes banned truthful, nonmisleading speech and that the state had failed to meet the heightened burden to justify the complete ban. In reaching this conclusion Stevens joined by Kennedy, Souter, and Ginsburg argued against the underlying theory of *Posadas*. "[W]e are now persuaded that *Posadas* erroneously performed the First Amendment analysis. . . . [W]e conclude that a state legislature does not have the broad discretion to suppress truthful, nonmisleading information for paternalistic purposes that the *Posadas* majority was willing to tolerate" (at 1511). The Court appears to be moving in a direction of protecting commercial speech based on the informational worth of the specific message. At least some members of it would establish two levels of review that are triggered by the informational worth of the particular speech. They would rigorously review the government encroachment if the particular speech has informational value for the consumer, such as product availability, price, and content. A "consumer's interest in the free flow of commercial information . . . may be as keen, if not keener by far, than his interest in the day's most urgent political debate." (*Virginia Pharmacy Board* 1976; 425 U.S. at 763). If, however, the speech misleads, deceives, aggressively promotes the product or if the government action requires the disclosure of information that would benefit the consumer, they would apply a less rigorous review.

In light of its decision in *Liquormart*, the Court vacated and remanded for further consideration two Baltimore cases in which the Fourth Circuit had upheld two separate ordinances prohibiting alcohol and cigarette advertising on billboards in designated areas (*Anheuser-Busch, Inc. v. Schmoke* 1995, 1996; *Penn Advertising of Baltimore, Inc. v. Mayor of Baltimore* 1995, 1996). In each case, the circuit court found that the legislature could reasonably have concluded that the means selected (prohibiting billboard advertising) would advance its ends (reducing consumption of alcohol and cigarettes among minors). It stated, "It is not necessary . . . to prove conclusively that the correlation in fact exists, or that the steps undertaken will solve the problem" (*Anheuser-Busch, Inc. v. Schmoke* 1995; 63 F.3d, at 1314; *Penn Advertising of Baltimore, Inc. v. Mayor of Baltimore* 1995; 63 F.3d, at 1325). In addition, the court indicated it would tolerate regulations that are marginally more restrictive than necessary, for "only where a regulation is 'substantially excessive, disregarding far less restrictive and more precise means' will the regulation be invalidated" (*Anheuser-Busch, Inc. v. Schmoke* 1995; 63 F.3d, at 1315). Thus, the Fourth Circuit seems willing to give the legislature some latitude when it seeks to protect the health, safety, and welfare of the public unless the regulation at issue is found to be part of a wholly irrational scheme and unable to achieve the legislature's proffered purpose. At least a portion of the Supreme Court in view of its decision to vacate and remand the cases appears to require an inquiry into the informational worth of the speech before a restriction can be held constitutional. Because the Court offered no explanation for its decisions in these two cases, it remains to be seen how *Liquormart* will impact public health initiatives such as those in Baltimore.

The Four-Part Test

When determining whether a regulation of commercial speech is protected by the First Amendment, the Supreme Court established a four-part test (*Central Hudson Gas & Electric Corp. v. Public Service Comm'n. of New York* 1980). First, for commercial speech to be protected by the First Amendment, it must concern a lawful activity and not be misleading. Second, the government interest asserted must be substantial. Third, the regulation of commercial speech must directly advance the government interest asserted. Fourth, the regulation must be no more extensive than necessary to serve the government's interest.

1. Is cigarette advertising lawful and not deceptive or fraudulent?

Most cigarette advertisements deserve constitutional protection because they concern a lawful activity and are not deceptive or fraudulent. The Supreme Court's concern with "inherently misleading" advertising is directed toward messages that tend to encourage fraud, overreaching, or confusion (*Ohralik v. Ohio State Bar Assoc.* 1978). Glamorous advertising, projecting images of smokers or drinkers as "successful, fun-loving people, without warning of the dangers" are *not* synonymous with *misleading* advertisements (*Oklahoma Telecasters Ass'n v. Crisp* 1983; *Capitol Cities Cable, Inc. v. Crisp* 1984).

Advertisements that portray *unlawful* activities such as smoking by children or drinking while operating a motor vehicle do not deserve constitutional protection. Targeting children with advertisements would similarly be unlawful. The problem for antitobacco campaigners is to prove that advertisements that present images particularly attractive to children, such as cartoon characters, are intended to promote smoking by children and adolescents.

The line between misleading claims and visual associations of the product with sport, adventure, or sex is not always clear. Yet, the courts rarely find advertisements misleading, provided they do not make any specifically false claims.

2. Is the government interest substantial?

Given the strong epidemiologic evidence associating smoking with lung cancer, heart disease, and other causes of morbidity and mortality, no court would deny that the state has a compelling interest in reducing smoking. The state has a direct *parens patriae* interest in protecting individuals from harming themselves.

3. Does the regulation directly benefit the public health?

The third prong of the *Central Hudson* test should be a significant hurdle in cigarette or alcoholic beverage advertising cases. *Central Hudson* requires that the regulation clearly achieve the public health goal, and not be an "ineffective" or "remote" method. Before

Posadas, lower courts carefully searched for empirical evidence showing a link between alcoholic beverage consumption and advertising. Virtually all courts found such a link despite the absence of scientifically rigorous studies. The courts appear to have accepted a reasonable belief and have not required an objective scientific assessment. The Supreme Court fostered this acceptance of legislative opinion over scientific evidence in *Posadas*. The Court refused to review the strength of the legislature's findings but accepted its "belief" that there was a direct and immediate connection between gambling advertising and an increase in crime, prostitution, and corruption. Although it did not directly overrule *Posadas*, the Court seems to bring to an end such deference and introduces a more rigorous review of government actions for speech that contains informational value for the consumer, such as "when a State entirely prohibits the dissemination of truthful, nonmisleading commercial messages for reasons unrelated to the preservation of a fair bargaining process" (*44 Liquormart, Inc. v. Rhode Island*; 116 S.Ct. at 1499).

In vacating and remanding the Baltimore cases in light of *Liquormart*, the Court seems to be asking for more than simply a strong cultural belief in the association of advertising and consumption of alcoholic beverages or cigarettes in order to uphold strict regulation of commercial speech. It appears that courts may look to informational worth of the message in determining whether the limitations on commercial speech promote the goals of the state with a "reasonable fit" (*44 Liquormart, Inc. v. Rhode Island*; 116 S.Ct. at 1510).

4. Is the regulation of advertising more restrictive than necessary?

The government must not merely show that its regulation directly achieves a public health purpose but also that the means used are no more extensive than necessary to achieve that purpose. Even before *Posadas*, courts tended to accept legislative judgments that restrictions on alcoholic beverage advertisements were no broader than necessary to pursue the public health goal of impeding stimulation of consumer demand (*Dunagin v. City of Oxford, Miss.* 1983, 1984; *Queensgate Investment Co. v. Liquor Control Comm'n.* 1982).

Because restrictions or bans on advertising affect First Amendment rights, it would be reasonable to assume that the fourth prong of *Central Hudson* required the regulation to be the least restrictive alternative. Yet, the Supreme Court in *Fox III* made clear that the regulation of commercial speech need not be the least restrictive to achieve the desired end but only a "reasonable fit" between the means and ends (*Board of Trustees of the State University of New York v. Fox* 1989).

The Court is shifting away from this deferential approach to legislative restrictions upon commercial speech. In *Liquormart*, the justices seem to apply a stricter version of this fourth prong. Justice O'Connor's concurrence expresses this trend for at least four justices, but it also echoes the manner in which Justices Stevens, Kennedy, and Ginsburg discuss the prong. "[W]e declined to accept at face value the proffered jurisdiction for the State's regulation, but examined carefully the relationship between the asserted goal and the speech restriction used to reach that goal. The closer look that we have required since *Posadas* comports better with the purpose of the analysis set out in *Central Hudson*, by requiring the State to show that the speech restriction directly advances its interest and is narrowly tailored" (*44 Liquormart, Inc. v. Rhode Island*; 116 S.Ct. at 1522). Thus, it appears that the informational worth of the speech may drive the rigor with which the Court examines restrictions on commercial speech.

Assuming that regulation of cigarette advertising would impede consumer demand, the question remains whether other reasonable means could be used to achieve the goal as well or better. Manufacturers and broadcasters point to other less extensive time, place, and manner restrictions, such as disclaimers, stronger warnings, or counteradvertising. Again, the courts never searched for less restrictive alternatives in a serious way before *Liquormart*. The decision to vacate and remand the Baltimore cases may also be a direction, albeit an unclear one, to the lower courts to examine the possibility of less restrictive alternatives.

The Importance of Sound Public Health Data to Justify Regulation of Advertising

The fact that regulation of advertising of cigarettes would probably be upheld does not mean that it would represent sound public policy. From a policy perspective the question remains, What data exist to demonstrate the relative efficacy of various public health strategies to reduce consumption? Only by reference to reasonable scientific judgments is it possible to distinguish rationally between the policies of banning all commercial advertising, banning certain content, or requiring warnings or counteradvertising. Sound public policy is measured by carefully balancing the public health efficacy of advertising with the costs to society in abridgement of constitutional freedoms. The branches of government, including the judiciary, should not succumb to secular values as a substitute for hard data in assessing the need for public health regulation. If public health regulation were itself without cost, it might be possible to justify regulation on the basis of values alone. The reality, however, is that regulation of advertising directly interferes with another core value: freedom of expression.

The moral indignation against manufacturers of hazardous products is fueled by the belief that advertisements are designed to increase overall consumption and not, as the industry asserts, only to develop brand loyalty. A public opinion poll conducted on behalf of the Bureau of Alcohol, Tobacco and Firearms (BATF) found that 80 percent of respondents believe that alcohol advertising is a major contributor to underage drinking (Opinion Research Corporation 1988, 14).

Public health organizations point to evidence that consumers show increased recognition and/or more favorable attitudes toward products that are heavily advertised. One prominent tobacco researcher concludes that a strong presumptive case favors the existence of a causal link between advertising and smoking, but the politics of the situation precludes a resolution (Warner 1986). Most studies rely on the measurement of advertising recognition, experimental studies of adolescents' reactions to advertising imagery, and the self-perceived influence of advertising on smokers (Chapman and Fitzgerald 1982; Aitken and Eadie 1990; Armstrong, DeKlerk, Shean, Dunn, and Dolin 1990). Others point to the indirect effect of tobacco advertising on smoking behavior.

> Indirect mechanisms would include the influence of cigarette advertising revenues in discouraging media coverage of issues related to smoking and disease, and the possible effect of advertising, by its mere existence, in fostering the notion that smoking is socially acceptable or at least "not really all that bad" (Davis 1987).

Despite claims of the scientific power of these and other studies, the connection between advertising and consumption is far from clear. The fact that a consumer recognizes a particular advertised product or has favorable attitudes toward it does not mean that he or she smokes or drinks *because* of the advertising. A study, for example, showing brand logo recognition of "Old Joe" Camel has been much cited in the popular press, reinforcing the secular value against smoking and tobacco advertising. The AMA and Surgeon General, in part, relied on this study in their call for the voluntary withdrawal of this advertising campaign by the manufacturer and media. Approximately 30 percent of three-year-old children correctly matched Old Joe with a picture of a cigarette, compared with 91.3 percent of six-year-old children. In this study, the authors themselves decline to suggest any causal relationship between the advertising and smoking by young people: "It is obviously impossible to predict how the exposure of children to environmental tobacco advertising might influence their later smoking behavior" (Fischer, Schwartz, Richards, and Goldstein 1991).

Social Costs and Burdens of Advertising Restrictions

Few people in the public health community would lament the silencing of the tobacco industry. The industry spent more than $4 billion in 1991 promoting a product that is "the leading cause of premature death, a product so pervasive and lethal that it causes more deaths than the combined total caused by all illicit drugs and alcohol, all accidents, and all homicides and suicides" (Lynch and Bonnie 1994; Warner 1987). The advertising campaigns themselves are insidious, with cute but harmful associations with beautiful, active lifestyles. What possible social value exists in allowing such a product to be promoted?

The powerful expression of secular morality directed against the tobacco industry is understandable. Yet, the defense of free expression ought not to collapse entirely when the speaker and the message are despised. To be sure, the government would have the power, perhaps the duty, to restrict further or prohibit advertising if sufficient evidence existed to demonstrate a clear association between the content of the commercial speech and the consumption of tobacco products. The scientific evidence, however, is equivocal, and must be balanced with the countervailing value of free expression. The *Central Hudson* test, if conscientiously applied, provides a balance between "the impact of the challenged regulations on first amendment values against the seriousness of the evil that the state seeks to mitigate or prevent, the extent to which the regulation advances the state's interest, and the extent to which the interest might have been furthered by less intrusive means" (Shiffrin 1983).

A ban on cigarette advertising would impact on First Amendment values. A ban or restriction is content-based, which is considered under general First Amendment theory to be one of the most significant violations of free expression. The ban presumably would not allow alternative forms of communication or even tolerate communication with adequate warnings. A ban could include all advertising of the product, including more positive public health messages, such as "don't drink and drive" or "don't sell tobacco to young people." The ban might similarly include messages more difficult to assess, such as "our beer has a lower alcohol content than others" or "our cigarettes have lower tar and nicotine than others." Alcoholic beverage manufacturers probably spend more money on safe drinking messages than all health departments put together.

Any content-based restriction adopts a highly paternalistic approach that "the only way [the state] could enable its citizens to find their self-interest is to deny them information that is neither false nor misleading." Justice Blackmun called for an alternative approach to a ban on commercial speech: "to assume that . . . information is not in itself harmful, that people will perceive their own best interests if only they are well enough informed, and that the best means to that end is to open the channels of communication rather than to close them." The choice, said Blackmun, "is not ours to make or the state's. It is precisely the kind of choice, between the dangers of suppressing information, and the dangers of its misuse if it is freely available, that the First Amendment makes for us" (*Virginia State Board of Pharmacy v. Virginia Consumer Council* 1976).

The evil of smoking seems to distinguish this product from others. Laurence Tribe (1988) aptly observes that "even when the victims of an anti-advertising policy are less sympathetic and the policy's objectives more compelling, the Court has insisted that commercial speech merits First Amendment protection" (893). For example, the Court struck down a local regulation of commercial speech intended to stem the flight of white homeowners from a racially integrated neighborhood. The ban on speech was demonstrably necessary to achieve a compelling government interest, but the method suffered from the fatal flaw of "restricting the free flow of truthful information" (*Linmark Associates, Inc., v. Township of Willingboro* 1977).

The fact that the tobacco industry is using its wealth to buy the right to communicate and that it stands to profit from the advertisements similarly provides little justification for a ban. A person who stands to profit from speech has no less a right to communicate than a person who has nonpecuniary motivations. The commercial free speech doctrine is designed to protect not only the rights of advertisers but also the rights of consumers. Many citizens have a more abiding interest in the quality and price of a product or service than in the most compelling political issue of the day.

The final distinction between cigarette advertising and other commercial speech, recognized by Justice Rehnquist in *Posadas*, is that the state could completely ban the manufacture and sale of cigarettes so that it could also prohibit speech encouraging its sale. This "greater power includes the lesser" analysis is similarly flawed. The government may have the power to ban all sorts of activities, such as abortion services. It would seriously dilute the First Amendment if government truly had the power to silence all truthful speech about a good or service that it could but chose not to ban. The fact is that the government has not attempted to make the manufacture and sale of cigarettes unlawful. The First Amendment has long required the state to regulate speech "with a far lighter touch" than it regulates unsafe products (Tribe 1988, 903). The court in *Liquormart* agreed that the *Posadas* reasoning is flawed. "Further consideration persuades us that the 'greater-includes-the-lesser' argument should be rejected for the additional and more important reason that it is inconsistent with both logic and well-settled doctrine" (*44 Liquormart, Inc. v. Rhode Island*; 116 S.Ct. at 1512). Thus, the stability of the "greater-includes-the-lesser" reasoning appears to have been discarded.

The principal benefit that would demonstrably outweigh the constitutional burdens of a ban on advertising would be a clear improvement in the health of the public. As future research finds a more definite link between advertising and smoking, the balance will certainly shift. Such evidence would allow society to develop a policy of restrictions on speech, understanding the diminution of personal freedoms but confidently asserting an equal or greater benefit in lives saved.

In the meantime, following a different model—widely accepted by both the public health and civil liberties communities—would serve society well. That model is a policy of counterspeech. A counterspeech policy would establish a comprehensive public health campaign on the serious health risks of smoking. The policy could require the tobacco industry itself to produce or fund the campaign, such as under the old fairness doctrine; a tax could be levied on the sale of the product with the proceeds used to develop effective anti-smoking messages, such as in California; or all advertising would have to be accompanied by a series of stern warnings as in the Cigarette Labeling Act or Senate Bill 664 that would require warnings on alcoholic beverage advertising. Counteradvertising could perhaps target the misleading images produced by the industry, rendering them less effective.

This counteradvertising policy meets legal, civil liberties, and public health concerns. From a legal perspective it represents a less restrictive alternative to a ban on speech, which finds support in the *Central Hudson* test. From a civil libertarian perspective, it satisfies the dogma that the best antidote to bad speech is more speech. From a public health perspective, perhaps the best evidence of behavior change exists for a policy based upon well-targeted and effective public health information. Exposing the dangers of cigarette smoking through thoughtful and well-funded public health campaigns can serve the public interest without interfering with core constitutional values, and without pandering to the secular morality most popular at the time.

Involuntary Smoking

When Surgeon General Luther Terry first published his seminal report on the causal connection between smoking and serious morbidity and mortality in 1964, he was able to support his conclusions with a number of strong epidemiological studies (Advisory Committee to the Surgeon General of the Public Health Service 1964). The 1964 report (and subsequent annual reports of the surgeon general) have led to a number of policies designed to reduce the level of smoking in the United States. The most notable policy change was the Cigarette Labeling and Advertising Act of 1965, requiring warning labels on all cigarette packages (Gostin, Brandt, and Cleary 1991). The act was amended in 1970 and 1984, requiring a stricter series of warnings and a comprehensive education campaign. This process represents a classic approach to health policy: observations of a major health problem, careful epidemiologic studies for causal factors, and policy development to increase the public's knowledge of the risk and to reduce behavior associated with the risk.

The contemporary history of scientific investigation and policy implementation relating to involuntary (or passive) smoking followed a different path. Involuntary smoking occurs when "nonsmokers are exposed to the tobacco smoke of smokers in enclosed environments" (Fielding and Phenow 1988).

The impetus for scientific study of involuntary smoking was not the observation that nonsmokers exposed to environmental tobacco smoke (ETS) had higher levels of morbidity or mortality but, rather, the increasingly intense secular value that smokers were becoming a public nuisance. The scientific investigations that ensued purported to be neutral assessments of the health consequences, but they had significant design defects, were based upon moral (as well as scientific) assumptions, and had squarely in mind a set of preconceived policies the investigators hoped the research would support. The Secretary of Health and Human Services illustrated the confounding motivations of the scientific community in his letter of transmittal to the president and to Congress in the first surgeon general's report on passive smoking in 1986 (U.S. Department of Health and Human Services 1986). The secretary called attention to the increased concern for protecting the health and well-being of nonsmokers, and the growing number of laws restricting smoking in public places. In some ways it was remarkable that forty states and the District of Columbia had laws in place restricting smoking in public buildings and in the workplace *before* the first Surgeon General's report on the health effects of involuntary smoking.

The Secretary's transmittal letter had a distinctly moral tone: "As a physician I believe that parents should refrain from smoking around small children"; and "the choice to smoke should not interfere with the nonsmokers' choice for an environment free of tobacco smoke." Notably, these are "should" phrases, not necessarily public health observations based upon sound epidemiologic data.

The data that did exist would have supported preventing the parent or spouse from smoking in the home because of the intensive long-term exposure to ETS (Janerich, Thompson, Varela, et al. 1990). Yet, no such law was proposed, and would probably be held to be an unconstitutional invasion of privacy. The public health data, however, could not reasonably support the main policy proposal endorsed in the report: comprehensive restrictions on smokers at work and in public places. Restrictions on workplace smoking could be challenged as overly broad. Although long-term exposure in confined workplace settings certainly poses a health risk, more temporary and less intense exposures may not.

The scientific conclusions reached in the surgeon general's report on involuntary smoking appeared less rigorous than in previous reports. The main conclusion was that "involuntary smoking is a cause of disease, including lung cancer in healthy smokers." The studies established a causal connection in certain cases, but the report failed to state clearly the conditions that must exist in order to create a significant health risk. At what level of exposure does the risk occur? How serious a risk exists compared with other environmental risks, such as automobile emissions? What kinds of involuntary smoking or what settings pose the risk? Intense and prolonged exposure to ETS, such as constantly living or working in a smoke-filled environment almost certainly poses a health risk. It does not necessarily follow, however, that mild or intermittent exposure, such as in a public building or restaurant entails a significant health risk.

The Surgeon General's second conclusion was that simple separation of smokers from nonsmokers within the same airspace may reduce but does not eliminate exposure of nonsmokers to ETS. This, of course, is a self-evident but largely meaningless statement— namely, that a person will breath in smoke at a reduced level the further he or she is from the source of the smoke. The Surgeon General's statement implies there is a significant *health* hazard of being separated in the same airspace, although it says only there is *exposure*. The report does not tell the reader, presumably because the data do not support it, that such indirect, intermittent exposure poses a health problem. The statement seems calculated to achieve a policy result cloaked in the name of public health.

A comprehensive review of involuntary smoking research by Fielding and Phenow (1988) concludes that there may be a causal effect between involuntary inhalation of tobacco smoke and the risk of lung cancer. Yet the authors point out that of fifteen case-control investigations, only six achieved a statistically significant result; only one of the three prospective studies reporting a slightly higher risk of lung cancer associated with ETS attained statistically significant results. "To date, studies examining the hypothesis that passive smoking increases the risk of lung cancer have had defects in design, methods or analysis." More important, most of the studies involved prolonged and intense exposure to ETS through living or working constantly with a smoker in a confined space. Because the dose of tobacco smoke is important for active smokers, the hypothesis that extremely low and intermittent exposure to ETS poses a significant public health threat is yet to be demonstrated.

Restricting Smoking in Public Places, at Work, and at Home

The combined research and media reports on ETS have had a profound impact on public tolerance of, and political action against, smokers (National Research Council 1986). Public opinion and policy developments have been formed, at least in part, around the assumption that a clear public health rationale existed for excluding (not merely separating) smokers from all kinds of public environments. Opinion polls indicate 90 percent of the public believes secondhand smoke is harmful, and 80–85 percent favors restrictions on smoking in public places (Ban urged 1992; Jacobson, Wasserman, and Raube 1992). Nonsmokers have become increasingly unwilling to tolerate ETS, and many see smokers as inconsiderate, even immoral, for risking the health of others, particularly children. These are the so-called innocent victims of tobacco smoke, as if those who do smoke are morally blameworthy. The very term *involuntary smoker* suggests a form of coercion or wrongdoing perpetrated by the smoker on vulnerable (or passive) recipients. This conception has charged the political atmosphere, and has led to greater regulation not of manufacturers but of smokers themselves.

By 1990, 45 states and the District of Columbia, together with 500 counties or cities, had enacted statutes or ordinances restricting smoking (Jacobson, Wasserman, and Raube 1992; Rogotti and Pashos 1991). The laws limited smoking in government buildings, transportation, restaurants, workplaces, and public places such as hospitals, cultural facilities, schools, and libraries. Ten states and 165 cities had comprehensive laws restricting smoking. The most restrictive ordinances proposed would completely ban smoking in all offices and restaurants (Elliott 1991). In many areas of the country persons who are incarcerated in prisons and jails, hospitalized in public or private hospitals, or attending a college or university are restricted from smoking (Cigarette smoking 1992; Joseph and O'Neil 1992). The restriction may apply across the entire facility or entire grounds, with or without any designated smoking area. Some of these laws are specifically endorsed by the Centers for Disease Control (Cigarette smoking 1992).

Federal regulation of smoking, other than the airline smoking ban, has been more limited. The possibility of more pervasive federal regulation of smoking in public places has been proposed (Horowitz 1991). A coalition of public health groups (including the American Heart Association, American Lung Association, and American Cancer Society) released a report in 1992 urging the Environmental Protection Agency and Department of Health and Human Services to ban ETS from work and public places as an environmental toxin (Health coalition urges 1992). The EPA has not explicitly issued an order, but it has recommended that all companies and agencies operating public buildings ban smoking or use ventilation (Hilts 1993). In 1994 the Occupational Health and Safety Administration (OSHA) issued proposed regulations that would significantly restrict smoking in the workplace (59 Fed. Reg. 15968 1994).

Even in the absence of regulation, nonsmokers are bringing litigation to ensure smoke-free public places. For example, parents of children with asthma have filed lawsuits to seek a ban on smoking in fast-food restaurants under the Americans with Disabilities Act (Johnson 1993). Prisoners' litigation received a boost from the Supreme Court's decision in *Helling v. McKinney* (1993). The Court allowed an inmate's lawsuit to proceed, based upon the claim that he had an Eighth Amendment right not to be subjected to high concentrations of ETS.

Laws enacted in the name of public health go beyond restrictions or exclusion from smoking in public places. Some statutes make smokers ineligible for certain government jobs or positions. Massachusetts law, for example, states that "no person who smokes any tobacco product shall be eligible for appointment as a police officer or fire fighter . . . and no person so appointed shall continue in such office or position if such person thereafter smokes any tobacco products" (Mass. Acts 1987). Similar provisions apply to employment involving the care, supervision, or custody of "prisoners, criminally insane persons, or defective delinquents" (Annotated Laws of Mass. 1992).

Some employers who have already established workplace policies banning all smoking have gone further. They have banned *any* smoking by employees anywhere in the vicinity of the workplace, in the car on the way to work, or even in the privacy of an employee's home. Although employers may justify this on the basis of employee health or potential burdens on the health benefits plan, some have made no secret of their moral disapproval of the behavior.

Public Health versus Personal Freedoms

Restrictive laws and policies have become a priority of the anti-tobacco coalition, including medical and public health organizations. A RAND study concluded that to "regain the initiative, antitobacco advocates will need to shift the legislative emphasis to a public health debate over smoking's health hazards" (Jacobson, Wasserman, and Raube 1992). The report recommended a strategy including key legislators committed to the antitobacco movement, a cohesive antitobacco coalition, and the active involvement of medical and public health organizations.

The antitobacco coalition is resisting the tobacco industry's way of framing the debate as one involving personal freedoms and smokers' rights. There remains good reason to distrust campaigns for the freedom and rights of smokers conducted or financed by cigarette manufacturers. Industry action in this regard has ranged from paid advertisements supporting smokers' rights, financing smokers' groups, and lobbying for smokers' rights legislation to ubiquitous campaigns celebrating the birth of the Constitution and Bill of Rights. Understandable antipathy to the public advocacy and political lobbying of the tobacco industry ought not prevent a balanced and sensitive examination of smokers—many of whom are seriously physically and psychologically dependent on tobacco products.

As with the case of advertising discussed above, the courts have been highly deferential to restrictions on smoking. Legal challenges to governmental and private restrictions on smoking in public places have been, for the most part, unsuccessful. The comprehensive New York City Indoor Air Act was upheld as constitutional (*Fagan v. Axelrod* 1990). Even when the Department of the Army placed a designated smoking area far from army headquarters, requiring a long walk, the courts upheld the restriction (In re *Department of the Army Headquarters et al. v. Local 1770, American Federation of Government Employees* 1990). Citing the "very strong" evidence of the health consequences of ETS, one court upheld a total ban on smoking in the workplace without a designated smoking area.

It is unclear whether the courts will take on employers who terminate workers for smoking at home in the absence of any adverse impact on their ability to perform their jobs. Because the decisions of a private employer are not deemed "state action," there may be no recourse to constitutional safeguards. Relief under disability law such as the Americans with Disabilities Act (ADA) may be possible but is not promising. The ADA certainly covers purely private employers, but courts probably would not find smoking to be a disability. If it could be demonstrated that the employer perceived the smoker as being disabled, the protection of the ADA might become available.

A realistic assessment of the public health objective remains the most important component of policy assessment. In cases where the restrictive law, policy, or practice is designed to protect nonsmokers from ETS of an intensive and/or prolonged exposure, there is a strong public health interest. In such cases the rights and freedoms of smokers can be restricted to the extent necessary to achieve the objective. A decision, for example, by an employer to curtail smoking within a relatively enclosed work space protects employees from intensive and prolonged exposure. Designating an area for smoking that does not significantly interfere with common work spaces does not detract from the public health goal, while providing decent treatment to the smoker.

Questions of equity also arise. Consider a university policy that bans smoking entirely except in a person's private office. This allows the professor to smoke if she or he chooses but grants little respect to the nonprofessional worker.

In some cases the policy appears based upon moral disapproval of the smoker rather than the health of others. A state that decrees that no one who smokes can hold certain positions or an employer who prohibits workers from smoking at home cannot assert that the policy is based upon sound public health grounds. In such cases, it is difficult to point to any legitimate interest for banning smoking.

Some policies do not rely on strong public health evidence but may have other reasonable grounds. Restrictions on smoking in public places such as restaurants, theaters, and libraries are not supported by a coherent body of scientific research. Nonetheless, smoking in these public areas can reasonably be regarded as a public nuisance. In such cases, because the public interest is hardly compelling, some designated separate area for smokers would be warranted.

Balanced against the public interest are the legitimate interests of smokers. So long as government does not ban smoking, it ought not to allow severe restrictions on their privacy or freedoms in the absence of a reasonable public health interest. The most severe restrictions on smokers impose on their own free time and private space. Decisions that prevent smoking in the home, in a car, or in an open, uncrowded place are unnecessarily intrusive. In cases where the smoker is merely inconvenienced, such as by requiring him or her to smoke in a designated area, his or her assertion of "rights" becomes weak.

Conclusion

It may be that my attempt to reconcile the rights of smokers and nonsmokers will be regarded as wrongheaded from the perspective of both public health and secular morality. Yet, forcing the public health community to demonstrate that there is a significant threat to the public health and that the means used will achieve the objective appears reasonable, even (perhaps especially) in a climate that is understandably hostile to smoking and smokers. I prefer to reject an authoritarian or coercive approach. Many people in the public health community understand, and advocate, a nonpunitive approach to other addictions, such as alcohol or drug dependency. That humane approach deserves consideration in the realm of tobacco addiction. By limiting coercive interventions to those necessary for the public health and by relying on an imaginative and truly comprehensive health education campaign, tobacco use can be dramatically reduced without an inordinate cost to our political principles.

Notes

I want to thank Allan Brandt for his contributions to the thinking in this paper and to Megan Troy and Kathleen J. Lester for their research assistance. The paper is based on an article on cigarette advertising written by Brandt and me (1993). Criteria for evaluating a ban on the advertisement of cigarettes: balancing public health benefits with constitutional burdens. *Journal of the American Medical Association* 269:904–9.

1. The reduction is to be accomplished within seven years of the date of publication of the final rule.

2. RJR is marketing two new varieties of Salem "each with marketing strategies strikingly similar to its ill-fated Uptown brand."
3. The FAAA allowed the disclosure of alcohol content on wine and spirits and permitted brewers to indicate high alcohol content through the use of the term "malt liquor." (*Rubin v. Coors Brewing Co.* 1995).

The government could have limited the alcohol content of beers, prohibited advertising that emphasizes alcohol strength, or limited the labeling to only malt liquors. (*Rubin v. Coors Brewing Co.* 1995; 115 S.Ct. at 1593).

References

59 Fed. Reg. 15968 (1994).

60 Fed. Reg. 41314 (1995) (to be codified at 21 C.F.R. pt. 801, et al.).

44 Liquormart, Inc., v. Rhode Island, 116 S.Ct. 1495 (1996).

Advisory Committee to the Surgeon General of the Public Health Service. 1964. *Smoking and health: Report of the advisory committee to the surgeon general of the public health service*. Public Health Service Publication 1103. Washington, D.C.: Office of the Surgeon General, U.S. Department of Health, Education, and Welfare.

Aitken, P., and D. Eadie 1990. Reinforcing effects of cigarette advertising on underage smoking. *British Journal of Addiction* 85:399–412.

Altman, D. 1987. How an unhealthy product is sold: Cigarette advertising in magazines 1960–1985. *Journal of Communications* 37:95–106.

Anheuser-Busch, Inc. v. Schmoke, 63 F.3d 1305 (4th Cir.) 1995, *Vacated and remanded*, _U.S._, 116 S. Ct. 2575 (1996).

Annotated Laws of Mass., chap. 27, sec. 2 1992.

Armstrong, B., N. DeKlerk, R. Shean, D. Dunn, and P. Dolin. 1990. Influence of education and advertising on the uptake of smoking by children. *Medical Journal of Australia* 152:117–24.

Auerbach, S. 1993. FTC staff takes aim at Joe Camel: Reynolds denies ad campaign is aimed at enticing teens to smoke. *Washington Post*, August 12, D9.

Ban urged on secondhand smoke in public places. 1992. *New York Times*, June 11, A20.

Bigelow v. Virginia, 421 U.S. 809, 826 (1975).

Board of Trustees of the State University of New York v. Fox (*Fox* III), 492 U.S. 469 (1989).

Capitol Broadcasting Company v. Acting Attorney General, 405 U.S. 1000

(1972) (mem.) aff'd sub nom., *Capitol Broadcasting Co. v. Mitchell*, 333 F. Supp. 582 (D.D.C. 1971).

Capitol Broadcasting Company v. Mitchell, 333 F. Supp. 582, 585 (D.D.C.) 1971, aff'd, 405 U.S. 1000 (1972).

Central Hudson Gas & Electric Corp. v. Public Service Comm'n. of New York, 447 U.S. 557 (1980).

Chapman, S., and B. Fitzgerald. 1982. Brand preference and advertising in adolescent smokers: Some implications for health promotion. *American Journal of Public Health* 72:491–94.

Cigarette smoking: Bans in county jails. 1992. *Journal of the American Medical Association* 267:2013–14.

Comment. 1987. Alcoholic beverage advertising on the airwaves: Alternatives to a ban or counteradvertising. *UCLA Law Review* 34:1139–93.

Dagnoli, J. 1988. RJR aims new ads at young smokers. *Advertising Age* 59 (July 11): 2.

———. 1990. RJR's new smoke looks Uptown. *Advertising Age* 61 (June 25): 6.

Davis, R. 1987. Current trends in cigarette advertising and marketing. *New England Journal of Medicine* 316:725–32.

Dunagin v. City of Oxford, Miss., 718 F.2d 738, 751 (5th Cir. 1983) (en banc), cert. denied, 467 U.S. 1259 (1984).

Editorial. 1990. The downing of Uptown. *Advertising Age* 61 (January 29): 32.

Elliott, C. 1991. Anti-smoking law gets tentative OK. *Los Angeles Times*, April 11, A3.

Elliot, S. 1992. Top health official demands abolition of 'Joe Camel' ads. *New York Times* March 10, D1, D21.

———. 1993. The media business: Advertising—27 attorneys general oppose Joe Camel. *New York Times* September 22, D21.

Fagan v. Axelrod, 550 NYS 2d 552 (1990).

Fielding, J., and K. Phenow. 1988. Health effects of involuntary smoking. *New England Journal of Medicine* 319:1452–60.

Fischer, P., M. Schwartz, J. Richards, and A. Goldstein. 1991. Brand logo recognition by children aged 3 to 6 years: Mickey Mouse and Old Joe the Camel. *Journal of the American Medical Association* 266:3145–48.

Gostin, L., A. Brandt, and P. Cleary. 1991. Tobacco liability and public health policy. *Journal of the American Medical Association* 266:3178–82.

Health coalition urges smoking ban, citing research on secondhand smoke. 1992. *Daily Labor Report*, June 11, A8.

Helling v. McKinney, 113 S.Ct. 2475 (1993).

Hilts, P. 1993. U.S. issues guidelines to protect nonsmokers. *New York Times*, July 22, A.14.

Horowitz, A. 1991. Terminating the passive paradox: A proposal for federal regulation of environmental tobacco smoke. *American University Law Review* (fall).

In re Department of the Army Headquarters et al. v. Local 1770, American Federation of Government Employees. Case No. 90, FSIP 117, Federal Service Impasses Panel (December 27, 1990) 1990 FSIP LEXIS 57.

Jacobson, P., J. Wasserman, and K. Raube. 1992. The political evolution of anti-smoking legislation. Santa Monica: Rand.

Janerich, D., W. Thompson, L. Varela, et al. 1990. Lung cancer and exposure to tobacco smoke in the household. *New England Journal of Medicine* 323:632–36.

Johnson, K. 1993. Lawsuits seek to ban smoking in fast-food restaurants. *New York Times*, April 3, 28.

Joseph, A., and P. O'Neil. 1992. The department of veterans affairs smoke free policy. *Journal of the American Medical Association* 267:87–90.

Kessler, L. 1989. Women's magazines coverage of smoking related health hazards. *Journalism Quarterly*, summer, 316–22.

Killroy, D. (Gen. Counsel FCC). Senate, 101st Cong., June 15 and 21, 1989. 1990. *Advertising alcohol abuse.* Washington, D.C.: Government Printing Office.

Leading Cases. 1986. *Harvard Law Review* 100:172–82.

Ledwith, F. 1984. Does tobacco sports sponsorship on television act as advertising to children? *Health Education Journal* 43:85–88.

Linmark Associates, Inc., v. Township of Willingboro, 431 U.S. 85, 97 (1977).

Loken, B., and B. Howard-Pitney. 1988. Effectiveness of cigarette advertising on women: An experimental study. *Journal of Applied Psychology* 73:378–82.

Lynch, B. S., and R. J. Bonnie, eds., Institute of Medicine. 1994. *Growing up tobacco free.* Washington, D.C.: National Academy.

Mangini v. R. J. Reynolds Tobacco Co., 17 Cal. App. 4th 354 (1993), *aff'd*, 7 Cal. 4th 1057, *cert. denied*, 115 S.Ct. 577 (1994).

Mass. Acts, 1987, chap. 697, sec. 101A.

National Research Council, Committee on Passive Smoking. 1986. *Environmental tobacco smoke: measuring exposures and assessing health effects.* Washington, D.C.: National Academy.

Ohralik v. Ohio State Bar Ass'n., 436 U.S. 447, 462 (1978).

Ohralik v. Ohio State Bar Ass'n., 436 U.S. 447, 456 (1978) *quoted with approval* in *Board Trustees of the State University of New York v. Fox*, 492 U.S. 469 (1989).

Oklahoma Telecasters Ass'n. v. Crisp, 699 F.2d 490, 500, (10th Cir. 1983), *rev'd on other grounds sub nom.*, *Capitol Cities Cable, Inc. v. Crisp*, 467 U.S. 691 (1984).

Old Joe is paying off for Camel. 1990. *New York Times*, August 7, D17.

Opinion Research Corporation. 1988. Final report of findings of research study of the public opinion concerning warning labels on containers of alcoholic beverages—conducted for BATF, vol. 1 (December): 14.

Penn Advertising of Baltimore, Inc. v. Mayor of Baltimore, 63 F.3d 1318 (4th Cir.) 1995, *vacated and remanded*, _U.S._, 116 S. Ct. 2575 (1996).

Posadas de Puerto Rico v. Tourism Company of Puerto Rico, 478 U.S. 328 (1986).

Proposals fail at Phillip Morris. 1991. *New York Times*, April 26, D2.

Queensgate Investment Co. v. Liquor Control Comm'n., 433 N.E.2d 138 (Ohio 1982).

R.J. Reynolds Tobacco Company. 1984. We don't advertise to children. *Time Magazine* 91 (April 9).

Rogotti, N., and C. Pashos. 1991. No smoking laws in the United States: An analysis of state and city actions to limit smoking in public places and workplaces. *Journal of the American Medical Association* 266:3162–67.

Rubin v. Coors Brewing Co., 115 S.Ct. 1585 (1995).

Shiffrin, S. 1983. The First Amendment and economic regulation: Away from a general theory of the First Amendment. *Northwestern University Law Review* 78:1212, 1252.

Tribe, L. 1988. *American constitutional law*. 2d ed. Mineola, N.Y.: Foundation Press.

U.S. Department of Health and Human Services, Public Health Service, Centers for Disease Control. 1986. *The health consequences of involuntary smoking: A report of the surgeon general*. Washington, D.C.: U.S. Department of Health and Human Services, Public Health Service, Centers for Disease Control.

Valentine v. Chreatensen, 316 U.S. 52 (1942).

Villarosa, L. 1991. Caution: Tobacco ads may be hazardous to your editorial freedom. *Harvard Public Health Review* 2:18–21.

Virginia State Board of Pharmacy v. Virginia Citizens Consumer Council, 425 U.S. 748 (1976).

Warner, K. 1986. *Selling smoke: Cigarette advertising and public health*. Washington, D.C.: American Public Health Association.

————. 1987. A ban on the promotion of tobacco products. *New England Journal of Medicine* 316(12): 745–47.

Lifestyle Correctness and the New Secular Morality

Howard M. Leichter

Susan Sontag had it only half right; wellness, as well as illness, is metaphor in American society. Although obviously prized in its own right, good health now represents more than merely a state of physical (and perhaps mental) well-being. For many Americans, especially the more affluent, it symbolizes a secular state of grace. As such, good health constitutes affirmation of a life lived virtuously. Furthermore, there is now a canon that, like the elaborate system of 650 dietary rules and abominations of the Torah, defines who are the Chosen—*and who are not*. We live in an age in which the keepers of the canon—the moral elite who exhort us to embrace low-fat, high-fiber diets, metabolic workouts, aerobic stepping, stress management, fitness center memberships, and at least eight glasses of designer-label water a day—can help determine our social and economic success.

None of this, of course, is new. Earlier in this century H. L. Mencken (1985) observed that "the whole hygienic art, indeed, resolves itself into an ethical exhortation" (269). Periodically in our history, for reasons examined below, Americans have pursued fitness and wellness with a missionary zeal, and equated them with a sacred and/or secular state of grace. Each such crusade has been accompanied by its own set of prescribed rituals or proscribed activities. In the past, however, these movements were restricted, in the main, to the political, social, or religious fringes of society (Whorton 1982). Certainly, nineteenth-century vegetarians, best represented by Sylvester Graham of cracker fame, communitarians, and hydrotherapists had relatively few adherents and little national impact. Furthermore, I think one could argue that even the more visible and active facets of the nineteenth-century purity crusade, namely, the temperance and antiprostitution movements, engaged and affected fewer people, and people who were less geographically and socially diverse, than the current wellness movement. Today lifestyle correctness, or the belief that there is a set of demonstrably health-enhancing and -protecting behaviors over which the individual has considerable control, has moved into the mainstream: U.S. presidents and corporate leaders jog, the media reports on every new health-enhancing and illness-avoiding breakthrough, restaurant menus identify healthy meal choices (which are endorsed by the American Heart Association), and large numbers of public and private employers require that potential and current employees adopt health-promoting lifestyle practices as a condition of employment, retention, and eligibility for employee benefits.

Furthermore, it is not surprising, given the social and political costs associated with being behaviorally incorrect, that popular concern with health and healthy living is, at least reportedly, widespread: nearly three-fourths of all Americans report that they are either somewhat concerned (38 percent) or very concerned (34 percent) about the effect of their diet on their health, and more than 60 percent say they are somewhat or very worried that they or someone in their family will experience a catastrophic illness (Gallup 1991, 35, 159). The number of Americans who report that they engage in some daily activity to keep physically fit increased from 21 percent in 1961 to 44 percent in 1985, and to 67 percent in 1990. These indicators, combined with the fact that a 1985 Gallup poll found that 84 percent of Americans mentioned good health as among the values they prized the most (Gallup 1989, 36), confirm what observers here and abroad view as our national preoccupation with health. (See Crawford 1980, 365; Potter 1983, 1140.)

The question for the public health establishment is: What are we to make of this new-time religion? Surely, we can all applaud efforts that encourage more prudent lifestyle choices, and especially those that are unambiguously associated with decreased morbidity and premature mortality (for example, stop smoking, consume alcohol in moderation and abstain when driving a motor vehicle, do not use psychotropic drugs, practice safe sex). Yet, there is, or at least should be, some discomfort over what I have chosen to call the lifestyle correctness movement. The problem emerges from the fact that by equating certain types of behavior with virtue and others with vice, the secular moralists—dare I say the lifestyle correctness police?—threaten to undermine the critical task of educating the public in general, but various socially and economically vulnerable groups in particular, to the very real dangers lurking behind everyday behavioral choices. By using the vocabulary of religion or morality, the zealots of wellness have created an atmosphere that, as a number of commentators have noted, is often self-righteous, punitive, exclusionary, imperious, evangelical, and elitist in tone (see, for example, Allegrante and Green 1981; Barsky 1988; Carlyon 1984; Stone 1989).

My purpose in this chapter is to inventory the reasons that health promotion has achieved the status of a moral imperative. I think it is important this be done in order to demonstrate the obvious but critical point that like all such ideologies, the lifestyle correctness movement serves the interests of various groups in our society, not the least of which are those who define and guard the canon. One of the most troubling consequences of the movement is that it is socially discriminatory and exclusionary. In this regard, the highly detailed rituals associated with lifestyle correctness serve the same purpose as the biblical dietary and sexual prescriptions and proscriptions which were less public health measures than they were rules for defining the path to spiritual salvation and for distinguishing the ancient Israelites from their neighbors. In short, what I am suggesting is that the new secular morality is only partly about health and a good deal about individual and collective social position, status, and image. Finally, I will argue that the pursuit of a correct lifestyle holds out the promise of salvation not only to individuals but corporations and even governments.

I would add here that the arguments presented below take the form more of hypotheses to be tested than empirically validated propositions. I have no survey evidence, for example, documenting that the lifestyle correctness movement has led to social and economic discrimination or lower-class isolation. At best, what can be done at this point is to identify relationships and urge empirical verification.

The Costs of Incorrectness

An understanding of why health and healthy lifestyles have come to occupy so sanctified a position in the American hierarchy of values begins with the obvious point that both good health and putatively virtuous lifestyle choices are important instrumental values. For example, failure to adopt correct lifestyle practices might lead to being turned down for an insurance policy, or a job, or admission to school. In addition, anecdotal and survey evidence suggest that the social and economic costs to those practicing health-harming behavior are quite high. We know that there is increasing social and economic hostility toward smokers. For example, in 1990 Gallup found that smokers faced antagonism from nonsmokers in both the workplace and social settings: 29 percent of employers who were nonsmokers indicated that they would be less likely to hire a smoker than a nonsmoker, and 22 percent of all nonsmokers said they had less respect for smokers than nonsmokers (Gallup 1990b, 22).

Perhaps most alarming is the fact that lifestyle choices have become a precondition for gaining and retaining employment, or enjoying company benefits: the Cable News Network (CNN) will not hire smokers; U-Haul, and Baker Hughes, Inc., of Houston, Texas, fine employees who smoke *while not on* the job; and one company, Ford Meter Box Company of Wabash, Indiana, fired an employee when she tested positive, in a urine test, for nicotine. Like CNN, Ford Meter Box Company does not allow employees to smoke on or off the job (*Houston Chronicle*, April 7, 1991). It is not only smokers, however, who need be concerned. Some companies, including U-Haul and Hershey Food Corporation, penalize employees, usually in the form of increased health insurance copayments, who are overweight.

Civil libertarians and other social advocacy groups have resisted some of these efforts. For example, there was widespread criticism of a decision by Circle K Corporation, the nation's second-largest convenience chain, not to offer medical insurance coverage to employees who had apparently made irresponsible "personal lifestyle decisions" (for example, people with AIDS, or who had attempted suicide, or who had drug- or alcohol-abuse-related illnesses). One week after the decision was made public, Circle K announced it was "temporarily" suspending the plan: the revocation came after adverse publicity and protests from the Human Rights Campaign, a gay advocacy group.

Many of the efforts to penalize lifestyle choices are justified in economic terms. Employers argue that greater employee prudence will lead to lower health care costs, as well as increased productivity through reduced absenteeism and job-related accidents. Among the most enthusiastic corporate advocates of monitoring lifestyle practices and penalizing those who engage in "modifiable risks" is the insurance industry. Beginning in the 1980s (Stone 1986, 676–78), insurance companies began pushing for risk-rated, rather than community- or experiential-rated, insurance premiums. Briefly, risk-rating involves basing "premiums on modifiable lifestyle behaviors thought to place the individual at risk for illness and attendant costs. It adjusts an individual's share of premium according to lifestyle, in effect shifting the responsibility for a variety of potential medical problems to the individual" (Risk-related 1990, 1). Critics of risk rating argue that it is contrary to the fundamental principle upon which insurance is based, namely, spreading risk across an entire population. Furthermore, they point out that the notion of "at-risk behavior" is notoriously imprecise (for example, there is no medical consensus on what is considered optimal body fat or what is a safe level of daily alcohol consumption); that it does not take environmental factors into account; and that the relationship among risky behavior, job performance, and ill health is complex and uncertain (see Terry 1991, 5, 8–9). Nevertheless, the notion of making the sinner pay for his or her transgressions dovetails nicely with the secular morality movement.

Neither punitive nor exclusionary employment practices are restricted, of course, to private enterprise. Several municipalities have banned smokers from serving as firefighters, and the City of Athens, Georgia briefly refused to hire people whose cholesterol levels were in the worst quartile nationally (*USA TODAY*, May 13, 1991). Furthermore, as McGuire (1984, 300–301) reminds us, it is by no means unprecedented for government to intervene and require people to behave prudently when they might not otherwise do so. He points to the example of requiring inoculations as a condition for school admission as one case of requiring "health promoting behaviors as a condition for the receipt of services."

The potential expansiveness and invasiveness of health-status and personal-habit monitoring, whether for purposes of insurance, employment, or even the selection of marriage partners, is only beginning to be realized. Employers, insurers, government, and others now have available the powerful tool of genetic profiling and screening to help identify people who are predisposed to a whole range of illnesses, diseases, or other socially undesirable characteristics. The *New York Times* (April 22, 1992) reported on a study by the Office of Technology Assessment that found 5 percent of Fortune 500 companies already use genetic profiling of employees, and that an additional fifty-five companies in the group indicated that they might adopt the procedure by 1994. Unlike medical screening in the past, which sought to identify potential employees with preexisting medical conditions, current screening practices seek to identify merely the predisposition toward such illnesses or diseases.

All of this has not gone unchallenged: Michigan has banned discrimination against people on account of weight; twenty-eight states have "smokers' rights bills," prohibiting discriminatory practices against smokers in hiring, compensation, and work conditions (Janofsky 1994); thirteen states currently prohibit insurance companies from denying coverage based upon genetic testing (Sardella 1995); and seven states (Colorado, Kentucky, Oregon, Rhode Island, South Carolina, Tennessee, and Virginia) have banned general lifestyle discrimination. The Oregon law, for example, declares, "It is an unlawful employment practice for any employer to subject, directly or indirectly, any employee or prospective employee to any breathalyzer test, polygraph examination, psychological stress test, genetic screening or brain-wave test" (*Oregon Revised Statutes* 659.227, 51–265). In addition, the 1990 Americans with Disabilities Act extends federal protection against discrimination in housing and employment to persons with AIDS or who are HIV-positive. These recent efforts to protect individuals from the health vigilantes join a series of earlier legal protections afforded by state fair employment statutes and Section 504 of the 1973 federal Rehabilitation Act, all of which seek to protect workers from discrimination based upon some preexisting health condition.

Finally, it should be noted that victims of corporate lifestyle correctness policies have not sat idly by. Overweight employees fired by Xerox and Agency Rent-A-Car successfully challenged their dismissals in court; and in a highly publicized case involving Milwaukee-based Johnson Controls, Inc., the largest automobile battery manufacturer in the country, the U.S. Supreme Court ruled in 1991 that the company could not exclude women of childbearing age from jobs in which they were exposed to lead (*New York Times*, March 21, 1991).

In sum, both the "wages of sin" and the capriciousness of heredity threaten to impose enormous social, political, and economic costs on individuals who pursue lifestyles that involve socially defined unacceptable risks. It is no wonder that health, healthy habits, and even physical attractiveness have become so important in American society. The question that remains is *why* good health, the appearance of good health, and the pursuit of health-enhancing behavior have become so important to individuals and corporate America. It is to that story that I now turn.

The Healthy Life: Our National Preoccupation

At the outset I should note that I am not going to repeat the now-standard story about how rising health care costs, combined with the discovery that the leading causes of illness and premature death lay in lifestyle-related behavior, have led governments in Western, industrial nations to elevate health promotion through lifestyle modification to a rhetorically honored place in national health care policies.[1] This story, which I have told elsewhere (Leichter 1991), is, of course, an important one. It does not, however, explain the ardor with which individuals have embraced health promotion through all sorts of health-promoting activities. None of the fitness-conscious joggers, vegetarians, yoga fans, or health club members whom I know do what they do in order to help rein in galloping health care costs. Let me suggest some alternatives to the "money-drives-health" explanation for the wellness movement.

"The Times They Are A-Changin' "

Perceptions and values about wellness, disease, and health promotion often reflect broad social trends and concerns. As a number of scholars have noted, during times of rapid and dislocating social and political change, Americans historically have turned inward and become preoccupied with their own physical well-being.

> In the first half of the nineteenth century, Jacksonian America entered a period of geographic mobility, rapid industrialization, and political upheaval. Beginning in the 1830s and 1840s, a popular health movement arose, partly in response to this social turmoil and rapid change. When it seems that there was little the individual could do to control the massive social, political, and economic upheaval, people sought something they could control. And many thought they found it in health (Barsky 1988, 143).

Some scholars have identified both the Jacksonian and Progressive eras as periods of social and political ferment that were accompanied by what James Whorton (1982) calls "radical schemes of hygiene" and "health extremism" (11; see also Huntington 1974, 188). My purpose here is not to review these earlier manifestations of wellness zealousness but to underscore the parallel between these earlier periods and our own time. I think a case can be made that the 1960s, the cradle of the current lifestyle correctness movement, and the following decades provided many of the same socially and politically dislocating experiences, and resulted in many of the same individual and collective responses that occurred in the earlier eras.[2] Compare, for example, Barsky's above description of the reaction to social turmoil in Jacksonian America to Christopher Lasch's account of the response to the sixties: "After the political turmoil of the sixties, Americans have retreated to purely personal preoccupations. Having no hope of improving their lives in any of the ways that matter, people have convinced themselves that what matters is psychic self-improvement" (Lasch 1978, 4). Lasch then goes on to describe how this improvement will occur: jogging, eating healthy foods, engaging the wisdom of the East, and so on.

There appears to be, then, an existential basis for our current national preoccupation with wellness that is reminiscent of previous periods of national turmoil and their immediate aftermath. What, then, are the forces that account for the tendency of individuals in times of social or political stress to turn inward to find salvation or at least solace in their own bodies? One explanation, explicit in the comments of Barsky and Lasch, is that when other aspects of life seem to be tumbling out of control, people try to reclaim a sense of power over which they are uniquely sovereign, namely, their own bodies (Stein 1982, 41).

Rob Crawford makes a similar point:

> For a generation which experienced the political motion and excitement of the 1960s, the turn inward toward self-cultivation can be partly understood as a reaction to the disappointment and political impotence experienced in the 1970s. Redefining the problem as self-change and preoccupying oneself with keeping healthy is one way to cope with that disillusionment (Crawford 1980, 377).

However vaguely or precisely felt the anxiety may be, self-improvement through health promotion is, in this interpretation, a major coping mechanism of our times.

The desire to assert control over one's life through improved physical fitness and attractiveness is especially noticeable, and often tragic, among an estimated 1 to 2 percent of all young women (that is, ages twelve to twenty-five) in the United States who suffer from anorexia. The disease, which is characterized by starvation or near-starvation in order to achieve a slender figure, is most common among upper- and middle-class white females. It is often the attempt to deal with both traditional and more modern role expectations. As Rolls, Federoff, and Guthrie (1991, 138) explain it, "The idealization of the thin female form and pressures on women to compete and perform well, yet be attractive and feminine, all contribute to the social pressures on women that could put them at risk for an eating disorder."

Thus, over the past few decades middle- and upper-class Americans have taken any number of exotic and banal paths in search of self-control over that portion of their destinies where some degree of control seemed within reach, namely, their physical condition. These efforts have included self-awareness and stress-reduction experiences (for example, yoga, primal scream, gestalt, tai chi), encounter sessions, holistic and other nontraditional medical approaches, exercise, nutrition management, neotemperance, biofeedback, changes in sexual practices, and so on.

On the Death of God and the Decline of the Family

Several years ago in an important article dealing with the growth of the health care industry in the United States, Victor Fuchs identified three nonmedical factors that have contributed to that growth: "the growth of government, the decline in importance of the family, and the weakening of traditional religion" (Fuchs 1979, 10). Of the three, the two that are most relevant to this discussion are the weakening of the family and religion. Evidence for the weakening of these two supporting social institutions is compelling. In 1952, 75 percent of the respondents to a Gallup Poll indicated that religion was "very important to them"; by 1978 the figure had declined to 52 percent, although by 1991 it was up to 57 percent (Gallup 1991, 238) Similarly, between 1952 and 1990 the divorce rate in this country nearly doubled: from 2.5 per 1,000 people to 4.7. Fuchs's point was that the family and religion historically have offered the kind of comfort care that now must be provided in or by hospitals, nursing homes, and physicians.

I argue, however, that there have been two additional, interrelated, consequences of the decline in the comforting role of the family, church, and other traditional social-support networks. The first is increased anxiety about our health. "The social institutions that in the past helped people to bear suffering and cope with sickness are in decline. Declines in the neighborhood, the extended family, and the religious community, and our estrangement from each, are a source of cultural hypochondria" (Barsky 1988, 221). The consequences of what Barsky calls "our troubled quest for wellness," are particularly evident in our increased anxiety over the prospects of aging and dying. "Obviously men have always feared death and longed to live forever. Yet the fear of death takes on new intensity in a society that has deprived itself of religion and shows little interest in posterity" (Lasch 1978, 209).

The second consequence of the decline in social-support systems that alleviate the anxiety associated with illness, aging, and death is, of course, that people have become preoccupied with avoiding or, in the case of aging and death, forestalling as long as possible, these conditions. Moreover, many of us believe that if we can just slow down the hands of time, then we can postpone the dreadful prospects of those diseases that plague the elderly. This appears to be an especially compelling and rational response in light of the seeming inability of modern medicine to deal with so many of the illnesses that threaten us not only in old age but throughout life (for example, cancer, heart disease, Alzheimer's disease). We see ourselves, in a sense, as the instruments of our own salvation. The less we can count upon others to alleviate our anxieties or to cure our illnesses, the more we believe that we must rely upon our own devices. As the early-twentieth-century antimedical propagandist Anne Riley Hale proclaimed, "The Kingdom of Health, like the Kingdom of Heaven, is within you" (quoted in Whorton 1982, 4). It is hardly surprising, then, that books that promise to help us stem the tide of aging enjoy such popularity. Who would not be seduced by the promise offered in Stuart Berger's book *Forever Young: 20 Years Younger in 20 Weeks* ("Dr. Berger's Step-by-Step Rejuvenating Program") (Berger 1989)?

A Little Knowledge is a Frightening Thing

The anxiety that many Americans feel about their physical well-being is fueled not only by the sense of individual and collective impotence and isolation we feel in the face of a seemingly infinite number of health-threatening forces but also by the enormous amount of knowledge that is at our disposal to keep those dangers omnipresent in our minds. Susan Baur in her book on hypochondria in the United States refers to "the steadily increasing amount of publicly disseminated medical information that encourages us to monitor our bodies for signs of disease. Television programs and magazine articles have increasingly focused attention on the dangers of our simplest habits" (Baur 1988, 138). Thus, health terrorism is compounded by the fact that at no time in our history have we had more visible reminders and examples of the consequences of either self-inflicted illnesses and diseases or those that are merely the result of biological capriciousness (Barsky 1988).

Political Values and Self-Absorption in Health

Yet another explanation for the self-absorption that characterizes the health-related behavior of many Americans is the notion that such behavior is consistent with a bundle of both persistent and transient cultural and political values of our society. A postindustrial value orientation is dominated by a relative decline in economic and material concerns, and a relative increase in emphasis on what Inglehart (1977) calls "higher order needs," and what Huntington (1974, 164) describes as "a new 'postbourgeois' value structure concerned with the quality of life and humanistic values." Among the values that contribute to an improved quality of life is good health, and the means of maintaining and regaining this state. People and governments in postindustrial societies, therefore, place a high value on health and health care issues.

Just how that value is realized is, of course, a function of the particular postindustrial society involved, and the idiosyncratic or transient political forces at work at any given time in that society. In the case of the United States, for example, the postbourgeois attachment to health has been superimposed not only upon values associated with the national and personal state of anxiety described above but also upon our historical attachment to rugged individualism. Although some may see the current inclination of self-absorption as narcissistic, others, especially conservatives, tend to view it in a more benevolent light. In this view, individual responsibility for health is consistent with American folklore concerning the "frontier" and its emphasis on self-help and self-sufficiency.

This latter view was revitalized beginning in the politically and socially conservative 1980s. This is of particular importance to an understanding of secular morality and lifestyle correctness because not only does American conservatism emphasize self-help, but, unlike its British cousin, it also often does so with a heavy religious and moral tone. The prominence of religion, especially in the American Bible Belt, has helped to invest lifestyle and health debates in this country with a great deal of moral posturing. "Those who are well and those who engage in the right behavior are righteous. Those who are ill are assumed to be off the right path and are modern-day sinners" (Brownell 1991, 304).

This moralism has been most evident in discussions about AIDS, but is also present in concerns over alcohol and other drug use. A number of sources, for example, suggest that we have entered a new era of temperance—the third in our history—that began in the early to mid-1980s (*New York Times*, October 1, 1985, March 15, 1989, January 1, 1991; *Business Week*, February 25, 1985, 113). Evidence of neotemperance can be seen in both self-reported drinking behavior and actual consumption (*New York Times*, January 1, 1991). The new sobriety derives from a number of factors, one of which has its roots in the growth of Protestant fundamentalism.

The abstemiousness is often applied by conservatives to lifestyle in general. Newt Gingrich (R-Georgia), current speaker of the House, for example, has urged that "we must shape a vision of personal responsibility, so that people take care of themselves by watching their diets and habits. We may want to reward people who do not need health care" (Gingrich 1984, 66). This view of rewarding the "virtuous" and, at least implicitly, punishing the miscreants is what Allegrante and Green (1981) called the "dark side" of the Reagan administration's view on health and individual responsibility. "It is a side that could preach an elite moralism about health while failing to recognize (or ignoring) the political, economic, and environmental forces that shape and reinforce unhealthy behavior" (1528). It is easy to see how readily such a view can lead to enshrining a canon of a morally correct lifestyle.

The Business of Wellness

Although I have tried to underscore the noneconomic motivations behind the new secular morality in health, no discussion of the lifestyle and wellness movement could possibly be complete without the obligatory acknowledgment that there are indeed substantial pecuniary interests in elevating the pursuit of health to a position of prominence in the lives of Americans. Although it is probably impossible to put a precise price tag on the total private and corporate investment in fitness, wellness, and physical attractiveness—how much of the $5 billion athletic shoe market represents an investment in fitness and how much of it is a fashion statement?—it is a multibillion-dollar-a-year enterprise. For instance, in 1990 Americans spent $1.8 billion on home exercise machines, $3.5 billion on vitamins, $33 billion on dieting, and $44 billion on sporting goods equipment. Getting Americans to believe in wellness, physical fitness, and personal attractiveness is a very lucrative business indeed!

"An Index of Our Civilization"

The text of the wellness movement has been that adopting more healthy lifestyles will lead to longer, healthier, and more enriching lives.[3] There is, however, a subtext to the movement that has little to do with health and a great deal to do with social status. It is this dimension of the wellness movement that has infused it with a sense of moralism, or more appropriately, moral posturing, that I have chosen to call lifestyle correctness.

Throughout history cultures have established rituals relating to personal habits involving food and drink, sexual relations, personal hygiene and grooming, clothing, birth, and death. The purpose, or at least interpretation, of these rituals has varied. One traditional view of the Judaic dietary laws outlined in Leviticus 11 and Deuteronomy 14 and advocated by the medieval physician Maimonides was that they were primitive rules of public health and personal hygiene. Hence, it was long assumed that such admonitions and prohibitions dealing with diet (for example, do not eat pork) were based upon the dangers that these foods posed to human health. More recent interpretations, however, suggest that this analysis is erroneous and that these laws had little, if anything, to do with health (Levine 1989, 248).

Instead, the biblical scholar Baruch Levine has argued that the abominations of Leviticus are part of an elaborate set of rules and rituals intended to establish the distinctiveness and, hence, holiness, of the people of Israel. This, I think, is made clear in Leviticus 20:24–26:

> I am the Lord your God: I have made a clear separation between you and the nations, and you are to make a clear separation between clean beasts and unclean beasts and between unclean and clean birds. You must not contaminate yourselves through beast or bird or anything that creeps on the ground, for I have made a clear separation between them and you, declaring them unclean. *You must be holy to me, because I the Lord am holy. I have made a clear separation between you and the heathen, that you may belong to me.* (*Revised English Bible* 1989; my emphasis)

As Levine (1989, 248) explains,

> Required along with avoidance of improper sexual unions, which would corrupt the family of Israel, and avoidance of pagan worship, which would alienate Israel from God, is the avoidance of unfit food. By such avoidance, Israelites are kept from bestiality; their humanness is enhanced. Such a pure people deserves to live in its own land, unmolested.

"If you faithfully obey the Lord your God by diligently observing all his commandments which I lay on you this day, then the Lord your God will raise you high above all nations of the earth" (Deut. 28:1). The Bible tells us that failure to follow God's commandments and statutes leads to quite another path: boils, tumors, scabs, itch, wasting disease, recurrent fever, and ague, just to name a few of the delights in store for the lawbreaker.

What I am suggesting is that what we are seeing today in the health and wellness movement is an analogous, if considerably less structured, effort to set and protect social boundaries by defining acceptable and unacceptable lifestyles. Just as "pre-modern societies patrolled their boundaries with dramatic rituals of inclusion and exclusion" (Turner 1984, 224), so too do modern societies. Referring to cigarette smoking, Sherwin Feinhandler (1986, 183) has noted that "people tend to evaluate their personal association with others according to whether the others are inside or outside of various social boundaries. . . . Tobacco has served to exclude people from, or to distinguish, groups—to maintain boundaries."

From a contemporary perspective, the notion of an "elect" people who follow a behaviorally correct lifestyle is in my judgment especially invidious because it is a status that is all but inaccessible to the most vulnerable segments of society. Theoretically, of course, unlike the ancient Israelites, one need not be born into the group of the correct lifestyle to be eligible for protected status. Presumably anyone can achieve membership through good deeds—for example, give up smoking, exercise regularly, limit intake of fatty foods, do not engage in unprotected sex, or share intravenous needles. Yet, as a practical matter, there is enormous overlap between lifestyle correctness and middle- and upper-class socioeconomic status. Muriel Gillick, in her marvelous article on jogging, that quintessential hallmark of lifestyle correctness and the pursuit of the moral life, notes that although jogging has expanded from its initial base of primarily middle-aged men concerned about heart disease, it is still largely reserved for the better educated and more affluent. She notes that "the search for fitness remains largely the province of a particular [that is, upper] class" (Gillick 1984, 379). Consumer-purchase data on fitness gear supports Gillick's observation. For example, 9 percent of all exercise machines were purchased by the lowest income group, compared to 45 percent by the highest income households (U.S. Bureau of the Census 1992, 242).

The socially restricted and exclusive nature of the fitness and wellness movement is evident in other areas as well. For example, a *New York Times* (March 18, 1992) headline announced, "As the Rich Get Leaner, The Poor Get French Fries." The article went on to note that "whether by limited finances or personal preference, health concerns [with regard to nutrition] are a great divider between the haves and have-nots today." The assumption that all are equally eligible and capable of following a healthy lifestyle, an assumption that is especially prevalent among conservatives, recalls the ironic and cynical comment by Anatole France (1894): "The law, in its majestic equality, forbids the rich as well as the poor to sleep under bridges, to beg in the streets, and to steal bread."

One final point about the use of wellness as a social discriminator. The practice has spread from individual relationships to collective ones as well. There is an increased sense that wellness and fitness are good for the corporate image, or what Peter Conrad (1990, 493) calls the "corporate culture." Such a position began, not surprisingly, in the health care industry (for example, hospitals, insurance companies, HMOs) but now includes most of the nation's major corporations.

Interestingly enough, the idea of a collective wellness image has even reached into the corridors of state public policy. Deane Neubauer has described "the emergence of a 'health culture'" in the state of Hawaii. Neubauer says that the state has adopted the unofficial title of "Hawaii, the Health State," and that this "health culture" emerges from a supportive natural, social, and economic environment, including "a benign climate and environment which in comparative terms is relatively free of 'environmental insults'; a highly trained and plentiful health care workforce . . ." (Neubauer 1992, 148–49). Hawaii, in other words, has adopted the posture of lifestyle correctness and the air of moral superiority and social distance associated with adopting the canon, in part to distinguish it from other states with which it competes for business and tourism.

The Casualties and Consequences of Correctness

Unlike its political cousin, the lifestyle correctness movement is only just beginning to inflame passions across the American landscape. One reason for this retarded divisiveness may be that many of its victims reside not in the hallowed halls of the academy but in far more modest surroundings. The wellness movement, however, is not a no-fault enterprise; there are casualties and culprits of lifestyle correctness. In a society in which the divide between the classes already has reached dangerous proportions, the lifestyle correctness movement threatens to widen that distance still further. It can do so in at least three ways.

First, as I have already suggested, there is the danger that those who are most likely to engage in unhealthy behavior are going to suffer from not merely the deleterious health consequences of their imprudence but also the attending economic deprivations. Second, the wellness movement, with its expensive paraphernalia, programs, and priestly class of health promotion and fitness gurus, introduces yet one more area in which the poor are excluded from the privileges and practices of middle- and upper-class American life. Third, the wellness movement threatens to polarize further race and class in the United States because of its success. As middle- and upper-class Americans adopt more healthy lifestyles, they, and the policymakers who serve their interests, may lose interest in, and decline to support, programs for those who remain trapped in conditions where modifying injurious lifestyle practices is problematic at best. Dr. Mitchell S. Rosenthal, president of Phoenix House Foundation, a drug treatment and education organization in New York, recently made this point with regard to drug abuse, but it could apply just as easily to alcohol and tobacco use: "The danger is that we will have a shrinking political interest in the problem and the most vulnerable and high risk populations will not get the kind of services they need" (*New York Times*, January 1, 1991).

Finally, there is another sense in which the success of the wellness movement may divert health-promoting resources from where they are most needed. John Brant ruminates over the possibility that in another time, perhaps some of the personal fitness trainers currently servicing privileged society would be in public schools, YMCAs, or community centers helping a larger number and more diverse group of people (Brant 1989, 24–25). It may well be that wellness in the United States today is being wasted on the well.

Notes

1. A study by the American Medical Association (1993) concluded that "premature death and disease are caused primarily by lifestyle factors. Of the two million American deaths each year, half are premature deaths, in the sense that they could have been postponed." Among the lifestyle factors reviewed are alcohol, tobacco, and drug use, excessive weight, and violence (11–16).

2. There have been no efforts, to my knowledge, empirically to delineate periods of social chaos or anomie. Hence, the designation of an era as one of "social turmoil and rapid change" is admittedly imprecise and subjective. I think there are few who dispute the assertion, however, that the 1960s was such a period. For example, Angus Campbell (1981) reports that between 1957 and 1972 the percentage of Americans describing themselves as "very happy" declined from 35 percent to 24 percent (29).

3. The quotation in the heading is from Edward Devine, a nineteenth-century purity reformer (quoted in Pivar 1973, 269).

References

Allegrante, J. P., and L. W. Green. 1981. Sounding board: When health policy becomes victim blaming. *New England Journal of Medicine* 305(25): 1528–29.

American Medical Association. 1993. *Factors contributing to the health care cost problem*. Chicago: American Medical Association.

Barsky, A. J. 1988. *Worried sick: Our troubled quest for wellness.* Boston: Little, Brown.

Baur, S. 1988. *Hypochondria: Woeful imaginings.* Berkeley: University of California Press.

Berger, S. M. 1989. *Forever young: 20 years younger in 20 weeks.* New York: Morrow.

Brant, J. 1989. To each his own. *Outside,* 23–25.

Brownell, K. D. 1991. Personal responsibility and control over our bodies: When expectation exceeds reality. *Health Psychology* 10:303–10.

Campbell, A. 1981. *The sense of well-being in America.* New York: McGraw-Hill.

Carlyon, W. H. 1984. Disease prevention/health promotion—Bridging the gap to wellness. *Health Values* 8:27–30.

Conrad, P. 1990. Wellness in the work place: Potentials and pitfalls of work-site health promotion. In *The sociology of health and illness,* edited by P. Conrad and R. Kern. New York: St. Martin's Press.

Crawford, R. 1980. Healthism and the medicalization of everyday life. *International Journal of Health Services* 10(3): 365–88.

Feinhandler, S. J. 1986. The social role of smoking. In *Smoking and society: Toward a more balanced assessment,* edited by R. D. Tollison. Lexington, Mass.: Lexington Books.

France, A. 1894. *Le Lys Rouge.* Paris: Calmann-L'evy.

Fuchs, V. R. 1979. The economics of health in a post-industrial society. *Public Interest,* 3–20.

Gallup, G., Jr. 1989. Public value intangible assets more than material possessions. *The Gallup Report,* 282/283, (March/April): 36.

———. 1990a. 1989 Gallup leisure audit. *Gallup Poll Monthly,* 295 (April), 27–30.

———. 1990b. Many Americans favor restrictions on smoking in public places. *Gallup Poll Monthly,* 298 (July), 19–27.

———. 1991. *The Gallup Poll: Public opinion, 1991.* Wilmington, Del.: Scholarly Resources.

Gillick, M. R. 1984. Jogging and the moral life. *Journal of Health Politics, Policy, and Law* 9 (fall): 369–87.

Gingrich, N. 1984. The best health care for everyone. *Policy Review* 29, (summer): 66–70.

Huntington, S. P. 1974. Postindustrial politics: How benign will it be? *Comparative Politics* 6 (January): 163–92.

Inglehart, R. 1976. The nature of value change in post-industrial societies.

In *Politics and the future of industrial society*, edited by L. Lindberg. New York: McKay.

Janofsky, M. 1994. Smokers need not apply, say firms; new laws dampen zeal. *Commercial Appeal* (Online), May 1, final ed., sec. A, 51. Available: NEXIS Library: NEWS File: CURNWS.

Lasch, C. 1978. *The culture of narcissism: American life in an age of diminishing expectations*. New York: Norton.

Leichter, H. M. 1991. *Free to be foolish*. Princeton: Princeton University Press.

Levine, B. A. 1989. *Leviticus*. New York: Jewish Publication Society.

McGuire, W. J. 1984. Public communication as a strategy for inducing health-promoting behavioral change. *Preventive Medicine* 13:299–319.

Mencken, H. L. 1985. *Prejudices: Third series*. New York: Octagon Books.

Neubauer, D. 1992. Hawaii: The health state. In *Health policy reform in America*, edited by H. M. Leichter. Armonk: M. E. Sharpe.

Pivar, D. J. 1973. *Purity crusade: Sexual morality and social control 1868–1900*. Westport, Conn.: Greenwood.

Potter, C. 1983. Showdown for health vigilantes. *Health and Social Services Journal*, September 22, 1140–41.

The revised English Bible with apocrypha. 1989. London: Oxford University Press: Cambridge University Press.

Risk-related health insurance: Incentives for healthy lifestyles. 1990. *The New York Business Group on Health, Inc. Discussion Paper* 10(1): 1–7.

Rolls, B. J., I. C. Fedoroff, and J. F. Guthrie. 1991. Gender differences in eating behavior and body weight regulation. *Health Psychology* 10:133–42.

Sardella, S. 1995. Genetic discrimination. *Boston Herald* (Online), September 24, 1st ed., magazine sec., 6. Available: NEXIS Library: NEWS File: CURNWS.

Stein, H. F. 1982. "Health" and "wellness" a euphemism: The cultural context of insidious Draconean health policy. *Continuing Education for the Family Physician* 16:33–44.

Stone, D. A. 1986. The resistible rise of preventive medicine. *Journal of Health Politics, Policy and Law* 11(4): 671–96.

———. 1989. At risk in the welfare state. *Social Research* 56(3): 591–633.

Terry, P. E. 1991. A dangerous innovation. *HealthAction Managers*, February 25, 1–9.

Turner, B. S. 1984. *The body and society: Explorations in social theory.* Oxford: Basil Blackwell.

U.S. Bureau of the Census. 1992. *Statistical abstract of the United States, 1992.* Washington, D.C.: Government Printing Office.

Whorton, J. C. 1982. *Crusades for fitness: The history of American health reformers.* Princeton: Princeton University Press.

Moralization

Paul Rozin

Within any culture, at a particular time, there is some consensus about the activities that fall into the moral domain, and those that fall outside it. This rough dichotomy is far from stable: moral status for an activity may ebb and flow over time. This paper deals with the changes in which an activity that was previously outside the moral domain enters into it. The process will be called moralization. It is quite common in both cultural evolution and individual development. It affects both the course of history and individual lives, and is of particular relevance to the understanding of attitudes toward health and the body. Because moralization has not been previously framed as a specific phenomenon, it has not been a focus of scholarly investigation and analysis.

In this chapter, I will first consider some definitions and follow with a discussion of the significance of moralization. I will then consider the parallel processes of cultural and individual moralization and deal with the moral emotions, particularly disgust, and their role in the process of moralization. Next, I will consider the processes through which moralization in individuals occurs. Then, I will consider the human predisposition to make moral interpretations of significant events, followed by a consideration of the factors that seem to promote moralization.

Throughout the chapter, I will focus on moralization of health-related issues, although I believe that moralization extends well beyond the health domain. In each section, I will illustrate the principles discussed, using the example of the moralization of meat consumption in the United States: that is, the increasingly prevalent belief in the United States (and other countries) that eating meat is immoral.

Some Definitions

I will define moralization as the acquisition of moral qualities by objects and activities that were previously morally neutral. Examples of this process at work at the level of culture in the United States include the moralization of slavery in the eighteenth and nineteenth centuries, and the moralization of cigarette smoking in the late twentieth century (Katz 1997). Because there is both an ebb and a flow in moral categorization, there must be an inverse process, which I will call amoralization. In the United States, this has happened for many individuals with respect to attitudes toward homosexuality. A particular species of amoralization is sometimes called medicalization; in these cases, an illness that originally was linked with moral failings loses some of this moral loading and comes squarely into the domain of medicine. Many aspects of mental illness, including alcoholism, have made some of this journey in the twentieth century.

For present purposes, something is in the moral domain if the term *ought* (or *ought not*) applies to it. Another gloss holds that if something is in the moral domain for person A, then A is concerned that other people hold and behave according to the position held by A. These criteria are exemplified in the contrast between pure "moral" (or "ecological") and "health" vegetarians, a subset of all vegetarians. Pure moral vegetarians avoid eating meat only because of the moral implications (killing animals, wasting resources, and so on), whereas pure health vegetarians avoid eating meat on the grounds that it is unhealthy (Amato and Partridge 1989; Rozin, Markwith, and Stoess 1997). In contrast to health vegetarians, moral vegetarians attach an "ought" to avoiding meat and are concerned that others eat meat. We might say that for moral vegetarians, the eating of meat enters into the domain of values, whereas for health vegetarians, it is a matter of mere preference. Of course, this distinction has its limits; it is a major premise of this book that health issues typically have a moral component (see Katz's discussion of secular morality in this volume).

The Significance and Consequences of Moralization

Moralization and Institutional Mobilization

At the level of culture, there are major consequences of moralization. Once moralization has occurred in a substantial part or in an especially powerful or influential segment of the population, the forces of government and major institutions align with it, quickening the pace of further moralization. In the contemporary United States, communication media, laws, courts, charitable institutions, universities, and granting agencies openly support the spread of consensus moral positions. In science, there has been a motivated attempt to discover third-party effects (passive smoking and sidestream smoke) to support opposition to smoking on moral grounds (Gostin 1997; Katz 1997). Gostin notes that the courts have been willing to accept limits on cigarette advertising without evidence that it is effective in encouraging smoking. Gusfield (1997) reports that with the moralization of alcohol abuse, statistics on alcohol-related automobile deaths are skewed by scientists, public health officials, and others to maximize the number. Accidents in which either driver is legally intoxicated are classified as alcohol-related. Most clearly, laws are passed forbidding moralized activities like smoking, and penalties for violation may be increased.

Institutional mobilization may serve as justification for moral censure of those who violate the now-regulated activity. In the United States today, one can approach and censure a smoker in many circumstances, whereas such a behavior, twenty years ago, would have been considered rude.

Moralization and Parent-Child Transmission

Moralization increases the likelihood of transmission of attitudes, preferences, and habits across generations. The transmission process, from parent and others to child may be different for values (including moral matters) and preferences. Two studies (Cavalli-Sforza, Feldman, Chen, and Dornbusch 1982; Rozin 1991) suggest that transmission of values (for example, attitudes toward abortion or drugs) from parent to child is much more effective than transmission of preferences (for example, food or music tastes). Transmission of preferences across generations is poor (parent-child correlations in the 0 to 0.3 range, compared to 0.3 to 0.6 for values).

Moralization and Internalization

When an individual chooses outcome A over outcome B, we say there is a preference for A. Attribution of a preference to a person is

essentially a matter of observing behavior. The reasons for the occurrence of a preference are many (Damon 1983; Kelman 1958;
McCauley, Rozin, and Schwartz 1997; and Rozin and Vollmecke
1986, in relation to food choice). At the extremes, the choice may
be made habitually (without thought) or it may result from a careful, "rational" consideration of costs and benefits for each option.
However, the motivation of many preferences lies between these extremes. Some of these preferences can be described as "compliant"
or "extrinsic"; that is, they are motivated by some end extrinsic to
the items being chosen. One might choose cottage cheese over
cream cheese because the former is lower in calories (serving the end
of weight control) or one might stop at red lights because of the fear
of receiving a ticket. Other preferences can be thought to result
from intrinsic forces; these are called internalized preferences. Internalized preferences or behaviors occur for their own sake
(Kelman 1958; Lepper 1980; Deci and Ryan 1985). Common internalized activities are participating in or watching sports, playing a
musical instrument, scholarship for most academics, and eating
one's favorite foods. The same behavior may be internalized in one
person and performed under compliance for another. For example,
some people exercise because they love to do so (it has been internalized), and others find it unpleasant but do so in compliance with
their long-term health goals.

We do not know much about what causes a behavior or a preference to be internalized. We need no account of behavior motivated by compliance; someone who is afraid of dying will comply
with requests to wear a safety belt and not eat wild mushrooms she
finds in the fields. The puzzle for psychology is why some of these
activities become internalized in some people. In general, it seems
that subtle social influences play an important role in internalization (Lepper 1980; Deci and Ryan 1985; McCauley et al. 1997).

Internalization is important because behaviors or preferences
that are internalized and, hence, liked for their own sake, tend to
endure, even under conditions of stress or in the face of information that argues against them. They are woven into the self. The
compliant exerciser will stop exercising if he is highly stressed or if
the latest medical wisdom indicates that exercise really does not
improve health. This is not so for the exerciser who has internalized exercise.

Moral values are often referred to as internalized. They are or
become a part of the self. It is reasonable to suppose that preferences and behaviors that are somehow attached to internalized val-

ues will themselves function as internalized. An action that is performed in the service of a value is likely to be more resilient and durable. One reason for this is that moral linkage may encourage a hedonic shift. In other words, an object or activity that is aligned with one's moral views may come to be liked, and one that is in violation of such views may come to be disliked.

A compliant vegetarian believes she derives health benefits from meat avoidance but is tempted by the aroma of meat and is fighting the tendency to eat it. Under stress (strong hunger or problems in her life) she is likely to succumb, and she is probably on the lookout for information that will absolve meat of its health-damaging properties. The moral vegetarian, on the other hand, cannot imagine that she will change her mind and decide that killing animals for food is acceptable, and she is looking for confirmation of her meat avoidance, not a reason to stop it. Often enough (see below), the moral meat avoider experiences a hedonic shift and actually comes to dislike or be disgusted by meat. Now she is not even tempted to consume meat. This opportune result internalizes the meat avoidance. Such a hedonic shift may be less likely in health-oriented vegetarians (Rozin, Markwith, and Stoess, 1997).

Parallels between Historico-Cultural and Individual Moralization

Culture-wide moralization of a particular entity would usually come about as a result of the growth of a large or politically powerful collection of individuals who accept and promote such a moralization. When the influence of such a group reaches a critical level, a culture-wide acceptance, by law or common consensus may occur. After this happens, children will regularly acquire these new values. The same factors that cause a shift in moralization at the cultural level may also act at the individual level. Insofar as this is true, the study of the psychology of internalization may inform attempts to understand moralization in a cultural-historical context, just as the historical record may inform those interested in the psychological processes operating in the individual.

This parallel may exist for meat avoidance, in that the justifications offered by cultures and religions that avoid meat overlap heavily with the justifications offered by individuals (in nonvegetarian cultures) who are becoming vegetarians.

Emotion and Moralization: The Moral Emotions

Robert Frank (1988) proposes that one function of emotions is to keep us on a biologically and culturally adaptive track. In his view the "emotion" of love is a way of reducing infidelity and helping to secure a monogamous relation. A number of emotions can be thought of as in the service of socialization, and hence vehicles for relating morality to behaviors and preferences. Unpleasant emotions such as embarrassment, shame, guilt, and disgust direct behavior by causing us to avoid doing things that will arouse them, and by causing us to cease doing things that have already aroused them. These emotions are elicited primarily by situations dictated by our socialization experience.

The emotion of disgust, which seems to have originated as a form of food rejection, has expanded, through cultural evolution, so that elicitors in many cultures include moral or quasi-moral violations (Rozin, Haidt, and McCauley 1993). A powerful feature of disgust is contamination (negative contagion): when disgusting things simply touch other entities, those entities become undesirable. It is probably universal that people reject wearing clothing that has previously been worn by an offensive other person (a stranger, a disliked person, a despicable public figure) or eating food that has been prepared or sampled by such a person (see Rozin and Nemeroff 1990 for a review). This feature of disgust effectively removes a person from disgust elicitors or things that have contacted them.

Disgust evolves, in culture and in individual development, from an emotion that deals with potential harm to the body from foods to one that deals with potential harm to the soul. In the end, disgust is a powerful tool for negative socialization; a very effective way to get people to avoid something and to have this avoidance internalized is to make the entity disgusting.

Among educated persons in American culture, disgust is at least superficially accounted for in relation to the risk of disease and filth, and we do not explicitly acknowledge it as a moral emotion. In other cultures, the domains in which disgust is elicited are more explicitly moral. In general, in more traditional cultures and in lower social classes, people are more willing to attribute immorality to disgusting activities (Haidt, Koller, and Dias 1992). This may be because morality in the developed Western cultures, at least among the elite, is restricted to violations of individual rights. Shweder and associates (1997), in this volume, have suggested that the rights-violation moral system is only one of three moral codes that exist across cultures. They point out that in Hindu India, the two moral codes of community and divinity (including purity and pollution) are more dominant than the Western code of autonomy (rights violations). Disgust seems to be an emotion that links into the divinity code; hence, in a culture in which the divinity code is active, disgust becomes a moral emotion. A similar argument can be made for the moralization of anger with respect to the autonomy code, and contempt with respect to the community code (Rozin, Lowery, Imada, and Haidt 1997).

Insofar as disgust is involved with purity/pollution violations, it is an emotion particularly involved with both morality and body/health issues. That is, moralization may promote disgust. Health vegetarians are less likely to find meat disgusting than are moral vegetarians (Rozin, Markwith, and Stoess 1997). With the moralization of smoking, we see an increase in disgust responses to cigarettes, smokers, and cigarette ashes than previously found (Rozin and Singh, 1997). Moral concerns about smoking show a higher correlation with the experience of disgust to smoking or cigarettes than do beliefs about the health effects of smoking.

Modes of Moralization

How does moralization occur at the individual level? I propose that there are two orthogonal dimensions to this problem. One is whether the cause of the change is primarily cognitive or affective. Cognitive causes imply a primary role for knowledge and information in the process of moralization. Cognitive changes are principled or reasoned. Affective causes indicate a primary role for emotional events, such as the co-occurrence of an activity with an emotionally/morally meaningful event. Affective changes are less reasoned and principled. The second dimension of moralization has to do with whether the moral issue is new for the target person ("moral expansion") or whether an existing moral issue is extended to a new entity ("moral piggybacking"). These two dimensions generate four possible modes of moralization. I will use examples from the study of meat avoidance to illustrate different aspects of moralization, citing individual examples from our own unpublished study on the origins of vegetarianism or from Amato and Partridge's (1989) excellent book on this same subject.

Moral Piggybacking

Moral piggybacking is the extension of an existing moral principle to a new object/activity. In this case, I will assume that the person in question has already decided that killing animals is immoral but has yet to "apply" this principle to eating.

Affective route. A subject reports on the onset of meat avoidance: "Visited McDonald's meat packing plant and experience was too much; the stench, the blood, the stale air, the flesh—left such a mark that I could not even imagine eating red meat."

Cognitive route. One subject stopped eating gelatine desserts on finding out that gelatine had an animal origin. Another "began not to be able to forget the tortures and abuses which preceded the production of food" that he was eating. The general expansion of vegetarianism from a red meat base (Dwyer, Mayer, Kandel, & Mayer 1973; Amato and Partridge 1989; Rozin, Markwith, and Stoess 1997) proceeds along the same lines; for example, the realization that a distinction between mammals and fish cannot be maintained.

Moral Expansion

This mode involves creation of a new moral domain.

Affective. One example from our data base cites the experience of watching the slaughter of seals in the Arctic, which caused the person, in an emotional context, to believe that the killing of animals by humans is immoral.

Cognitive. One of the most common causes of vegetarianism is exposure to reasoned arguments about animal rights and the cruelty of the treatment of animals raised to be food for humans. Peter Singer's (1975) *Animal Liberation* has created many vegetarians by establishing a moral principle.

Once moralization has begun, it often moves ahead with the force that a moral justification can motivate. Red meat avoidance often proceeds to a wider spectrum of animal-food avoidances, and the degree of moral commitment tends to increase. Social psychologists have shown that people strive for cognitive consistency and try to resolve apparent contradictions in their attitudes and behaviors. Furthermore, it has been shown (for example, Frey 1986) that when people take a strong and irrevocable position, they tend to selectively seek and process information in such a way as to reinforce this position. Although a mere preference for A over B would be unlikely to invoke such selectivity, a moral position is quite likely to. For these reasons, vegetarians of long standing usually offer many reasons for their meat avoidance. In particular, there is a tendency for moral vegetarians to offer more reasons for their vegetarianism than do health vegetarians (Rozin, Markwith, and Stoess 1997).

Food, Vegetarianism, and Moralization

It is no accident that vegetarianism has been a convenient exemplar for illustrating moralization. The food domain is predisposed to moralization. In many cultures, diet is linked to health, and health to morality. In the history of Western culture, there have been tendencies to see both the animal aspects of humans and the experience of pleasure as immoral activities. Eating and food are both major sources of pleasures and properties we share with animals. In the cultural evolution of disgust, we have posited that in the stage following disgust to foods based on their nature and origin, reminders of our animal nature (death, inappropriate sex, violations of the body boundaries) become the next set of disgust elicitors (Rozin, Haidt, and McCauley 1993). Later, as we have said, disgust elicitors expand further, into the explicitly moral domain. Food is also central to Shweder and associates' (1997) divinity (purity/pollution) moral code. It is not surprising that four of the chapters in this book (Belasco, Courtwright, Gusfield, and Mintz) have ingestion as a major concern. Our interaction with food involves the intimate act of taking something that is outside the self and incorporating it into the self. This accounts, at least in part, for the strong feelings about eating. Such feelings are accentuated by the widespread belief that "you are what you eat" (see Nemeroff and Rozin 1989; Rozin 1990 for elaborations). "You are what you eat" provides a potentially powerful link between food practices and moral issues. There is widespread explicit acknowledgement of this belief in traditional societies. Frazer (1890/1959), in the *Golden Bough*, states that an individual in a traditional culture "commonly believes that by eating the flesh of an animal or man, he acquires not only the physical but even the moral and intellectual qualities which are characteristic of that animal or man" (573). "You are what you eat" was also a common belief in premodern Europe (Thomas 1983). The importance of this belief is that the conjunction of animals being considered morally loaded entities and the "you are what you eat" principle opens food and eating to moral considerations.

The "you are what you eat" principle makes intuitive sense. It is generally true that when we mix two entities, the resultant product has properties of both entities. Modern knowledge of digestion and the common molecular constituents of all foods renders the principle invalid, but this is both a modern and a counterintuitive idea. We (Nemeroff and Rozin 1989) have found evidence for a widespread, unacknowledged belief in "you are what you eat" among American college students. Indirect measures indicate that these students believe that eating animals makes one more animal-like, and that specific properties of ingested animals are transmitted to the person who eats them.

There are other features of food that make food a rich area for cultural elaboration of meanings (Douglas 1966; Gusfield 1992). The centrality of body functions in symbolization and metaphor (Lakoff and Johnson 1980) provide one avenue of elaboration. The fact that food is typically shared by humans, and that there is often a complex path, involving numbers of people, from the raw material to the final product, allows many opportunities for invasion by moral issues. Origins of foods become important materials for moral feelings. Note the Hindu concern about eating foods previously contacted by people of lower social/purity statuses (Appadurai 1981); rejections of sugar in European history because of the association with slavery (Mintz 1985, 1997); and rejection of foods by contemporary Americans because of associations with killing animals or immoral labor practices (Belasco 1997).

In short, food is a source of sustenance and pleasure, and a social and moral vehicle. Appadurai (1981) refers to food, in the Hindu context, as a "condensed biomoral substance." These combined forces are well represented in Mintz's (1997) statement that one should forgo sugar "for others, for self, and for God."

A small percentage of reasons offered by individuals to account for their vegetarianism is that ingestion of animal foods will increase the tendency to behave like animals. The Hebrew animal prohibitions have been interpreted as a means of avoiding the passage of animal properties to humans (Grunfeld 1972/1982). The belief in transmigration of souls in ancient Greece provided a basis for a belief in "you are what you eat" and constituted one of the justifications for meat avoidance (Barkas 1975).

Searching for Meaning:
The Human Inclination toward Invoking Moral Violations to Account for Illness and Misfortune

Humans search for meaning for their experiences in the world, perhaps especially their misfortunes. Rosenberg notes, with respect to the acceptance of germ theory, a reluctance of Americans to accept randomness as an account for who gets a disease. Moral accounts are natural and satisfying alternatives to randomness. "We honor randomness in the abstract, but seek to manage it in practice, to constrain misfortune in reassuring frameworks of meaning" (Rosenberg 1997, 35). Shweder and associates (1997) begin their analysis of the moral meanings of illness with the statement "Wherever one looks on the globe, it appears that human beings want to be edified by their miseries" (119). They add later that "For most people of the world, there are no faultless deaths" (130). And finally, they note the central place of moral-misfortune links in the Hindu belief systems: "In India the human tendency to interpret fortune and misfortune in terms of spiritual or moral merit and debt is institutionalized in the widespread cultural doctrine of karma" (150).

In a cross-cultural survey of beliefs about illness, Murdock (1980) reports that the predominant theory of the cause of disease is moral; people who violate some moral principle become ill (see also data presented in Shweder et al. 1997). Moral accounts of illness are much more common than contagion accounts, which occur in only 49 of 139 cultures surveyed. In Western culture, as recently as the mid-nineteenth century in the United States, the medical profession attributed cholera to moral or quasi-moral defects characteristic of the lower classes who accounted for the great majority of cases (Rosenberg 1962).

Children in Western cultures also frequently make moral attributions for illness. Contagion/germ accounts of illness are uncommon in children until the age of about seven years (Bibace and Walsh 1979; Nagy 1953). Indeed, a prominent account of illness by children is moral, in the form of what Piaget (1932/1965) has called immanent justice: illness as a form of punishment for a misdemeanor. This may well be fostered by parent claims (even though they may "know" better) that some illness in a child (particularly an accident or a cold) is a result of careless or otherwise faulty behavior.

Some Americans explicitly believe in a moral component to illness. For example, some believe that AIDS is God's punishment for sin. Sontag (1977) has described a history of moral beliefs about illness in Americans. But many contemporary educated adults, raised in the Western tradition, hold that health and morals are essentially independent entities. However, just as with denials by these same people of the "you are what you eat" principle, there is clear evidence that traditional views lurk just below the surface. Most Americans express reluctance about wearing a sweater that has been previously worn by a person with AIDS (Rozin, Markwith, and McCauley 1994). This reluctance is typically justified in terms of a minimal risk of contracting AIDS. However, the response of most people to the same sweater after it has been sterilized is almost as negative as the response to the unsterilized sweater. This suggests a moral as well as health-risk cause for aversion, and is confirmed by the fact that most people are also reluctant to wear a sweater previously worn by a healthy convicted murderer (even after thorough laundering and sterilization) (Rozin, Markwith, and McCauley 1994).

Recently, Stein and Nemeroff (1995) have demonstrated a striking link between eating "health" foods and morality, in a study on American college students. Students made a variety of personality and character ratings on the basis of vignettes describing a college student. Subjects read either vignette A or B, which were identical, except that in A, the student was described as regularly eating "steak, hamburgers, French fries, doughnuts and double-fudge ice cream sundaes," and in B, the regularly eaten foods were "fruit (especially oranges), salad, homemade whole-wheat bread, chicken and potatoes." The subjects eating the "healthy" foods were rated substantially higher on a morality measure, based on a combination of judgments on individual scales contrasting terms such as immoral/virtuous, unethical/ethical, and considerate/inconsiderate.

Factors That Promote or Discourage Moralization

As Gordon (1997) points out, we use the term *moralistic* to describe inappropriate introduction of moral discourse into discussion about some event. The term itself suggests that there is disagreement, within cultures, about the moral status of certain events. Some things that could be moralized are not, and some "moralization movements" fail. This raises the question, what promotes and what discourages moralization? There are many behaviors that are neither universally classified as moral or immoral nor clearly outside the realm of morality. What determines whether they are amor-alized or moralized? Are the factors that promote amoralization the same as those that promote moralization? The chapters in this volume, as they consider the linkage between morality and health, one domain of moralization, provide many examples of failure and success in moralization. Using materials that bridge diverse periods of history, domains of human activity and cultures, I propose some regularities in the relationship between morality and health. These regularities are likely to be relevant to the general issue of moralization, in a framework larger than just morality and health.

1. Protestantism—Evangelical Self-Discipline and Control

Protestantism is commonly invoked, in the chapters in this volume, as a factor promoting moralization in the health-behavior domain. Thomas (1997) notes that "implicit in Protestantism was the doctrine that the human body had been given to man by God, and that it was therefore a religious duty to take all reasonable steps to preserve it" (18). In particular, in the United States, evangelical Protestantism focuses on self-discipline and control (Courtwright 1997). Rugged individualism and control of and responsibility for one's body are central themes in many versions of Protestantism (Courtwright 1997; Leichter 1997; Thomas 1997). In the contemporary American scene, many efforts at moralization may grow out of the early Puritan spirit. Gusfield (1997) refers to latent Puritanism in the debates over prohibition of alcohol consumption, and notes that in general it is Protestants who seek abolition and Catholics who support moderation. Successful temperance movements occurred only in the United States, England, and Scandinavia, all predominantly Protestant countries.

2. Harm to Children

Perceived harm to the health of children is a particularly powerful mobilizer of moral forces, at least in Western cultures (see comments by Belasco 1997). A. Kleinman (personal communication) notes that in China, the elderly may occupy this same privileged position with respect to the engagement of moral issues. Harm to children from drugs (Courtwright 1997), or alcohol (through driving, fetal alcohol syndrome, or early intoxication; Gusfield 1997) is explicitly mentioned as a force for moral mobilization. The recent passive-smoking debate has been intensified by invocation of harm caused by parents' smoking to their children, and attention to AIDS and crack babies has mobilized opposition. Pictures in the mass media of children wounded in military action or of starving children from Third World countries have, in recent decades, produced indignation and mobilized action.

There are many reasons that harm to children may be especially potent, at least for Westerners. First is the natural sympathy we have for children, and hence our strong emotional reaction when we encounter a harmed child. Second, children are often thought of as pure and innocent. Third, they are thought of as helpless, defenseless victims of the actions of others. Fourth, from a more economic view, children have much more life to live, so that a child death involves a much larger reduction in life expectancy than an adult death. In short, there are abundant reasons for the saliency of children's health and welfare.

3. Stigmatized, Marginalized, or Minority Groups

Moralization seems to be facilitated if the group primarily associated with the target activity is already stigmatized or marginalized or is a minority group. This has occurred for leprosy, syphilis, plague, and cholera at different historical moments; in all of these cases, the more susceptible lower classes were already stigmatized groups (Rosenberg 1962; 1997; Thomas 1997). Thomas (1997) explicitly recognizes this factor, in stating: "Readiness to impose a moral interpretation upon sickness was greater when the malady was particularly associated with some marginal or deviant sector of society" (25).

This principle is illustrated by the impetus to illegalization of drugs in the early twentieth century in the United States by the association of opium smoking with Chinese laborers (Courtwright 1997); and the focus of the moral responsibility for teenage and out-of-wedlock pregnancies on the less politically powerful mothers (Gordon 1997). Furthermore, in recent times in the United States, out-of-wedlock and teenage pregnancy have been strongly associated, in the public mind, with minority (particularly African-American) and impoverished segments of the population. On the other hand, certain privileged groups, such as meatpackers, manufacturers of highly refined foods, and cigarette manufacturers, have been subject to considerable moral condemnation over the course of this century in the United States.

4. Fit with Existing Practices and Predispositions

A moral-health link is facilitated if the behaviors promoted by the moral link are already practiced for other reasons. On the other hand, a prior moral link may itself function as a predisposition for the acceptance of ideas or activities subsequently justified for a non-moral reason. Tomes's (1997) analysis of the advent of germ theory is a particularly apt illustration of both of these points. Sanitary practices were already in force as a result of the sanitarian movement (Tomes 1997), and the death rate due to infectious disease was already declining before germ theory was accepted (Brandt 1997). In the face of the debate about prevention of tuberculosis, practices like spitting that had previousy been thought to be only disgusting or ill-bred became threats to public health (Tomes 1997). Existing linkages between contagion and uncleanliness in the popular mind, under the impact of germ theory, were extended to dusting, coughing, plate sharing. Hygienic precautions practiced only during epidemics became general. The developing idea of resistance to infection gave support to personal regimens already promoted by nineteenth-century American health reformers (Belasco 1997; Tomes 1997).

For the case of germ theory and infectious disease, it seems that prior moralization predisposed to the acceptance of medical advice. The cleanliness-godliness link is implicit in Jewish and Christian teaching (Thomas 1997); again, prior to germ theory, Thomas (1997) notes a gradual increase in cleanliness, manifested as increased use of soap and increased frequency of bathing, in eighteenth- and nineteenth-century England. Presumably, the principal motivation for such activities was to appear more upper-class and less animal-like (Elias 1939/1978).

Food and sex, because of their animal/biological quality, and their direct stimulation of pleasure, may be domains that are predisposed to moralization. Gluttony and promiscuity are moralized in many cultures at many historical times, and there is a certain re-spect (moral value) attributed to voluntary starvation or reduction in food intake and celibacy.

The opposite side of the predisposition coin is the discouraging effect of inconvenience in preventing adoptions of morally "desir-able" changes (Belasco 1997). In this regard, Belasco suggests that substitutions work better than reductions or prohibitions.

5. Favorable Short-Term Benefit-Cost Ratio

Moralization often entails abandonment of certain activities. It is obviously easier to give up something that one is not strongly at-tached to. Generally, people don't want to pay a lot for virtue. The attachment can result from the pleasure produced by the activity, the fear of the consequences of loss of the activity (for example, ad-dictive withdrawal), or the fact that the activity in question is inti-mately interwoven with the daily cycle of activities. Cigarette smoking is an example of all of these things because it produces great pleasure and fear of the consequence of withdrawal, and is of-ten a habitual act related to other activities, including social inter-action, eating, and drinking coffee. In many individuals and cultural groups, drinking of alcohol and drug use may engage the same set of "attachments." Another example is Fletcherism, the nineteenth-century American health movement that encouraged people to do endless chewing of their food to facilitate ingestion and eliminate defecation (Belasco 1997; Whorton 1982). Multihour, tedious mealtimes were too much of an imposition, providing further evi-dence for Belasco's assertion that inconvenience can be a barrier to moralization.

6. Potential for Accretion of Reasons

The addition of a moral component to an attitude or behavior mobilizes institutional and psychological processes that serve to strengthen adherence (or abandonment). The moral dimension in-duces both an implicit and explicit "search" for additional justifi-cations. People are probably more concerned about apparent contradictions or uniqueness in values that they maintain than they are about corresponding contradictions or uniquenesses in preferences. (The contradiction between eating meat and believing that animals have a right to live is more likely to engage action than the contradiction between disliking bitter tastes but liking coffee.) Mere preferences are simply less central to the self. Hence, people are probably more likely to do cognitive work to produce consistency in values than in preferences, and to reinforce these values with rationales for their adoption. Striking examples include the multiple motives that developed for alcohol prohibition: moral issues related to the public order, moral issues having to do with loss of self-control, and health concerns (Gusfield 1997). Opposition to alcohol use in the United States became favored by different people in different contexts in the early twentieth century: it appealed to politically concerned people, who worried about irresponsibility in the electorate; churches' concern for purity in their members; and employers seeking a disciplined work force (Gusfield 1997). The addition of a moral component to an attitude or behavior promotes an opportunism, an active search for reasons: the link of sugar to slavery, to luxury and excess, to the threatening beverages of tea, coffee, and chocolate all conspired to produce moral opposition to sugar (Mintz 1997).

In the contemporary scene, accretion of reasons is a clear consequence of the moralization of cigarette smoking. There is a developing sense that cigarette residues (smoke, butts, ashes) are disgusting (Rozin and Singh, 1997), and a motivated attempt to discover third-party effects (passive smoking and sidestream smoke; Gostin 1997; Katz 1997). Returning to vegetarianism, as mentioned previously, moral vegetarians have, on average, more different reasons for avoiding meat than do health vegetarians (Rozin, Markwith, and Stoess 1997).

7. Vulnerable Periods

There may well be times when moralization is more likely, what we might call windows of moralization susceptibility. Three authors in this book independently suggest that chaotic times or cultural crises may promote moralization. Brandt (1997) notes that in times of chaos, desire for individual control over the body becomes paramount. Gusfield (1997), in reference to growing social disorder in the United States in the early nineteenth century, notes that the weakening of institutions encourages self-control. Leichter (1997) holds that in times of rapid sociopolitical change, Americans turn inward and become preoccupied with their own well-being. He cites the turmoil of the 1960s, in association with attempts to reclaim control over body. These body and control concerns and their moral implications may be accentuated in the context of Protestantism as a dominant religion. Perhaps the same theme is at work in recent suggestions that the increase in eating disorders in the United States involves a desire for something to control in a life somewhat out of control.

8. Confusion and Lack of Understanding about Disease Causation

It is sobering to realize that prior to the twentieth century, physicians had little understanding of the cause of different diseases, and little they could do in the way of effective treatment. Rosenberg (1997) points out that the idea of specific disease entities with different, specific causes arose in the later nineteenth century. Mechanic (1997) notes that even today, only a minority of patient complaints can be definitively diagnosed and treated by modern physicians. He further notes that "when confirmed medical models don't fit, one gets a heavy dose of social judgment often disguised as diagnosis." The point is that it is easier for moral issues to invade matters of health when there is uncertainty about causation. Though the microbe was moralized (Tomes 1997), germ theory did present a challenge to the moralization of infectious diseases.

Brandt (1997), Leichter (1997), and Rosenberg (1997) note that in spite of the major advances in medical science in the past fifty years, changes in the disease spectrum and attitudes toward illness have maintained an environment in which moralization of illness is frequent and easy. The predominance of chronic diseases places us in a domain where there is complex, difficult to understand, multiple causation, and where lifestyle can be easily invoked as a contributor to causation. And the development of the idea of risk factors, treated as if they themselves are diseases, provides ample opportunities to invoke individual responsibility and hence moral factors in the etiology of this newly expanded notion of disease. Both physicians and nonphysicians dislike multicausation and probabilistic accounts. The field is wide open for moralization.

9. The Rise of Secular Morality

The decline of religion in the middle to late twentieth century has coincided with the rise of modern medical science, and particularly the field of epidemiology. This change stimulated Katz (1997) to define secular morality, based in large part on principles and facts that flow out of epidemiological research. Epidemiological findings become more plentiful and public every year. These findings do not have any inherent moral character, but in the context of a "risk-factor-is-disease" mentality, they provide great opportunities for moralization. As we come to know more and more risk factors, and as these invoke more and more features of life that are nominally under our own control, the opportunities for moralization multiply.

Katz (1997) points to the importance of charismatic and powerful figures in the development of secular morality. Everett Koop is his principal example. There is no doubt that such figures can have major influences: we are reminded of Sylvester Graham and Upton Sinclair (Belasco 1997). Although charismatic figures may not be a necessary part of moralization, they surely can be an important part of the success of a moralization movement.

Conclusions

I have tried to make a case for the reality and importance of the process of moralization, specifically as it pertains to the domain of health. Of course, moralization is not categorical. In an individual or in a culture, an object or activity may be partially moralized, and this is no doubt often a step toward complete moralization. We are witnessing the process of moralization in contemporary American society with respect to eating meat and cigarette smoking. It is notable that religion is probably the major force for moralization in traditional societies, and was probably the major force in Western societies until recent times. The emphasis in modern Western societies has shifted more to a harm/rights/justice framework with the emergence of what Katz (1997) has called secular morality.

This "autonomy" framework focusses on the individual. In many contemporary cultures, the individual is not the obvious or the only "unit" in moral discourse; local groups and interpersonal processes are often the central entities (Kleinman and Kleinman 1997; Shweder et al. 1997).

Although I have concentrated on moralization, the inverse process of amoralization may be as important. This process may share many of the predispositions for moralization but may have some of its own special causes. Surely, amoralization is related to the process of medicalization, which has occurred in the United States for various aspects of alcohol abuse and with respect to most types of mental disorders. However, there may be something special about moralization, because it may reflect the power of the moral domain as a simple and satisfying account for misfortune in our species.

I hope to engage the interests of some scholars in the process of moralization, in the hope that we will better understand the conditions under which it occurs, what determines its "success," and the processes involved, at both the individual and culture-wide level. Such an enterprise will require the cooperation of historians, anthropologists, sociologists, and psychologists.

Note

Thanks to the Whitehall Foundation and the John D. and Catherine T. MacArthur Foundation for supporting some of the research and conceptual development presented in this paper. Thanks to Deidre Byrnes for comments on the manuscript and to Clark McCauley, Barry Schwartz, and Richard Shweder for fruitful discussions of some of the issues treated in this paper.

References

Amato, P. R., and S. A. Partridge. 1989. *The new vegetarians*. New York: Plenum.

Barkas, J. 1975. *The vegetable passion*. New York: Scribner.

Belasco, W. 1997. Food, morality, and social reform. In *Morality and health*, edited by A. Brandt and P. Rozin. New York: Routledge.

Bibace, R., and M. E. Walsh. 1979. Developmental stages in children's conception of illness. In *Health psychology: A handbook*, edited by N. E. Adler et al. San Francisco: Jossey-Bass.

Brandt, A. 1997. Behavior, disease, and health in twentieth century America: The moral valence of individual risk. In *Morality and health*, edited by A. Brandt and P. Rozin. New York: Routledge.

Cavalli-Sforza, L. L., M. W. Feldman, K. H. Chen, and S. M. Dornbusch. 1982. Theory and observation in cultural transmission. *Science* 218:19–27.

Courtwright, D. 1997. Morality, religion, and drug use. In *Morality and health*, edited by A. Brandt and P. Rozin. New York: Routledge.

Damon, W. 1983. *Social and personality development*. New York: Norton.

Deci, E. L., and R. M. Ryan. 1985. *Intrinsic motivation and self-determination in human behavior*. New York: Plenum.

Douglas, M. 1966. *Purity and danger*. London: Routledge and Kegan-Paul.

Dwyer, J. T., L. D. v. H. Mayer, R. F. Kandel, and J. Mayer. 1973. The "new" vegetarians: Who are they? *Journal of the American Dietetic Association* 62:503–9.

Elias, N. 1939/1978. *The history of manners: The civilizing process*. Translated by E. Jephcott. vol. 1. New York: Pantheon Books.

Frank, R. H. 1988. *Passions within reason: The strategic role of the emotions*. New York: Norton.

Frazer, J. G. 1890/1959. *The golden bough: A study in magic and religion*. New York: Macmillan. Reprint of 1922 abridged edition, edited by T. H. Gaster; original work published 1890.

Frey, D. 1986. Recent research on selective exposure to information. In *Advances in experimental social psychology*, edited by L. Berkowitz. vol. 19. New York: Academic Press.

Gordon, L. 1997. Teenage pregnancy and out-of-wedlock birth: Morals, moralism, experts. *Morality and health*, edited by A. Brandt and P. Rozin. New York: Routledge.

Gostin, L. 1997. The legal regulation of smoking (and smokers): Public health or secular morality. In *Morality and health*, edited by A. Brandt and P. Rozin. New York: Routledge.

Grunfeld, D. I. 1972/1982. *The Jewish dietary laws*. vol. 1, *Dietary laws regarding forbidden and permitted foods, with particular reference to meat and meat products*. 3d ed. London: Soncino Press.

Gusfield, J. 1992. Nature's body and metaphors of food. In *Cultivating differences: Symbolic boundaries and the making of inequality*, edited by M. Lamont and M. Fournier. Chicago: University of Chicago Press.

———. 1997. Alcohol in America: The entwined frames of health and morality. *Morality and health*, edited by A. Brandt and P. Rozin. New York: Routledge.

Haidt, J., S. H. Koller, and M. G. Dias. 1992. Disgust, disrespect and moral judgment in the U.S. and Brazil (Or, is it wrong to eat your dog?). *Journal of Personality and Social Psychology 65,* 613–628.

Katz, S. 1997. Secular morality. In *Morality and health,* edited by A. Brandt and P. Rozin. New York: Routledge.

Kelman, H. (1958). Compliance, identification and internalization: Three processes of opinion change. *Journal of Conflict Resolution* 2:51–60.

Kleinman, A., and J. Kleinman. 1997. Moral transformations of health and suffering in Chinese society. In *Morality and health,* edited by A. Brandt and P. Rozin. New York: Routledge.

Lakoff, G., and M. Johnson. 1980. *Metaphors we live by.* Chicago: University of Chicago Press.

Leichter, H. 1997. Lifestyle correctness and the new secular morality. In *Morality and health,* edited by A. Brandt and P. Rozin. New York: Routledge.

Lepper, M. R. 1980. Intrinsic and extrinsic motivation in children: detrimental effects of superfluous social controls. In *Minnesota Symposium on Child Psychology,* edited by W. A. Collins. Vol. 14. Hillsdale, N.J.: Lawrence Erlbaum.

McCauley, C. R., P. Rozin, and B. Schwartz. 1997. The origin and nature of preferences and values. Completed book manuscript.

Mechanic, P. 1997. The social context of health and disease and choices among health interventions. In *Morality and health,* edited by A. Brandt and P. Rozin. New York: Routledge.

Mintz, S. 1985. *Sweetness and power.* New York: Viking.

———. 1997. Sugar and morality. In *Morality and health,* edited by A. Brandt and P. Rozin. New York: Routledge.

Murdock, G. P. 1980. *Theories of illness: A world survey.* Pittsburgh: University of Pittsburgh Press.

Nagy, M. H. 1953. The representation of "germs" by children. *Journal of Genetic Psychology* 83:227–40.

Nemeroff, C. J., and P. Rozin. 1989. "You are what you eat." Applying the demand-free "impressions" technique to an unacknowledged belief. *Ethos: The Journal of Psychological Anthropology* 17:50–69.

Piaget, J. 1932/1965. *The moral judgment of the child.* Translated by M. Gabain. New York: Free Press.

Rosenberg, C. 1962. *The cholera years.* Chicago: University of Chicago Press.

———. 1997. Banishing risk: Continuity and change in the moral management of disease. In *Morality and health,* edited by A. Brandt and P. Rozin. New York: Routledge.

Rozin, P. 1990. Social and moral aspects of food and eating. In *The legacy of Solomon Asch: Essays in cognition and social psychology*, edited by I. Rock. Hillsdale, N.J.: Lawrence Erlbaum.

———. 1991. Family resemblance in food and other domains: The family paradox and the role of parental congruence. *Appetite* 16:93–102.

Rozin, P., J. Haidt, and C. R. McCauley. 1993. Disgust. In *Handbook of emotions*, edited by M. Lewis and J. Haviland. New York: Guilford.

Rozin, P., L. Lowery, S. Imada, and J. Haidt. 1996. The moral/emotion (CAD) triad hypothesis. A mapping between the other-directed moral emotions, disgust, contempt, and anger and Shweder's three universal moral codes.

Rozin, P., M. Markwith, and C. R. McCauley. 1994. The nature of aversion to indirect contacts with other persons: AIDS aversion as a composite of aversion to strangers, infection, moral taint, and misfortune. *Journal of Abnormal Psychology* 103:495–504.

Rozin, P., M. Markwith, and C. Stoess. 1997. Moralization: Becoming a vegetarian, the transformation of preferences into values and the recruitment of disgust. *Psychological Science* 8:67–73.

Rozin, P., and C. J. Nemeroff. 1990. The laws of sympathetic magic: A psychological analysis of similarity and contagion. In *Cultural Psychology: Essays on comparative human development*, edited by J. Stigler, G. Herdt, and R. A. Shweder. Cambridge: Cambridge University Press.

Rozin, P., and Singh, L. (1997). The moralization of cigarette smoking in America (submitted manuscript).

Rozin, P., and T. A. Vollmecke. 1986. Food likes and dislikes. *Annual Review of Nutrition* 6:433–56.

Shweder, R. A., N. Much, M. Mahaptra, and L. Park. 1997. The "big three" of morality (autonomy, community, divinity), and the "big three" explanations of suffering. In *Morality and health*, edited by A. Brandt and P. Rozin. New York: Routledge.

Singer, P. 1975. *Animal liberation*. New York: New York Review of Books.

Sontag, S. 1977. *Illness as metaphor*. New York: Farrar, Straus and Giroux.

Stein, R. I., and C. J. Nemeroff. 1995. Moral overtones of food: Judgments of others based on what they eat. *Personality and Social Psychology Bulletin* 21:480–90.

Thomas, K. 1983. *Man and the natural world*. New York: Pantheon Books.

———. 1997. Health and morality in early modern England. In *Morality and health*, edited by A. Brandt and P. Rozin. New York: Routledge.

Tomes, N. 1997. Moralizing the microbe: The germ theory and the moral construction of behavior in the late-nineteenth-century antituberculosis movement. In *Morality and health*, edited by A. Brandt and P. Rozin. New York: Routledge.

Contributors

Warren Belasco is Professor and Chair of American Studies at the University of Maryland, Baltimore County. He is the author of *Americans on the Road: From Autocamp to Motel* (1979); *Appetite for Change: How the Counterculture Took On the Food Industry* (1993); and numerous articles on the history, culture, and politics of food.

Allan M. Brandt is the Amalie Moses Kass Professor of the History of Medicine and Professor of the History of Science at Harvard University. Brandt is the author of *No Magic Bullet: A Social History of Venereal Disease in the United States since 1880* (1985). He has written on the social history of epidemic disease; the history of public health; and the history of human subject research among other topics. He is currently writing a book on the social and cultural history of cigarette smoking in the United States.

David T. Courtwright is a member of the Departments of History and Health Science at the University of North Florida. He is the author of *Dark Paradise: Opiate Addiction in America before 1940* (1982); *Addicts Who Survived: An Oral History of Narcotic Use in America, 1923–1965* (1989); and *Violent Land: Single Men and Social Disorder from the Frontier to the Inner City* (1996). He is currently researching the spread and regulation of psychoactive substances and other pleasurable commodities in the modern world.

Linda Gordon is the Florence Kelley Professor of History and Vilas Distinguished Research Professor at the University of Wisconsin. Her research focuses on the historical roots of contemporary policy debates, particularly as they concern gender and family issues. Her books include: *America's Working Women* (orig. 1976, revised ed. 1995); *Woman's Body, Woman's Right: A Social History of Birth*

Control in America (1976); and *Heroes of Their Own Lives: The Politics and History of Family Violence: Boston, 1880–1960* (1988). Her latest book is *Pitied But Not Entitled: Single Mothers and the History of Welfare, 1890–1935* (1994).

Lawrence O. Gostin is Professor of Law at Georgetown University Law Center, and the Co-Director of the Johns Hopkins/Georgetown University Program on Law and Public Health. Gostin is the Editor of the Health Law and Ethics section of the *Journal of the American Medical Association (JAMA)*, is a member of the Advisory Committee on HIV and STD Prevention of the U.S. Centers for Disease Control and Prevention, and was a member of the President's Task Force on National Health Care Reform. His most recent book is *Human Rights and Public Health in the AIDS Pandemic* (1997).

Joseph R. Gusfield is Professor Emeritus of Sociology at the University of California, San Diego. For twenty-four years he has taught at his present institution, and has written widely on developing nations, sociology of education, and political sociology. Among his books are *Symbolic Crusade: Status Politics and the American Temperance Movement* (1966); *Protest, Reform and Revolt* (1970); *The Culture and Public Problems: Drinking-Driving and the Symbolic Order*, and most recently, *Contested Meanings: The Construction of Alcohol Problems* (1996).

Solomon H. Katz is Professor of Physical Anthropology and Director of the Krogman Growth Center at the University of Pennsylvania and Children's Hospital of Philadelphia. Katz is Consulting Curator of Physical Anthropology at the University Museum of Archaeology and Anthropology, and is the author of several books including: *Biological Anthropology Readings from Scientific American* (1975); *African Food Systems in Crisis* (1989); and *Origins and Ancient History of Wine* (1995).

Arthur M. Kleinman is the Maude and Lillian Presley Professor of Medical Anthropology; Professor of Psychiatry and Chairman, Department of Social Medicine, Harvard Medical School; and Professor of Social Anthropology, Department of Anthropology, Harvard University. His major books include: *Writing at the Margin: Discourse Between Anthropology and Medicine* (1995); *World Mental Health: Problems and Priorities in Low Income Countries* (editor, 1995); *Patients and Healers in the Context of*

Culture (1980); *Social Origins of Distress and Disease* (1986); and *The Illness Narratives: Suffering, Healing and the Human Condition* (1988).

Joan Kleinman is a Research Associate in Social Medicine; Director of the *Circle on Social Experience in Chinese Society*; and Coordinator of the China Research Group Program in Medical Anthropology, Harvard University. She was co-convenor of a conference, *Changing Social Experiences in Chinese Societies*, held at Academia Sinica, Taipei, Taiwan (1996); and she presented a paper, *The Social Course of Suffering: Schizophrenia, Epilepsy and Other Chronic Conditions in Chinese Culture*, Taniguchi Foundation, Japan (1996).

Howard M. Leichter is Professor and Chairman of the Department of Political Science, Linfield College, and Clinical Professor of Public Health and Preventive Medicine, Oregon Health Sciences University. He is the author of several books and articles, including: *Free To Be Foolish: Politics and Health Promotion in the United States and Great Britain* (1991). Leichter is a member of the Board of Editors of the *Journal of Health Politics, Policy and Law*. He recently completed a Fulbright fellowship in Great Britain where he studied the changing role of the British Medical Association.

Manamohan Mahapatra is Professor of Anthropology at BJB College in Bhubaneswar, Orissa, India, and author of many books and essays about Oriya culture, including *Traditional Structure and Change in an Orissan Temple* (1981).

David Mechanic is the René Dubos University Professor of Behavioral Sciences and Director of the Institute for Health, Health Care Policy, and Aging Research at Rutgers University. His research and writings deal with social aspects of health and health care with a particular emphasis on patient perspectives. A member of the National Academy of Sciences, Mechanic has written or edited over 300 research articles and twenty-four books including: *Inescapable Decisions: The Imperatives of Health Reform* (1994); *From Advocacy to Allocation: The Evolving American Health Care System* (1986); and *Mental Health and Social Policy* (1969).

Sidney W. Mintz taught anthropology for nearly twenty-five years at Yale, and has been teaching at The Johns Hopkins University since 1975. Mintz has done fieldwork in Puerto Rico, Jamaica, Iran,

Haiti and Hong Kong. He is the T. H. Huxley Medalist of the Royal Anthropological Institute of Great Britain and Ireland (1994), and Distinguished Lecturer of the American Anthropological Association (1996). His publications include: *Worker in the Cane* (1960); *Caribbean Transformations* (1974); *Sweetness and Power* (1985); and *Tasting Food, Tasting Freedom* (1996).

Nancy C. Much is a researcher at the University of Chicago. Her papers on cultural psychology and philosophical anthropology include: "Cultural Psychology," in J. Smith, R. Harre, and L. Van Langenhove (eds.) *Rethinking Psychology* (1995); "How Psychologies 'Secrete' Moralities," (with R. Harre) in *New Ideas in Psychology*, vol. 12, no. 3 (1994); "Constructing Divinity" (with M. Mahapatra), in P. Stearns and R. Harre (eds.) *Discursive Psychology in Practice* (1995); "The Analysis of Discourse as Methodology for a Semiotic Psychology," in *American Behavioral Scientist*, vol. 36 (1992); and "Determinations of Meaning: Discourse and Moral Socialization" (with R. Shweder) in R.A. Shweder's *Thinking Through Cultures: Expeditions in Cultural Psychology* (1991).

Lawrence Park is a Ph.D. candidate in the Committee on Human Development at the University of Chicago. He is the recipient of an International Pre-Dissertation Fellowship from the Social Science Research Council for his research on Mental Health in China. He is a physician doing a medical internship at Massachusetts General Hospital.

Charles E. Rosenberg is the Janice and Julian Bers Professor of the History and Sociology of Science at the University of Pennsylvania. Rosenberg's research is in the areas of the history of heredity and genetics, psychiatry, disease and its social impact, and government support of scientific research and medical care. His publications include: *The Cholera Years* (1962); *The Trial of the Assassin Guiteau: Psychiatry and Law in the Gilded Age* (1968); *No Other Gods: On Science and American Social Thought* (1976); *The Care of Strangers: The Rise of America's Hospital System* (1987); and *Explaining Epidemics and Other Studies in the History of Medicine* (1992). At present, he is working on a study of changing concepts of disease, 1800–1990.

Paul Rozin is the Edmund J. and Louise W. Kahn Professor for Faculty Excellence at the University of Pennsylvania. He has written over 150 journal articles/chapters, dealing most recently with the development of food preferences and attitudes, food cravings, the nature and origin of the emotion of disgust, magical thinking, and cultural evolution, principally in the food domain. Current interests include cross-cultural studies of disgust and the role of food in life, vegetarianism, and the linkage between food attitudes or behaviors and moral issues.

Richard A. Shweder is a cultural anthropologist and Chair of the Committee on Human Development at the University of Chicago. He is the author of *Thinking Through Cultures: Expeditions in Cultural Psychology* (1991); as well as the editor or co-editor of several volumes including *Culture Theory: Essays on Mind, Self and Emotion* (1984); and *Metatheory in Social Science: Pluralisms and Subjectivities* (1986). Shweder has served as President of the Society for Psychological Anthropology, and is currently co-chair of the Social Science Research Council's Planning Committee on Culture, Health and Human Development.

Keith Thomas is President of Corpus Christi College, Oxford and was formerly Professor of Modern History and Fellow of St. John's College. He has written extensively on the social and intellectual history of the early modern period. His works include *Religion and the Decline of Magic* (1971); and *Man and the Natural World: Changing Attitudes in England 1500–1800* (1983). He is general editor of the Past Masters Series (Oxford University Press) and is currently President of the British Academy. He was knighted in 1988 for services to the study of history.

Nancy Tomes is an Associate Professor of History at the State University of New York at Stony Brook. She has written widely on the history of American psychiatry and public health. Her latest book, *The Gospel of Germs: Men, Women, and the Microbe in American Life, 1880–1930*, will be published by Harvard University Press in Spring 1998.

Index